Assisted Living Nursing

A Manual for Management and Practice

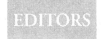 **EDITORS** Barbara Resnick, PhD, CRNP, FAAN
Ethel Mitty, EdD, RN

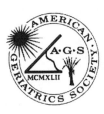

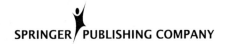
SPRINGER PUBLISHING COMPANY

New York

Springer Publishing Company, LLC
11 West 42nd Street
New York, NY 10036
www.springerpub.com

Acquisitions Editor: Allan Graubard
Project Manager: Mark Frazier
Cover design: TG Design
Composition: Apex CoVantage, LLC

Ebook ISBN: 978-0-8261-5739-3

11 / 5 4 3

The authors and the publisher of this Work have made every effort to use sources believed to be reliable to provide information that is accurate and compatible with the standards generally accepted at the time of publication. Because medical science is continually advancing, our knowledge base continues to expand. Therefore, as new information becomes available, changes in procedures become necessary. We recommend that the reader always consult current research and specific institutional policies before performing any clinical procedure. The authors and publisher shall not be liable for any special, consequential, or exemplary damages resulting, in whole or in part, from the readers' use of, or reliance on, the information contained in this book. The publisher has no responsibility for the persistence or accuracy of URLs for external or third-party Internet Web sites referred to in this publication and does not guarantee that any content on such Web sites is, or will remain, accurate or appropriate.

Library of Congress Cataloging-in-Publication Data
Assisted living nursing : a manual for management and practice /
Barbara Resnick, Ethel Mitty, editors.
       p. ; cm.
    Includes bibliographical references and index.
    ISBN 978-0-8261-5738-6 (alk. paper)
   1. Geriatric nursing—Handbooks, manuals, etc.   2. Congregate housing—Handbooks,
manuals, etc.   3. Geriatric nursing—Handbooks, manuals, etc.   I. Resnick, Barbara.
II. Mitty, Ethel L.
    [DNLM: 1. Geriatric Nursing—organization & administration.   2. Assisted Living
Facilities—organization & administration.   3. Geriatric Nursing—methods.
4. Homes for the Aged—organization & administration.   WY 152 A848 2009]
    RC954.3.A87   2009
    618.97'0231—dc22   2009014202

Printed in the United States of America by Gasch Printing

Special discounts on bulk quantities of our books are available to corporations, professional associations,
pharmaceutical companies, health care organizations, and other qualified groups.
If you are interested in a custom book, including chapters from more than one of our titles, we can provide
that service as well.

For details, please contact:
Special Sales Department, Springer Publishing Company, LLC
11 West 42nd Street, 15th Floor, New York, NY 10036-8002
Phone: 877-687-7476 or 212-431-4370; Fax: 212-941-7842
Email: sales@springerpub.com

To assisted living nurses who, by their years of unheralded work and dedication, made assisted living a reality for older adults

Contents

SECTION I

Management and Leadership

S E C T I O N   I I

Approach to the Resident

S E C T I O N   I I I

Syndromes

SECTION IV

Psychological Health

SECTION V

Diseases and Disorders

Contributors

Sumaira Z. Aasi, MD
Assistant Professor
Department of Dermatology
Yale University School of Medicine
New Haven, CT

Harold P. Adams, Jr., MD
Professor and Director
Division of Cerebrovascular Diseases, Department of Neurology
University of Iowa Hospitals and Clinics
Iowa City, IA

Reva N. Adler, MD
Medical Director, STAT Centre and At-Home Supports
Vancouver Hospital and Vancouver Community Health Services
Clinical Associate Professor, Division of Geriatric Medicine
University of British Columbia
Vancouver, BC

Marc Edward Agronin, MD
Director of Mental Health Services
Miami Jewish Home and Hospital for the Aged
Assistant Professor of Psychiatry
Miller School of Medicine at the University of Miami
Miami, FL

Cathy A. Alessi, MD
Associate Director
Clinical Programs: Geriatric Research, Education
    and Clinical Center, Sepulveda Division
Veterans Administration Greater Los Angeles Healthcare System
Professor, University of California, Los Angeles
Multicampus Program in Geriatric Medicine and Gerontology
Sepulveda, CA

Neil B. Alexander, MD
Professor, Division of Geriatric Medicine
Department of Internal Medicine
Research Professor, Institute of Gerontology

University of Michigan
Director, VA Ann Arbor Health Care System Geriatric
Research, Education and Clinical Center
Ann Arbor, MI

Wilbert S. Aronow, MD
Clinical Professor of Medicine
Divisions of Cardiology, Geriatrics, and Pulmonary/Critical Care
Westchester Medical Center and New York Medical College
Valhalla, NY
Adjunct Professor of Geriatrics and Adult Development
Mount Sinai School of Medicine
New York, NY

Priscilla Faith Bade, MD, MS
Associate Professor of Internal Medicine
University of South Dakota School of Medicine
Rapid City, SD

Caroline Blaum, MD
Associate Professor of Internal Medicine
Division of Geriatric Medicine
University of Michigan
Research Scientist, Ann Arbor DVAMC Geriatric Research,
Education and Clinical Center
Ann Arbor, MI

Harrison Bloom, MD
Senior Associate
International Longevity Center, USA
Associate Clinical Professor
Brookdale Department of Geriatrics and Adult Development
Mount Sinai School of Medicine
New York, NY

Andrea Brassard, DNSc, MPH, CRNP
Assistant Professor, Department of Nursing Education,
George Washington University
Washington, DC

David M. Buchner, MD, MPH
Chief, Physical Activity and Health Branch, Division of Nutrition
   and Physical Activity
Centers for Disease Control and Prevention
Atlanta, GA

Joan Gleba Carpenter, MN, RN, NP-C, ACHPN
Nurse Practitioner, Evercare
Berlin, MD

Erin L. Cassidy, PhD
Research Associate
Department of Psychiatry and Behavioral Sciences
Stanford University School of Medicine
Palo Alto, CA

Gurkamal Chatta, MD
Associate Professor of Medicine
Division of Hematology-Oncology
University of Pittsburgh
Pittsburgh, PA

Colleen Christmas, MD
Assistant Professor of Medicine
Division of Geriatric Medicine and Gerontology
The Johns Hopkins University School of Medicine
Baltimore, MD

Anne L. Coleman, MD, PhD
Professor of Ophthalmology and Epidemiology
Frances and Ray Stark Chair of Ophthalmology
Jules Stein Eye Institute
University of California, Los Angeles
Los Angeles, CA

G. Willy Davila, MD
Chairman, Department of Gynecology
Head, Section of Urogynecology and Reconstructive Pelvic Surgery
Cleveland Clinic Florida
Ft. Lauderdale, FL

Catherine E. DuBeau, MD
Associate Professor of Medicine
Section of Geriatrics
University of Chicago
Chicago, IL

E. Wesley Ely, MD, MPH
Associate Professor of Medicine
Associate Director of Aging Research
Tennessee Valley Geriatric Research, Education and Clinical Center
Allergy, Pulmonary and Critical Care
Vanderbilt University School of Medicine
Nashville, TN

William B. Ershler, MD
Director
Institute for Advanced Studies in Aging and Geriatric Medicine
Washington, DC

Sandi Flores, RN-C
Education Director, Community Education LLC
San Marcos, CA

Elizabeth Galik, PhD, ANP-BC
Assistant Professor, University of Maryland School of Nursing
Baltimore, MD

Angela Gentili, MD
Associate Professor of Internal Medicine
Director, Geriatrics Fellowship Training Program
VA Medical Center/Virginia Commonwealth University
Richmond, VA

Thomas M. Gill, MD
Associate Professor of Medicine
Yale University School of Medicine
New Haven, CT

Lisa J. Granville, MD
Professor and Associate Chair
Department of Geriatrics
Florida State University College of Medicine
Tallahassee, FL

David A. Gruenewald, MD
Associate Professor of Medicine
Division of Gerontology and Geriatric Medicine
Department of Medicine
University of Washington School of Medicine
Staff Physician, Geriatrics Research, Education and Clinical Center
VA Puget Sound Health Care System
Seattle, WA

Jennifer Hauf, GNP-BC
Nurse Practitioner, Stella Maris Nursing Facility
Timonium, MD

Kenneth W. Hepburn, PhD
Professor and Associate Dean for Research
Emory University
Atlanta, GA

Kevin Paul High, MD, MSc
Associate Professor of Medicine
Sections of Infectious Diseases and Hematology/Oncology
Wake Forest University School of Medicine
Winston Salem, NC

Jennifer Kapo, MD
Assistant Professor of Clinical Medicine
Division of Geriatrics

University of Pennsylvania
Philadelphia, PA

Gary J. Kennedy, MD
Professor of Psychiatry and Behavioral Science
Albert Einstein College of Medicine
Director, Division of Geriatric Psychiatry
Montefiore Medical Center
Bronx, NY

Douglas P. Kiel, MD, MPH
Associate Professor of Medicine
Harvard Medical School Division on Aging
Director, Medical Research
HRCA Research and Training Institute
Boston, MA

Maureen Kilby, ANP-BC
Nurse Practitioner, VA Medical System
Rising Sun, MD

Kurt Kroenke, MD
Professor of Medicine
Indiana University School of Medicine
Senior Scientist
Regenstrief Institute for Health Care
Indianapolis, IN

Melinda S. Lantz, MD
Director of Psychiatry
Jewish Home and Hospital
Assistant Professor, Department of Geriatrics and Adult Development
Mount Sinai School of Medicine
New York, NY

David A. Lipschitz, MD
Professor of Geriatrics
Chair, Donald W. Reynolds Department of Geriatrics
University of Arkansas for Medical Sciences
Little Rock, AR

Dan L. Longo, MD
Scientific Director
National Institute on Aging
Baltimore, MD

Courtney H. Lyder, ND
University of Virginia Medical Center Professor
Chairman, Department of Acute and Specialty Care
University of Virginia School of Nursing
Charlottesville, VA

Constantine G. Lyketsos, MD, MHS
Professor of Psychiatry and Behavioral Sciences
Co-Director, Division of Geriatric Psychiatry and Neuropsychiatry
The Johns Hopkins University and Hospital
Baltimore, MD

Anna M. Mago-Sisic, CRNP, CWOCN
Nurse Practitioner
Erickson Retirement Communities at Riderwood Village
Silver Spring, MD

Coleman O. Martin, MD
Clinical Associate
Department of Neurology
University of Iowa Hospitals and Clinics
Iowa City, IA

Alvin M. Matsumoto, MD
Professor, Department of Medicine
University of Washington School of Medicine
Division of Gerontology and Geriatric Medicine
Director, Clinical Research Unit
Associate Director, Geriatric Research, Education, and Clinical Center
VA Puget Sound Health Care System
Seattle, WA

Kathleen Michael, PhD, CRRN
Assistant Professor
University of Maryland
School of Nursing
Baltimore, MD

Thomas Mulligan, MD
Ruth S. Jewett Professor of Medicine
Chief, University of Florida Division of Geriatrics
Director, Geriatrics Research, Education and Clinical Center
North Florida/South Georgia Veterans Health System
Gainesville, FL

David W. Oslin, MD
Associate Professor
Geriatric and Addiction Psychiatry
University of Pennsylvania
Philadelphia, PA

Bradford L. Picot, DDS
Dentist
Spurgeon Webber III, DDS PA & Associates
Charlotte, NC

Sandra J. Fulton Picot, PhD, RN, FAAN, FGSA
Associate Professor, University of Maryland, Baltimore
Baltimore, MD

Karen M. Prestwood, MD
Associate Professor of Medicine
UConn Center on Aging
University of Connecticut Health Center
Farmington, CT

John W. Rachow, PhD, MD
Assistant Clinical Professor
Department of Medicine
University of Iowa College of Medicine
Iowa City, IA

Paula A. Rochon, MD, MPH
Associate Professor
Department of Medicine and Health Policy Management
    and Evaluation
University of Toronto
Senior Scientist and Assistant Director
Kunin-Lunenfeld Applied Research Unit
Baycrest Centre for Geriatric Care
Scientist, Institute for Clinical Evaluative Sciences
Toronto, ON

David Sarraf, MD
Assistant Clinical Professor of Ophthalmology
Jules Stein Eye Institute, UCLA School of Medicine
    and the Greater Los Angeles VA Healthcare Center
Assistant Professor of Ophthalmology
Martin L. King Medical Center/Charles R. Drew
University of Medicine
Los Angeles, CA

Susan Avillo Scherr, GNP-BC
Nurse Practitioner, Evercare
Baltimore, MD

Anne Scheve, MSN
Clinical Instructor, University of Maryland School of Nursing
Baltimore, MD

Todd P. Semla, MS, PharmD
Clinical Pharmacy Specialist
Department of Veterans Affairs
Pharmacy Benefits Management & Strategic Health Group
Hines, IL

Associate Professor
Department of Psychiatry and Behavioral Sciences
The Feinberg School of Medicine
Northwestern University
Chicago, IL

Kenneth Shay, DDS, MS
Director of Geriatric Programs
Office of Geriatrics and Extended Care
VA Central Office, Washington, DC
Adjunct Professor of Dentistry
University of Michigan School of Dentistry
Ann Arbor, MI

Javaid I. Sheikh, MD
Professor
Department of Psychiatry and Behavioral Sciences
Stanford University School of Medicine
Stanford, CA
Chief of Staff
VA Palo Alto Health Care System
Palo Alto, CA

Yael Sollins, BSN, Graduate Student
New York University
New York, NY

Mark Andrew Supiano, MD
Professor and Chief, Division of Geriatric Medicine
University of Utah Health Science Center
Director, Veterans Affairs Salt Lake City
Geriatric Research, Education and Clinical Center
Executive Director, University of Utah Center on Aging
Salt Lake City, UT

Krystal L. Thomas, GNP-BC
Nurse Practitioner, EMA Health Services
Easton, MD

George Triadafilopoulos, MD
Clinical Professor of Medicine
Division of Gastroenterology and Hepatology
Stanford University School of Medicine
Stanford, CA

Debra K. Weiner, MD
Associate Professor of Medicine, Psychiatry and Anesthesiology
University of Pittsburgh School of Medicine
Pittsburgh, PA

Assisted living is a residential long-term care option that provides housing, 24-hour oversight, personal care services, health related services, or a combination of these on an as-needed basis to vulnerable and medically, functionally, and cognitively impaired older adults. Assisted living is the fastest-growing senior housing option in the United States. Key philosophical tenets of assisted living are aging-in-place and maximizing the function and quality of life of the resident. The goal of the physical environment is a home-like atmosphere, pace, and place that specifically avoids the appearance of an institutional or medical facility.

Most assisted living residents are in their early 80s, require some assistance with at least two activities of daily living (ADLs), and demonstrate functional decline over time similar to that of nursing home residents. Assisted living residents have similar medical diagnoses and chronic illnesses and take approximately the same number of prescription medications as nursing home residents. Between 66% and 80% of assisted living residents suffer from dementia, depression, other psychiatric illness, or receive psychotropic medications, and approximately 25% of assisted living communities have a dedicated Alzheimer's or dementia unit. Many states permit and encourage assisted living facilities to admit or retain residents who meet the state's nursing home level of care; all states permit hospice care in the facility. At least 65% of residents need assistance with managing their medications. The older adult living in assisted living seeks a protective but not restrictive environment. The balance between autonomy and safety is constantly renegotiated, sometimes on a daily basis.

Seeking freedom of expression, self-determination, and personal growth, an assisted living resident benefits from nursing practice that maximizes their independence, dignity, and overall continued well-being. Yet, on-site licensed nursing varies substantially across and within states. Nurses may be present 24/7, or only on a periodic or on-call basis. Nursing oversight can include assuring appropriate placement, health promotion, identifying acute clinical problems quickly, and optimally managing physical and behavioral problems. A professional nurse in assisted living may have the responsibility for assessment of potential residents to determine their suitability and safety living in an assisted living environment as well as assessing change in condition to determine if a resident needs a higher level of care. When fully realized, the scope of practice of the nurse in assisted living resembles a combined role of administrator, wellness coordinator, and clinical expert, focused on health promotion and optimizing function. Nurses with special expertise in care of older adults increase the likelihood that assisted living residents will be able to age in place and more importantly do so with meaningful quality of life.

Relatively isolated from nursing and interdisciplinary colleagues, an assisted living nurse is an autonomous decision maker and manager of care, people, and systems. The guiding principles of assisted living nursing practice are a unique blend of gerontological and administrative nursing framed by person-directed care planning. Despite the growing body of knowledge about aging, persistent myths about aging erode optimism, outlook, and quality of life for the older adult. Hence, the assisted living nurse needs to be as informed about prevailing science and evidence-based practice as about the misperceptions about aging that work against the older adult's self-care abilities and independent decision making.

This book precisely fills the need for a text that informs assisted living nurses as to best practices in geriatric nursing care. Expert clinicians and managers share their knowledge, skills, and practices across the key domains of assisted living nursing leadership and care of the older adult. The tools, protocols, and tables that are an inherent part of every chapter provide effective strategies and resources that address what is known as to the science of nursing practice while keeping in mind the practicality needed in a busy residential and clinical environment. Nurses will find this book invaluable as they seek to shape care to assure that people age with dignity and quality of life.

Mathy Mezey, EdD, RN, FAAN
Professor Emerita, Senior Research Associate
Director, the Hartford Institute for Geriatric Nursing
New York University College of Nursing

Preface

Assisted living (AL) nursing is a unique domain of practice. It is holistic because it brings together—as no other domain of nursing practice can—people, health, environment, and psychosocial factors. The goal of assisted living nursing practice is to preserve (if not restore) an older adult's function, independence, and engagement with the environment and the people in it, and maximize the older adult's well-being and quality of living. Nursing practice in assisted living is guided by the older adult's (i.e., resident's) values and preferences, supporting them in their choices. The nurse or nursing role in the AL community requires nurses to have expertise in both gerontologic and administrative nursing. Nursing activities for residents in assisted living can include a variety of things such as wellness management, counseling, health education, chronic illness management and monitoring, and care at the end of life. Nurses in AL communities have the responsibility of educating, guiding, mentoring, and motivating the direct-care workers in these settings and in some cases the other nursing staff with whom they work. In addition, the nurse has a responsibility to the organization and the community to oversee quality assurance and improvement, cost-effective practices, and marketing. This book was written to provide nurses with the knowledge and skill to provide the level of combined gerontological and administrative expertise that is required of them in the AL community.

Specifically this book will provide AL nurses with evidence and research-based information and knowledge regarding nursing management and clinical practice, descriptions of components of ethical nursing practice explicated in each chapter, and a "refresher" for former long-term care nurses who wish to return to practice (a sorely needed workforce) as well as for nursing students or those new to the nursing workforce. Moreover, the book provides an introduction to this unique domain of nursing practice for nurses unfamiliar with the demands as well as the consummate satisfaction of assisted living nursing. This book can, and should, be used as a resource for the assisted living nurse interested in taking the American Assisted Living Nurses Association (AALNA) Assisted Living Nurse Certification exam.

Each chapter provides a theoretical, scientific, and/or conceptual base for the nursing acts that are recommended, whether clinical or managerial. Recommendations are research-based or borne out of the years of experience of expert clinicians in management or clinical practice. To the extent possible, each chapter suggests guidelines, protocols, and other nursing activities that will facilitate or enhance staff development and resident well-being. The book is divided into five sections: "Management and Leadership," "Approach to the Resident," "Syndromes," "Psychological Health," and "Diseases and Disorders." There is extensive cross-referencing in each chapter to other sections of the book or chapter as well as an Internet reference list for sources of information regarding care of the older adult including state and federal resources. Each chapter in Section I, "Management and Leadership," begins with a brief introduction that describes the specific content of the chapter. For example, Chapter 4, "Marketing, Quality, Consumer Choice, and Admission Agreements," discusses nursing's role in marketing, the preadmission evaluation, assessing nursing's marketing image, safety goals, satisfaction, and mechanisms of quality accreditation. The clinical chapters (Sections II–V) address age-related changes, disease etiology, symptom management, nursing assessment and intervention, and patient education. Overall this is a comprehensive source of both management and clinical information for every nurse working in the assisted living or long-term care environment.

This book reflects an interdisciplinary team of individuals including physicians, nurses, social workers, and dentists. Specifically, as coauthors of this work, we would like to thank the following: The American Geriatric Society for partnering with us on this endeavor; the individual contributors of the Geriatric Review Syllabus, which served as a basis for the clinical chapters; and the advanced practice nurses who were chapter coauthors. With deepest appreciation we thank Ardis O'Meara who completed the final editing and organization of this book.

Ethel Mitty
Barbara Resnick

It is with great pleasure and pride that I share with my colleagues the opportunity to introduce this comprehensive book covering the many critical areas of nursing care for those living in assisted living communities. This book, written by and for nurses across the spectrum of nurse providers (advanced practice nurses, delegating nurses, and the direct care workforce), covers all aspects of management as well as the many common clinical problems and syndromes we encounter among older adults. Further, this book proposes wonderful assessment and intervention material that will help the entire health care team keep residents within their AL communities through early recognition and management of acute illnesses. Kudos to our nursing colleagues for editing this publication and may it serve as the useful guide for AL residents across the country.

John B. Murphy, MD
President, American Geriatrics Society
Professor of Medicine and Family Medicine
Warren Alpert Medical School of Brown University

Management
and
Leadership

An assisted living (AL) nurse is both a manager and a clinician, a combined role that requires management as well as gerontological knowledge and leadership skills. The 13 chapters in this section of the book focus on managing nursing care and nursing staff in the context of AL nursing practice, AL philosophy, and regulations. The first chapter is an overview of the AL community population, their demographics, and the nature of AL nursing, including the scope and standards of AL nursing practice. Subsequent chapters address health care financing, marketing and service plan construction, theories of nursing, organizational culture, management theory, and leadership styles and responsibilities, such as staffing and assignments (workload), problem solving, change and conflict resolution, job descriptions, staff development and performance evaluation, reimbursement and budget, ethical and legal aspects of practice, and research and quality improvement. The content includes assessment and hands-on how-to guidelines.

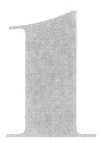

The Assisted Living Setting of Nursing Practice

Ethel Mitty

This chapter describes some key demographics of the older adult population in the United States that pertain to assisted living (AL) residents: life expectancy, socioeconomic status, literacy, trends in health and functional status, and elder mistreatment. The second half of the chapter addresses key concepts of AL: the notion of homeyness, resident independence and self-direction, and aging-in-place. It concludes with a description of the American Geriatrics Society position paper on AL, the scope and standards of practice, and principles of AL nursing.

AGING AND LIFE EXPECTANCY

The aging of the baby boomers (i.e., those born between 1946 and 1964), longevity differences within and between population groups, and increases in the old-old age group (i.e., over 85 years old) has created a significant shift in the composition of the older adult population in the United States. In 2007, about one in eight persons living in the United States was age 65 or older—approximately 13% or 37 million people. By 2030, one of every five persons (i.e., 20% or 71.5 million people) will be age 65 or older. The older adult U.S. population is predominantly White, but minority older adults are expected to increase. Life expectancy upon reaching age 65 is an average additional 18.7 years (20.0 years for females, 17.1 years for

males). The number of centenarians in the United States is growing and is expected to be over 800,000 by 2050.

Socioeconomic Status and Education

Overall, older adults are becoming better educated, better off financially (though ethnic minorities lag behind non-Latino White Americans), and are changing their living arrangements, especially with the growth of AL. In the early 1960s, 35% of people age 65 or older had incomes below the federal poverty level, and only 70% received Social Security pensions. Improvements in the Social Security system (e.g., cost-of-living-adjustments), Medicare, asset income, and government employee and private pension systems have significantly improved the economic well-being of older adults in the United States. In 2008, approximately 4.5 million older adults were Medicare and Medicaid beneficiaries (i.e., so-called dual eligibles); 95% of all older adults are Medicare beneficiaries. The effect of the national and worldwide economic downturn in fall 2008 on the economic well-being of current and future AL residents is unknown at the time of this publication. The forecast, however, is that older adults will be economically less well off than heretofore seen as a result of pension wipeouts, inability to sell their home, and so forth.

Older adults with more education are generally in better health and at lower risk of disability than those with low levels of educational attainment. Between 1970 and 2001, the percentage of older adults who completed high school increased from 28% to 76%; it is projected at 83% by 2030. Those with a bachelor's degree or more will have increased from the 2001 level of 15% to 24% by 2020. It is suggested that better-educated older adults will be more activist and informed health care consumers (i.e., adept at using the Internet to get information) and more demanding of the health care system.

Literacy and Health

Literacy is the ability to communicate and function in society. Limited health literacy is associated with increased use of emergency departments, increased rates of hospitalization (associated with medication mismanagement), and failure to take important diagnostic tests (e.g., mammograms). Among older adults in 2003, almost 70% had below basic literacy—lower than any other age group. *Functional illiteracy* is inability to read sufficiently well to function in the everyday; it signifies being at risk. *Health literacy* is the ability to understand and then act on health information; the basic skills are reading, numeracy, and writing (to a lesser extent). Numeracy skills are related to medication management: calculating when the next dose is due or the number of pills needed until it is time to order a refill. An AL resident who wishes to maintain his or her independence needs to be able to read and understand written and verbal information about his or her diagnosis/illness, test preparation, and treatment instructions; ask relevant questions; and manage problems that might arise in his or her care regimen.

An excuse for a missed appointment or medication—"I forgot where I put my glasses"—might be signaling limited literacy. The Test of Health Literacy in Adults (TOHLA; S-TOHLA, short version) includes numeracy items (e.g., figuring out when to take the medication next), when to take a medication on an empty stomach, and is available in Spanish. The TOHLA also tests comprehension of preparation instructions for a diagnostic test, such as what one can eat, the number of hours to be without food, and so forth. Assessment takes 10 minutes.

Using *plain language* does not mean dumbing down. Reading levels for surveys (e.g., satisfaction), interviews, and instructions should be set at sixth-grade but no higher than eighth-grade level. The notion of plain language holds that the information—written or verbal—should be understood on first reading or hearing it. The difficulty with this concept is that emotions, such as fear or anxiety, can block comprehension of even the most simply constructed sentence.

Written material for AL residents should use a 12-point (or greater) font size, sharp characters, and color contrast of print and page. Diagrams and illustrations should be representative of the AL resident. Here are some general guidelines for a document or program to deliver health education or information, such as the evacuation procedure:

- Clearly state the goal of the instructions/education, that is, the desired actions as well as those activities that are not desirable or recommended.
- Make no more than four major points in the document.
- Do not use pictures or diagrams that add little or nothing of importance.
- Avoid fancy script, italics, or use of all capital letters.
- Leave at least one inch between text segments; use headings and bullets when possible to avoid dense text.
- Do not mix positive and negative information (i.e., "go" and "stop") in the same paragraph.

The ability of older adults to access and use Internet information is unknown. Web text is purportedly written at a 10th-grade reading level or higher. Prior to suggesting that a resident go to the Web to get more information, assess their ability to search the Web efficiently—and comfortably.

To ascertain if the resident understood the information/instructions, do not ask: "Do you have any questions?" There is a natural inclination to say "no" to avoid embarrassment; the person has no questions and understood everything. Similarly, there is a natural face-saving inclination to respond "yes" to the question "Did you understand what you were told?" Rather, provide information or instruction in small bits and then use *rephrasing:* ask the resident to tell you in his or her own words (i.e., to rephrase) what you've just said. It is relatively easy to judge if the resident has understood the information and that it has been recalled correctly. A similar process is used in the process of obtaining informed consent for treatment and research participation. To ease the resident's anxiety about having to recall and rephrase, say something like, "I just gave you a lot of information. I am concerned that I didn't leave anything out that you need to know. Tell me in your own words what I said, about what you need to do, and so forth."

Trends in Health, Functional Status, and Disability

In 2006, about 40% of older adults felt that their health status was excellent or good. Minority older adults, overall, rated their health status as less good than White older adults. In that same year, about 84% of older adults had one or more chronic conditions (virtually unchanged from previous years). Hypertension was the most common medical diagnosis, followed by arthritis, cardiovascular disease, chronic obstructive pulmonary disease, and cancer. Although 80% of those 80 years of age or older report two or more chronic conditions, only 36% say that they are in fair or poor health. Almost two-thirds of community-dwelling older adults received an influenza vaccine in 2006; slightly over half reported that they received a pneumococcal vaccine. The number of AL residents who receive these vaccinations, and whether there are assisted living community (ALC) policies that address this, are unknown and not tracked by most states. As a nursing practice and infection control issues, this warrants examination.

Functional disability is associated with chronic disease and increases with age. Most community-residing older adults under the age of 85 report no difficulty in activities of daily living (ADL) or instrumental activities of daily living (IADL); fewer older adults age 85 and older report little or no difficulty. An admission assessment should ask about the onset and degree of difficulty in ADLs and IADLs.

On average, older adults have more contacts with health care professionals than do younger adults. Those who assess their health as fair or poor have twice as many contacts per year as those who report being in excellent or good health. Information about the resident's pattern of physician (or nurse practitioner) contact should be obtained, recorded, and folded into the service plan. This has import for the resident's feelings of safety and well-being. It bears noting, however, that older adults in 2005 had almost two times greater out-of-pocket medical expenses than younger adults—an increase of almost 60% since 1995. This speaks to the importance of health status monitoring by the AL nurse because some residents might not be refilling their medications in order to save some money.

There is a strong relationship between severe disability and self-report of being in fair or poor health. Data indicate an association between severe disability, low income, and limited educational attainment. Some studies suggest a decline in the proportion of older adults who are unable to do some activities (i.e., one or more ADLs or IADLs); other studies do not support this. Disability increases with age: 57% of the old-old report a significant disability, almost half of whom need assistance. Projection in disability trends are important with regard to increased life expectancy and whether these years will be disability free. For AL, this speaks to service and staffing needs as the residents age in place.

Data indicate that a higher educational level and being female (because of their increased life expectancy) are an advantage for disability-free years. The notion of *compression of morbidity* suggests that the period of disability prior to death will gradually shorten (compress) as the number of disability-free years (or active life expectancy) increases. Being less than 85 years old, in good nutritional status, and having good mobility are all associated with increased likelihood of restoration of basic ADL ability that might have been diminished after (possibly associated with) an acute health event. Given that many AL residences provide rehabilitation services or assist the resident in accessing them, the data from these studies is encouraging but clearly indicates the need for cost-effective service plans that recognize the high cost of rehabilitation therapy.

Elder Mistreatment

Elder mistreatment (EM) affects almost 13% of older adults in the United States and includes physical, financial, psychological, and sexual abuse or neglect; it also includes self-neglect. Given that AL residents have family members and friends age 65 and older, it is important to be aware of the red flags of abuse as well as barriers or resistance to disclosure of EM. In AL, self-neglect can be a first sign of clinical depression and/or cognitive dysfunction. Financial abuse can also occur to an AL resident. Women are more likely to report abuse of any kind, especially verbal mistreatment, than are men; both genders report equal rates of financial mistreatment.

Clues regarding exploitation, financial abuse, or misappropriation of property might be apparent if an AL resident describes changes in his or her testamentary will and seems unsure or unclear about it; describes changes in his or her buying or banking practices; describes being forced to sign a document; or describes improper enactment of a guardian, conservator, or power of attorney role, or check-cashing without permission. All states and the District of Columbia have Adult Protective Services (APS) to investigate allegations of EM. Calls about EM protect the identity of anyone making a complaint and can also be made anonymously.

Assessment tools for EM are widely available as are suggested questions or probes when talking with an older adult whom you think might be an EM victim:

- So, tell me, how are things at home?
- Has anyone tried to hurt you in any way?
- Has anyone tried to touch you without your permission?
- Has anyone used degrading or insulting (bad) language to you?

- Have you been made to do things you didn't want to do?
- Have you signed a paper that you didn't understand?
- Have you been missing some meals?
- Are you getting the assistance you need at home?

THE CONTEXT OF ASSISTED LIVING NURSING PRACTICE

The philosophy of AL is based on the industry's declaration that it is a different care model for long-term care than ever known before. AL is not like a skilled nursing facility, nor a retirement hotel, but is rather a unique hybrid. The data indicate that approximately 1 million older adults are living in about 30,000 ALCs. The very diversity of long-term care is one reason that there has yet to be a standardized definition of AL; descriptions, definitions, and licensure vary from state to state, provider-to-provider, and even between ALCs operated by a single provider. Models of AL include independent housing with services (free-standing market rate and low-income); purpose-built free-standing AL facility; nursing home/AL campuses or building(s); and continuing care retirement communities, or CCRCs (see Chapter 17, "The Continuum of Care" for CCRC discussion). The phrase *ALC* denotes various types of housing with services, a specific residence or facility that is licensed (or certified) to provide AL services. Some unique concepts pertain to AL residency.

Home Versus Room

AL is no longer a stopping point before moving in to a nursing home. The vision is that the AL residence is a community; each living unit is the resident's home; the nurse and care staff are invited guests. Residents are encouraged to personalize their units as well as their care. Many communities avoid the use of institutional-looking furnishings. Even the medication carts are sometimes difficult to identify; some look like lovely etageres and often are made of real wood.

The notion of homeyness or "at-homeness" implies the experience of home as much as it does a precise location. It can be construed as one aspect of quality of life, and, as such, it will vary among AL providers, residents, families, and staff. Two major concepts of home are *separation* and *connection*. Separation connotes safety and refuge, privacy, control and ownership, and personal imprinting. Connection means being cared for, reciprocity and relationships, rituals, continuity and meaningfulness, status, identity, and role. The Experi-

ence of Home (EOH) scale (Table 1.1) can be useful for monitoring quality of life in relationship to an AL residence's environment prior to and after making changes in the homelike environment. The simple question, "What makes you feel at home?" could be added to marketing, preadmission and periodic postadmission survey among residents in an ALC.

Resident Independence and Self-Direction

AL residents should be encouraged to continue their usual lifestyle as much as possible. In many ALCs, residents dine when they choose and even prepare meals in their homes, if equipped with kitchens (or a Pullman kitchen). It is not unusual for residents to direct much of their care. Often, the AL nurse has to obtain a physician's order for the resident to manage their own medications, or to change timing on medications to meet the resident's preferred schedule (see Chapter 10, "Medica-

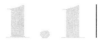   The Experience of Home Scale

Scale: SA = strongly agree; A = agree; N = neutral; D = disagree; SD = strongly disagree.

1. I feel at home here.
2. I can do what I want here.
3. This place feels cold and sterile.
4. I feel safe here.
5. I can be myself here.
6. I have my favorite places/spaces to spend time in here.
7. I have enough privacy to meet my needs here.
8. I feel cared for here.
9. I feel like an outsider here.
10. I am valued as a person here.
11. I feel isolated here.
12. I feel welcome here.
13. When I am away, I look forward to coming back to this place.
14. I feel cut off from my life here.
15. I feel a part of this place.

Note. This instrument is for internal use only; it cannot be published nor can the quality improvement data drawn from use of the instrument. Findings can be described and documented, however, with a view to comparing differences across time or before and after an innovation in the ALC.

tion Management"; Chapter 14, "Resident Assessment and Service Plan Construction," regarding decisional capacity).

Complexity of Care

AL promotes independence, but the reality is that many residents have complex medical care needs, including oversight. AL is not just for seniors who require occasional assistance with ADLs. Residents are receiving hospice care, have multiple comorbidities and, in some ALCs, have advanced dementia. Some ALCs rely extensively on outside therapies (e.g., occupational therapy, physical therapy) and home health care agencies.

Aging-in-Place

Aging-in-place and maximizing the function and quality of life of residents in an ALC is a key philosophical tenet of AL. The ALC's physical environment seeks to avoid the appearance of an institutional or medical-type of facility. Yet ALCs want to provide care to a vulnerable and medically, functionally, and cognitively impaired older adult population—many of whom require some assistance with ADLs and IADLs. Over time, AL residents decline functionally and look similar to nursing home residents.

AL residents are more likely to require assistance with bathing and dressing, are less likely to need help with toileting and locomotion, and are even less likely to need help with eating and transferring in comparison to nursing home residents. Many states permit and encourage ALCs to admit or retain residents who meet a nursing home level of care. On average, residents need assistance with 2.8 ADLs. Approximately 50%–75% of residents require assistance of some kind with their medication. Given the limited data, 66%–81% of residents suffer from dementia, depression, other psychiatric illnesses, or receive psychotropic medications.

Average length of stay is about 2 years; approximately 28% of residents will die in the ALC; 35% will transfer to a nursing home; 15% will be hospitalized and not return to the ALC. All states permit hospice services in ALCs. Almost 25% of ALCs have a dedicated Alzheimer's or dementia unit.

American Geriatrics Society Position Paper on Assisted Living

The American Geriatrics Society position paper consists of six principles that describe the benefits of AL and

providers' responsibilities. Developed for the purpose of guiding legislators, health care professionals, and consumers in the achievement of benefits/outcomes that should be expected of ALCs, the principles address:

- Providing complete information about an ALC's services to assure an appropriate match between a prospective resident and facility (i.e., disclosure);
- A holistic, culturally sensitive admission assessment in order to maintain the older adult's independent living and maximum function;
- Discussion of the plan of care with the resident, ALC, and family with regard to responsibility for each aspect of the plan;
- Staff knowledge and skills needed to competently provide care for older adults that includes signs of condition change, risk for falls, depression, and so forth; and
- Seamless transition between levels of care (see Chapter 17, "The Continuum of Care").

Interestingly, the principles address access to AL services or sites for older adults living in rural areas where the absence of such services is seen in the fact that nursing homes are admitting younger and less disabled older adults compared to urban-located ALCs.

SCOPE AND STANDARDS OF ASSISTED LIVING NURSING PRACTICE

The scope and standards of AL nursing practice describes the ethical obligations and duties of the AL nurse; guides the practice and conduct of the AL nurse; articulates the AL nurse's understanding of the profession's commitment to health care, nursing, and society; and assures timely identification of acute clinical problems to optimally manage physical and behavioral problems. The nursing role may be a joint role as administrator/wellness coordinator, generally overseeing residents' well-being, as well as being a clinician. An additional or independent role might be that of a consultant, reviewing health records and guiding unlicensed staff in optimization of residents' function and quality of life, monitoring residents' chronic illness status, or conducting assessment during an acute change of condition.

Principles of Assisted Living Nursing

AL nursing practice is holistic in that it seeks to optimize and maintain, if not improve, an older adult's function, independence, and engagement in order to maximize well-being and quality of life. AL nurses are guided by the residents' preferences, supporting them in their choices. Role activities include assessment and counseling, health education, clinician, medication management, and helping the older adult access the health care system. Principles of AL nursing embrace and support collaborating with the resident in planning, guiding, and managing his or her care; promoting and assisting the resident to maintain his or her maximum physical, mental, and psychosocial function and to reduce risk of infection and trauma, educating older adults about their options for quality of care and quality of living, maintaining and building practice skills and competencies, and advocacy in the public policy arena.

Scope of Practice

It is important to be aware of the scope of AL nursing practice with regard to the job description, performance evaluation, legal aspects of practice and accountability, and opportunity for career growth. The scope of AL nursing practice includes but is not limited to:

- Assessment: functional and mental status of the resident on admission, during and after acute changes in condition, and annually;
- Service/care planning: communication of the plan to the resident, family member/proxy, and other members of the health care team; oversight of care provided by assistive staff; recognition of deviation from the plan;
- Medication management: assessment of resident's ability for self-administration of meds; oversight of medication storage and administration (by other staff, including those who are not licensed);
- Development and oversight of health promotion and disease prevention programs: immunization, protocols for infectious disease management (e.g., influenza, herpes zoster, *C. difficile*, tuberculosis);
- Care that is focused on optimizing function;
- Determination of resident's decision-making capacity, identification of a surrogate health care decision maker, and establishment of end of life care preferences; and
- Staff development as relevant to the needs of the residents and for professional growth.

Standards of Practice

The standards of AL nursing practice, formulated by the American Assisted Living Nurses Association, are based on the American Nurses Association (ANA, 2001)

Standards of Gerontological Nursing Practice. Each standard contains description, rationale, and measurement criteria.

- Standards 1–4: Assessment, Diagnosis, Outcome Identification, Planning, Implementation, and Evaluation.
- Standards of Professional Performance include the *administrative and wellness coordinator roles* and refer to the expected professional role and behaviors of the AL nurse. These standards are a necessary component of certification of AL nursing as a specialty practice, are part of the scope and standards document, and consist of nine standards: quality of care, performance appraisal, education, collegiality, ethics, collaboration, health care consultant/educator of AL residents, research, and resource utilization.

Licensed Practical/Vocational Nurse Practice Standards

Virtually all states require the licensed practical/vocational nurse (LPN/LVN) to practice under the supervision of a registered nurse, advanced practice nurse, or physician. Given the diverse state regulations and statutes that direct AL programs and services among the states, the LPN/LVN is often the sole, as well as autonomous, decision maker and manager of care in ALCs. The LPN/LVN scope and standards and the LPN/LVN professional performance standards developed by the American Assisted Living Nurses Association use the same headings and address the same domains as the registered nurse document. The complete scope and standards of AL nursing practice for registered nurses and LPNs/LVNs is available on the Web site of the American Association of Assisted Living Nurses (http://www.alnursing.org).

RESOURCES

American Geriatrics Society. (2005). Assisted living facilities: American Geriatrics Society position paper. AGS Health Care Systems Committee. *Journal of American Geriatric Society, 53*(3), 536–537.

American Nurses Association. (2001). *Standards of gerontological nursing practice* (2nd ed.). Silver Spring, MD: Author.

Burdick, D., Rosenblatt, A., Samus, Q. M., Steele, C., Baker, A., Harper, M., et al. (2005). Predictors of functional impairment in residents of assisted living facilities: The Maryland Assisted Living Study. *The Journals of Gerontology Series A: Biological Sciences and Medical Sciences, 60*, 258–264.

Fonda, S., Clipp, E., & Maddox, G. (2002). Patterns in functioning among residents of an affordable assisted living housing facility. *Gerontologist 42*, 178–187.

Frytak, J., Kane, R. A., Finch, M. D., Kane, R. L., & Maude-Griffin, R. (2001). Outcome trajectories for assisted living and nursing facility residents in Oregon. *Health Services Research, 36,* 91–111.

Fulmer, T., & Greenberg, S. (2008). *Elder mistreatment and abuse.* Retrieved December 1, 2008, from http://www.consultgerirn. org/topics/elder_mistreatment_and_abuse/want_to_know_ more

Golant, S. (2004). Do impaired older persons with health care needs occupy U.S. assisted living facilities?: An analysis of six national studies. *The Journals of Gerontology, Series B: Psychological Sciences, 59B,* S68–S79.

Gruber-Baldini, A. L., Boustani, M., Sloane, P., & Zimmerman, S. (2004). Behavioral symptoms in residential care/assisted living facilities: Prevalence, risk factors, and medication management. *Journal of American Geriatrics Society, 52,* 1610–1617.

Mitty, E., & Flores, S. (2008). Health literacy and chronic illness management. *Geriatric Nursing, 29,* 230–235.

Molony, S. L., McDonald, D. D., & Palmisano-Mills, C. (2007). Psychometric testing of an instrument to measure the experience of home. *Research in Nursing and Health, 30,* 518–530.

Moore, J. (2000). Placing *home* in context. *Journal of Environmental Psychology, 20,* 207–217.

Morgan, L. A., Gruber-Baldini, A. L., & Magaziner, J. (2001). Resident characteristics. In S. Zimmerman, P. D. Sloane, & J. K. Echert (Eds.), *Assisted living. Needs, practices, and policies in residential care for the elderly* (pp. 144–172). Baltimore, MD: Johns Hopkins University Press.

National Center for Assisted Living. (2008). *Assisted living state regulatory review. 2008.* Washington, DC: Author.

National Center on Elder Abuse. (2005). *The basics: Major types of elder abuse.* Retrieved December 1, 2008, from http://www. elderabusecenter.org

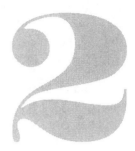

Public Policies, Assisted Living Models, and Regulations

Ethel Mitty

This chapter begins with an overview of key federal policies that affect assisted living (AL) residents: Supplementary Security Income (SSI); the Older Americans Act (OAA), which established the Administration on Aging (AOA); the Health Insurance Portability and Accountability Act (HIPAA), which established the privacy rule in health care (treatment and research); and the Patient Self-Determination Act (PSDA), which established the right and rules by which individuals could state their treatment wishes in a legal document. Various models of AL are described, as are the components of a mission statement useful to guide practice, orient new staff, and market the AL community (ALC). Nursing's fit with the mission of the AL organization and its role in strategic planning are discussed. The penultimate section, "Regulations and Oversight," discusses the aspects of a standardized admission assessment, disclosure, and the current state of AL survey or monitoring by state governments.

PUBLIC POLICIES

Supplemental Security Income (SSI)

SSI provides an older adult (such as an AL resident) with a monthly check based on the fact that he or she does not qualify for regular Social Security benefits or based on the fact that the Social Security benefits are inadequate. Individuals age 65 or older or younger persons who are blind and/or disabled are eligible if their income and assets are below a certain level. A means test is the gateway to access, but benefit levels can change yearly. The SSI program is linked to the Medicaid program, thereby entitling the older adult to have access, also, to health care benefits under Medicaid. Many ALC residents used to pay for their room and board costs but not their supportive or health care costs.

Older Americans Act (OAA)

The Older Americans Act (OAA) was enacted in 1965, the same year as Medicare (Title 18 of the Social Security Act [SSA] and Medicaid [Title 19 {SSA}]). The OAA seeks to maintain older adults in the least restricted environment by using home and community-based programs. The OAA established the Administration on Aging (AOA), which is within the Department of Health and Human Services and state-level agencies known as Area Agency on Aging (AAA). The seven different titles in the OAA provide grants for meals-on-wheels and congregate meal settings in order to combat poor nutrition related to poverty among older adults; employment placement; transportation assistance (e.g., dial-a-ride); senior centers and adult day care; in-home services; increased access to health care for rural and minority elders; grants to Native American groups;

protective services regarding elder mistreatment; and legal services. Reauthorized in 2006, the OAA is supporting demonstration programs related to aging-in-place (including aging in naturally occurring retirement communities [NORCs]) and developing mental health screening and treatment services. Access to OAA programs and services by ALCs or their residents varies among states but is worth knowing about!

Health Insurance Portability and Accountability Act (HIPAA)

Among the features of this act is the *privacy rule* that applies to covered entities, of which AL might be one, depending on the state. Because each state has different licensure rules for AL, the privacy rule may be applicable to the AL program based on how the ALC is reimbursed *and* how it transmits patient information. The privacy rule holds that electronically transmitted health information by a health care provider requires special protection of that information. The HIPAA contains 18 identifiers that could identify an individual: for example, medical record number, social security number, or demographic data. This has particular relevance in the conduct of research. For example, date of birth cannot be used in describing research participants 89 years of age or older. In some cases, a fax transmitted by telephone is not an electronic transmission, but if faxed via a computer, it is! Each state has its own interpretation.

It is very important to be aware of the restrictions on transmitting any resident information. The ALC should have specific policies in this regard. If an ALC does not consider itself a health care provider, then HIPAA's privacy rule does not apply. However, if hospice care is permitted in the ALC, it needs to be clarified if the hospice agency or the ALC is the health care provider. It bears noting that patients have to sign consent for their medical information to be shared with insurance companies, other payers, and so forth.

Patient Self-Determination Act (PSDA)

Passed as an amendment to the Omnibus Budget Reconciliation Act (OBRA) of 1990, the PSDA went into effect in December 1991. This act requires that all health care facilities that receive Medicare and/or Medicaid reimbursement (such as, hospitals, nursing homes, home health care, HMOs, and hospice) must inform their adult patients about their right to participate in, or direct, decisions about their health care; accept or refuse medical or surgical interventions; and prepare an advance directive (AD). An AL resident whose health care costs are covered by Medicaid or who is receiving skilled nursing services from a Medicare-approved provider is entitled to have this information and exert these rights.

ADs allow individuals to state in advance the kind of treatments/interventions that they want or do not want should they become unable to make or communicate their decisions or preferences. As such, ADs guide health care professionals, families, and substitute or surrogate decision makers about the person's wishes. In addition, an AD provides immunity for health care professionals when, in good faith, they follow the person's stated wishes (for example, treatment refusal).

There are two kinds of ADs: durable power of attorney for health care (DPAHC) or health care proxy (HCP) and living will (LW).

- HCP or DPAHC: The individual appoints someone he knows and trusts (i.e., the agent, proxy, or surrogate) to make health care treatment decisions for him if he is unable to do so or is unable to communicate his wishes.
- LW: Specific written instructions to health care providers about the life-sustaining interventions that an individual wants, wants to have used in a limited way, or does not want to prolong her life.

An *instructional* or *medical directive*, legal in virtually all states, identifies the specific intervention that is acceptable to the individual in particular situations (e.g., short-term ventilator support in event of brain trauma; blood transfusion to replace blood loss, etc.).

Oral ADs or a verbal directive consists of *clear and convincing evidence* of a person's wishes. This kind of directive is permitted in some states, but the legal rules vary. *Evidence* means that the person stated his wishes, consistently and unvaryingly over time, with regard to a specific medical situation.

The Five Wishes document consists of a HCP and LW but also speaks to a person's comfort interests and needs, how she wants to spend her last days, what she would like her family to know, whom she wants to forgive or whom she seeks forgiveness from, and what she would like said at her funeral. This is an intensive document, not to be completed in one sitting. Consider a small group meeting in the ALC for interested residents (and their families) to begin the discussion, including whom they can contact for the next step, if desired. The document is legally accepted in 40 states and is also available in Spanish.

The physician's order for life-sustaining treatment (POLST) may or may not be an AD; its status varies with states' health care association positions. Nevertheless, it is considered a legal document and represents a physician's (MD) or nurse practitioner's (NP) orders written after consultation with the patient about the kind of care he wants at the end of his life. POLST originated in Oregon and is spreading across the United States. A nurse or social worker can fill it out, but it must be signed by the MD or NP. It is helpful to have an AD in addition to the POLST, in order to guide clinicians, but it is not required. The POLST addresses desired intensity-of-intervention levels regarding cardiopulmonary resuscitation (CPR), comfort care, antibiotic use, and artificial administration of nutrition. It also indicates the goals of care, signatures of those with whom the orders were discussed, and when it was reviewed.

Location of the ADs, whether in the medical file or some other ALC file, varies by state and by ALC; there are few state mandates in this regard. Some ALCs post a sign on the inside of the resident's room door stating whether or not an AD exists and where it is located. This has been done, as well, with regard to do-not-resuscitate (DNR) orders (even though they are not considered an AD in the legal sense). All individuals are presumed to have the capacity to create an AD unless shown otherwise (see Chapter 14, "Resident Assessment and Service Plan Construction," for discussion of decision-making capacity). ADs should be reviewed annually and if there has been a significant change in condition.

Key Terms Related to Self-Determination

Conservator: appointed when the court finds that an individual is unable to properly and safely attend to her legal and/or financial matters. The conservator is not automatically the individual's HCP or agent.
Guardian: appointed by the court to act on another's behalf—and make decisions—when he is unable to attend to personal matters, such as health care, safety, and treatment decisions. As with conservatorship, guardians are not necessarily the legally designated HCPs/agents, yet they make health care decisions. States vary in this regard, however; there is lack of clarity, as well, on the legality of a guardian authorizing a DNR order.
Power of attorney (POA): similar to conservatorship, the court allows another person to act on behalf of an individual with regard to contracts, bills, access to banking and checking, and so forth. As a rule, the POA does not have the legal right to make health care treatment decisions.

MODELS OF ASSISTED LIVING

The concept of AL, right from the start in the 1970s, had three basic components: (a) a residential environment consisting of private space and community space shared by all residents, including dining, (b) a capacity to deliver personal and health-related services both scheduled and nonscheduled, and (c) an operational *philosophy* that supported resident autonomy, values, independence, and choice with regard to residents' preferred lifestyles. In marketing as well as in state regulations, the AL mission is to have an organization and structure that support these aims. The right to remain in the ALC and age in place tends to vary with regulations and individual provider decisions. Values embedded in the philosophy and mission include the ALC's focus on ability rather than disability (e.g., design features such as roll-in showers and tubs, adjustable closet features, etc.) and an intention to manage chronic illness as well as respond appropriately to acute illness. A key construct of AL—preservation of residents' self-esteem—constitute the ALC's philosophy, mission, and values and is embedded in its organizational style, structures, and processes.

Four different models of AL have emerged over time, each attempting to actualize an AL philosophy, mission, and values. These models can frame descriptions or expectations regarding nursing services and nursing's role in an ALC.

(1) *Hybrid model:* This model incorporates residential housing (sometimes purpose-built), available services, and a philosophy focused on resident choice. Attempting to move away from the nursing home image of dependent older adults, these hybrid AL operations avoided use of the word "facility" and substituted, instead, "residence," or "community." Phrases associated with health care, such as "admission and discharge" criteria were replaced by "move-in/move-out" language.

(2) *Hospitality model:* An outgrowth of hoteliers becoming housing providers, this model purveyed concierge-like hotel services and extensive, gracious public and private spaces. Hands-on personal or health care was not part of this model's mission or vision, although, of late, these ALCs are offering some health-related services. This model was likely responsible for suggesting that satisfaction surveys are a legitimate outcome measure of quality (of life).

(3) *Housing model:* This model originated in already-existing buildings where older adults had need for,

but difficulty accessing, personal and health-related services. In large part stimulated by states' Medicaid waivers to bring services to the domicile, this model set the highest standards regarding a home-like environment and how it could be measured (e.g., privacy and control over one's private space by locking the door, temperature control, personal furniture). In metropolitan areas, AL services are being provided in NORCs for some tenants.

(4) *Health care model:* An outgrowth of the nursing home sector, this model responded, in part, to the need for (nursing) health care supervision but not at the level provided by a skilled nursing home. Originally, these operations were compared to the pre-Medicaid nursing home older adult—that is, the person living in a board and care home or a so-called home for the aged. This model now has a distinct niche in the long-term care continuum (between independent housing and nursing home), forced the adoption of strict move-in/move-out criteria in virtually every state, and is credited for pushing forward the notion of clinical accountability and quality of care outcome measurement.

Mission and Philosophy

A *mission statement* has a present orientation; it states why a residence/facility/institution such as AL exists. The document is generally brief and should include a description or statement regarding the type of organization (e.g., if religiously affiliated, a teaching institution, for- or not-for-profit); the population that the facility (wishes to) serves; programs and services provided (broadly described); relationship with the external community; accountability and quality improvement responsibilities or initiatives; goals of service; and measurement of success (i.e., how the organization will know it has achieved what it set out to do).

Nursing does not need a separate mission statement, but the nursing service or practice—even if not an identified department in the ALC—should have a statement that describes what nursing at the ALC believes *and does* about achieving the ALC's mission. A nursing philosophy statement is more concrete than the ALC's mission statement and is useful in orienting staff to the ALC. It addresses nursing's beliefs about aging (including cultural sensitivity); resident rights; practice values/standards of care; accountability and quality improvement protocols; and education and evidence/research-based guidance of practice.

Strategic Planning

Most organizations have a strategic plan (SP), if only for the opportunity to think about where they have been and the direction in which they are heading. SPs should be reviewed annually, especially after a major shift in organization or ALC ownership and/or mission. The SP is written with a view to the organization's internal and external environment, desired customers (i.e., residents), and how the organization will meet their needs and serve their interests. The SP can also address risk reduction, especially if the ALC admits persons with significant dementia.

The nursing organization/service contributes to the SP in a very specific way by analyzing what nursing does well, what it does poorly; nursing's strengths and weaknesses; and nursing staffing needed to meet the ALC's goals. As a nursing manager contributing to SP development, it is important to be aware of trends in nursing education *and* practice (especially changes in entry-level practice and nurse delegation regulations) and changing demographics of older adults.

REGULATIONS AND OVERSIGHT

The challenge for many AL nurses is that the regulations have not necessarily kept pace with the presenting and emerging needs of older adults in ALCs (for example, insulin administration by nonlicensed staff). To be effective, AL nurses must have a strong working knowledge of regulation, as well as knowledge of how to work with the regulatory agency when residents' care needs are unique.

While some federal laws affect AL operations (see, for example, Chapter 3, "The Economics of Assisted Living"), regulations and oversight are primarily the responsibility of each respective state. Hence, there are differing terms regarding the types and levels of care and various settings in which AL services can be provided. For the provider as well as the consumer, this represents options as well as confusion. Virtually every state is continuing to create and/or revise its AL statutes and regulations. Since 2004, the states have been addressing the fact that frailer and sicker older adults are residing in ALCs—some by preference, others by state policies that encourage AL rather than nursing home residency. Most states have adopted the licensure term "assisted living," but about one-third of states use the term "residential care." Some states use these terms: "board and care," "home for the aged," "adult foster care," "enriched housing," and "personal care home." Several states have multiple levels of licensure, each serving a specific kind of resident or care need. Most states define AL in their regulations or statutes and identify the state agency responsible for AL monitoring/oversight. In 2008, 44 states had specific requirements for ALCs providing Alzheimer's/dementia care services.

All states require a pre- or on-admission assessment, but few states have a specific, *standardized admission assessment* form that the ALC is required to use. In those states, the document might be available on the state agency's Web site. Some states have a separate form to be used for those residents whose AL costs will, in part, be covered by Medicaid. In a few states, ALCs have the option to add their own data-collection instrument—or items—to the state-mandated form. Some states permit the ALC to use its own form, but it has to be approved by the state oversight agency. Virtually all states require physician clearance or approval for the older adult to live in an ALC. Most states require periodic review of the initial assessment data and when there has been a significant change in the resident's condition.

An increasing number of states require full *disclosure* to prospective residents regarding the ALC's services and costs, move-in/move-out policies, staffing, and so forth. Most states either identify the types of conditions or care needs that are permitted in the ALC, and/or those that are not permitted, and/or require move-out. Some states provide only very brief descriptions of permitted or prohibited conditions or needs. In many states, the ALC is guided by a brief regulatory statement that says, in effect, that a resident cannot (or should not) remain in the ALC if service needs are greater than what the ALC can provide or if the resident is unable to safely and independently evacuate the premises in event of a fire. Some states permit a medically unstable resident (i.e., one who needs skilled nursing care or monitoring) to remain in the ALC for a finite number of days—with or without getting the additional nursing care needed by paying for it privately.

In greater or lesser detail, states' AL regulations/statutes address:

- Medication management (i.e., use of unlicensed assistive personnel to administer or assist with medications; see Chapter 10, "Medication Management")

- Fire safety requirements
- Staffing requirements and training
- Administrator education/training and licensure
- Continuing education requirement for staff and/or administrator
- Bathroom and physical plant requirements
- Alzheimer's unit requirements, including state approval of the program and the number, type, and education of staff working in this program
- Resident rights and dispute resolution
- Criminal background check requirements
- Emergency preparedness
- Infection control standards (including food, nosocomial infection reporting, etc.)
- Medicaid coverage

Survey Oversight

There is no uniform survey content or process across all states. Some states describe what the survey will examine; other states do not conduct surveys. In many states, survey and oversight is under the aegis of a state office of quality assurance, but specific definitions or criteria might be lacking. Some states offer formal consultation and advisement by state surveyors for AL providers; others are revising their survey process and content. Surveys can be standard, abbreviated (i.e., if there have been no deficiencies or ombudsman reports since the past survey), or conducted by self-report. The content and manner of deficiency citations varies between states. Unlike nursing home citations, the deficiency citations do not speak to severity or resident endangerment, nor do they place a hold on admissions until the quality of care issue has been addressed.

RESOURCES

National Academy for State Health Policy. (2008). *Assisted living and resident care policies compendium, 2007.* Retrieved September 21, 2008, from www.aspe.hhs.gov/daltcp/reports/2007/07alcom1.pdf

National Center for Assisted Living. (2008). *Assisted living state regulatory review. 2008.* Washington, DC: Author.

Wilson, K. B. (2007). Historical evolution of assisted living in the United States, 1979 to the present. *The Gerontologist, 47*(special issue), 8–22.

The Economics of Assisted Living

Ethel Mitty

This chapter describes the financing and coverage of assisted living (AL) services by state and federal government. It describes Medicare and Medicaid programs, medical savings accounts (MSAs), the Program for All-inclusive Care of the Elderly (PACE), fee for service (FFS) arrangements, and the Balanced Budget Act of 1997.

MEDICARE

Medicare (Title 18, Social Security Act of 1965) is a social insurance entitlement program that provides health insurance coverage to persons age 65 or older (or younger, if they meet special criteria—e.g., if they are suffering end-stage renal disease or if they are receiving disability benefits via Social Security Disability or the Railroad Retirement Board). It is financed, in part, by payroll taxes imposed by the Federal Insurance Contributions Act (FICA) and the Self-Employment Contributions Act. The Medicare program has four components (A–D). Although the Medicare program is administered by the Centers for Medicare and Medicaid Services (CMS), the Social Security Administration determines Medicare eligibility.

Medicare Part A (Hospital Insurance)

Part A (hospital insurance) uses regional insurance companies known as *intermediaries* to pay hospitals, nursing homes, home-care agencies, and hospice programs

for the Medicare-covered services they provide. Older adults (and their spouses) who have had Medicare taxes deducted from their paychecks for at least 10 years are entitled to coverage through Part A without paying premiums. Others may be able to purchase Part A coverage depending on how long they had Medicare taxes deducted from their paycheck(s).

Hospital and nursing home reimbursement is based on a *prospective payment system*. In hospitals: diagnostic related groups (DRGs); in nursing homes: resource utilization groups (RUGs).

Hospice Medicare Benefit

Hospice Medicare Benefit (HMB), available under Part A, provides coverage for noncurative medical interventions and support services in a terminal illness. A physician must certify that the person is terminally ill with a life expectancy of 6 months or less. Medicare hospice is also available for persons suffering from dementia and meeting other criteria, as well (see Chapter 17, "The Continuum of Care"). An individual receiving hospice services is not required to be homebound. Hospital-based interventions to provide symptom relief (e.g., pain management, obstructed large bowel, pathological fracture) are generally Medicare covered. All states permit hospice care/services in assisted living communities (ALCs).

Most hospice costs/charges are covered at 100%; medications at 95% (5% co-pay). Many states' Medicaid programs will cover any additional costs related to hospice care that are not covered by Medicare and that the beneficiary cannot pay for. The HMB includes registered nurse (RN) visits as often as necessary 24/7 and as directed in the care plan, social work services (paperwork, referrals, advance directives assistance), skilled rehabilitation services as ordered by the physician, all medical and durable medical equipment (DME), respite care for the family, volunteer services, and spiritual and bereavement services. The patient must sign a statement that he or she chooses hospice care instead of standard Medicare benefits for the terminal illness, and the patient must receive care from a Medicare-approved hospice program. At any time, the patient can opt out of hospice care and return to his or her standard Medicare benefits.

The extent to which an ALC chooses to engage with a hospice agency or handle the paperwork and other arrangements is variable and often left to the resident or family to manage. Policies should be clear with regard to what the ALC will be responsible for and what the resident/family must manage. Medicare will not pay for any treatment or hospitalization that is not part of the plan of care for symptom management and pain control.

Medicare Part B (Medical Insurance)

Part B (medical insurance) uses regional insurance companies known as *carriers* to pay physicians, nurse practitioners, social workers, psychologists, rehabilitation therapists, home-care agencies, ambulances, outpatient facilities, laboratory and imaging facilities, and suppliers of DME for the Medicare-covered goods and services they provide. Eligibility for Part B coverage occurs at age 65 if the older adult is entitled to Part A coverage. The person must enroll in Part B and pay a monthly premium that can be deducted from his or her monthly Social Security check. Beneficiaries pay out-of-pocket for Part B monthly premiums and the Part B annual deductible, the deductible for Part A, and for co-insurance payments (usually 20%) for goods and services for which Medicare or other insurance pays only a portion. The patient may be billed by the physician for services not covered by Medicare. Physicians who do not participate in Medicare can bill patients directly for up to 15% more than 95% of Medicare's allowed amounts. Patients pay the physician and then submit their requests to Medicare for partial reimbursement (i.e., for 80% of 95% of the allowed amounts). Some physicians choose to enter into private contracts with older patients. Under these contracts, Medicare (and Medigap insurance plans) pay nothing; patients pay physicians the full amount of the fees specified by the contracts.

Physicians decide whether or not to participate in the FFS Medicare program.

In the interest of disclosure and ethical practice, the ALC should have guidelines with regard to these payment options for residents. This is particularly important if a new resident, for whatever reason (e.g., relocation to the ALC), has to obtain a new primary health care provider.

Medicare covers medically necessary outpatient physical therapy and DME if it is used in the beneficiary's home or an institution that is used as a home. Physical therapy is covered under Part B and requires physician approval of the plan of care *and* a Medicare-certified provider. DME is defined as equipment that can be used repeatedly, serves a medical purpose, and is appropriate for home use. As such, walkers, wheelchairs, and the like are considered DME.

Medicare does not cover periodic physical examinations, dental care, hearing aids, eyeglasses, foot care, orthopedic shoes, cosmetic surgery, care in foreign countries, or custodial long-term care at home or in nursing homes.

Medicare Part C (Medicare Advantage [MA])

Part of the Balanced Budget Act of 1997, this is an optional way to receive Medicare Parts A, B, and D. Originally known as Medicare + Choice, MA is a private health plan. Members pay a monthly premium in addition to their Part B monthly premium; the government pays the MA a fixed amount, monthly, for every member.

Medicare Part D (Prescription Drug Plan)

Part D is an optional plan available to Medicare Part A or B beneficiaries; it is also known as the Medicare Prescription Drug, Improvement and Modernization Act (2003, 2006). The beneficiary must enroll in a stand-alone prescription drug plan (PDP) or an MA plan with prescription drug coverage. Plans can choose which drugs or classes of drugs they will cover and at what level. Medicare specifically excludes from coverage such drugs as cough medicines, barbiturates, and benzodiazepines.

Medigap Supplemental Insurance

Medigap supplemental insurance plans are optional and cover Medicare Part A and Part B deductibles and co-insurance costs. These plans can also provide preventive care and other health-related goods and services but do not cover long-term care, dental care, eyeglasses, hearing aids, or private-duty nursing. Their applicability to AL appears limited.

Medicare HMOs

Medicare HMOs are health maintenance organizations (i.e., a group of providers) that enroll Medicare beneficiaries. It is a type of managed care service. The HMO contract with CMS specifies that the HMO will provide the beneficiary with at least the standard Medicare benefits in return for fixed monthly capitation payments. (*Capitation* is a prepayment for a group of patients [i.e., a population] based on the number of members [or enrollees] regardless of the amount—or costs—of care provided. The dollars provided are capped.) Enrollees must continue to pay their monthly Medicare Part B premiums and must obtain their health care from the HMO's provider network.

Every November, Medicare beneficiaries can choose to join any Medicare HMO operating in their area; they cannot be denied enrollment because of any health problems except end-stage renal disease. Members can leave the HMO at any time and go back to the FFS Medicare program. Every January, the HMOs can change their premiums, benefits, and provider networks—or can choose to discontinue their Medicare plans altogether. The ALC is constrained from directing a resident to a particular HMO. However, if a new resident has relocated to the ALC, information should be provided regarding the plans that are locally available.

Some older adults may have additional health insurance options through the Department of Veterans Affairs or through their (or their spouses') present or previous employer or union. Many older adults are dual beneficiaries: they qualify for Medicare and Medicaid.

MEDICAID

Medicaid (Title 19, Social Security Act of 1965) is a joint federal and state needs-based, means-tested, social welfare program that provides supplemental health insurance (including long-term custodial care in nursing homes and at home) to people of all ages who have low incomes and limited savings and resources. Administered by each state, Medicaid eligibility criteria and the benefit packages vary considerably from state to state. Most state Medicaid programs pay Medicare Part B premiums; some pay Medicare deductibles and co-insurance costs.

Several states have begun offering fixed capitation payments to managed-care organizations that are willing to provide Medicaid and Medicare benefits to residents who are dually eligible (for Medicaid and Medicare).

Assisted Living

This domain of the long-term care continuum is not considered a Medicare reimbursable care setting, such as acute care or a nursing home (for skilled nursing). There is nothing in the Medicare statute that speaks to paying for residency in an ALC. However, Medicare will pay for medically necessary care that is provided to a Medicare beneficiary in an ALC; such a residence is "home" in Medicare parlance. Home health services that an ALC provides its residents because such services are mandated by state law or are provided by private contract are *not* reimbursed by Medicare. Home health care services have to be medically reasonable and necessary, ordered by a primary care provider (such as physician or nurse practitioner), periodically reviewed by that provider, and provided by a Medicare-certified home health agency (CHHA).

Several states' Medicaid plans are reimbursing ALCs for the home care (i.e., health and supportive services) portion of the daily or monthly rate. This is done via three routes: the personal services are included as part of the state's home care Medicaid benefit, via the home and community-based services (HCBS) waiver of the federal Social Security Act, also known as the 1915© waiver program, or via Section 1115 waivers (i.e., demonstration programs). Some states use all three sources, although most states primarily use the HCBS waiver. The HCBS waiver allows states to extend Medicaid services not normally covered under the state's Medicaid plan to individuals who—if not for the waivered and received services—would likely be in a more costly setting, such as a nursing home. Personal care services provided via the HCBS waiver can include adult day care, personal emergency response systems, home-delivered meals, and adaptations in the home that would improve or maintain functionality and safety. States with an HCBS waiver can limit the number of individuals or the amount paid per unit of service or by locality or by certain groups; such authority is not permitted under normal Medicaid regulations. A critical difference between the waiver plan and the state Medicaid plan is that the Medicaid-waiver beneficiary must meet the state's nursing home level of care criteria. Among the regulations regarding the HCBS waiver is that states can set the eligibility level for Medicaid assistance, thus providing greater access to this kind of coverage for Medicaid beneficiaries. Social Security Disability Insurance can also be used to cover AL room and board costs.

CMS is conducting several demonstration projects. Provider and managed care contractors are being paid capitated monthly fees for case or disease management services for Medicare beneficiaries with specified chronic conditions, such as heart failure, diabetes mellitus, or other special needs. Some of these demonstrations are based on pay for performance (P4P): CMS will pay the capitation fees only if the contractor/provider achieves pre-agreed-to standards of performance, such as performing certain diagnostic tests (e.g., eye exams), achieving and maintaining appropriate blood levels for diabetics, and satisfying beneficiaries. Enrollment of AL residents is dependent on location of the demonstration site, not on whether they live in an ALC.

Program for All-Inclusive Care of the Elderly (PACE)

PACE is a capitated, community-based, long-term care program for dual eligibles whose care needs or disabilities meet eligibility requirements for nursing home admission and care. The PACE plan covers all costs associated with hospitalization, nursing home, or home care. There is no PACE presence in AL at this time.

RESOURCES

Center for Medicare Advocacy. (2003). Medicare and assisted living. *Healthcare Rights Review, 4*(1).

Emmer, S., Allendorf, L., & the Medicare Prescription Drug, Improvement, and Health Care Financing Administration. (2004). *2004 guide to health insurance for people with Medicare* (Pub. No. HCFA-02110). Rockville, MD: U.S. Government Printing Office.

Health Care Financing Administration. (2004). *Medicare and you 2005* (Pub. No. HCFA-10050). Rockville, MD: U.S. Government Printing Office.

Luchins, D. J., Hanrahan, P., & Murphy, K. (1997). Criteria for enrolling dementia patients in hospice. *Journal of the American Geriatrics Society, 45,* 1054–1059.

Modernization Act of 2003. (2004). *Journal of the American Geriatrics Society, 52*(6), 1013–1015.

Schonwetter, R. S., Han, B., Small, B. J., Martin, B., Tope, K., & Haley, W. E. (2003). Predictors of six-month survival among patients with dementia: An evaluation of hospice Medicare guidelines. *American Journal of Hospice and Palliative Care, 20*(2), 105–113.

Marketing, Quality, Consumer Choice, and Admission Agreements

Ethel Mitty

The assisted living (AL) nurse has a somewhat unique and under-appreciated role in marketing. Given the diverse models of AL described in Chapter 2, it is vitally important, financially as well as ethically, that the AL nurse is aware of marketing terminology and how the AL community (ALC) is represented in the marketplace. This chapter discusses, as well, notions of quality and satisfaction, admission agreements, models for aging-in-place (AIP), and negotiated risk agreements (NRAs).

In marketing parlance, an AL resident or family is a consumer, purchaser, buyer, or an end user. An ALC's marketing strategy (model or plan) is based on an assessment of current and future residents' needs, perceptions, and preferences *and* on what the ALC is capable of doing. *Market research* describes how and why consumers make certain choices. A *market niche*, identified by research, is an opportunity to meet a consumer need or demand that the ALC can provide. *Positioning* is based on market research; it shows what factors are attractive to potential buyers or users (e.g., dementia care services such as memory enhancement sessions). *Promotion* is a selling strategy that provides information through advertising and the like. *Market success* is noted by an ALC's waiting list for admission and requests for it to participate in community programs (e.g., health screening for hypertension). The gross domestic (or gross national) product (GDP/GNP), one of several

economic indicators, is a country's total final value of goods and services produced in a specific period of time (usually a calendar year). In 2006, the health care portion of the U.S. GDP was 16%, higher than in 2005 and in 1994 (when it was slightly over 14%). Most AL spaces in the facility are paid for privately, although some are reimbursed through long-term care insurance or a state's Medicaid waiver programs (See Chapter 3, "The Economics of Assisted Living"). Many ALCs have marketing directors. Yet the ability of an ALC to maintain full capacity relies on a team approach to marketing. This is unfamiliar territory to most AL nurses.

Marketing AL nursing itself has at least two purposes: to recruit staff and to attract residents (i.e., consumers). Nursing's role in marketing the ALC with regard to attracting residents and maintaining a full census resides in resident (and family or other responsible party) satisfaction—as ascertained through surveys, town hall meetings, and family service planning meetings. Nursing staff need to know the results of such surveys, not only to track negative trends but to set measurable goals that future surveys can assess. The AL nurse should be present at town hall meetings or *community nights* to directly respond to resident care issues as well as listen to the range and depth of resident concerns. Periodic review of the service plan (see Chapter 14) is another opportunity for the AL nurse to listen attentively to any care concerns or disappointments that residents or families have with service—and to respond accordingly.

Whereas inquiries about care, referrals, and leads are typically managed by the marketing person or the executive director of the ALC, marketing staff often bring nursing into the discussion relatively early—even before the older adult has made a decision whether or not to move into the ALC. Many ALCs have a *move-in packet* that includes a pre-assessment quasi-interview (about the person's sense of well-being and health), a physician screening tool, and a resident lifestyle questionnaire. It is important to have this information as soon as possible in order to make an informed recommendation or decision about the appropriate residence for this individual.

PRE-PLACEMENT/ADMISSION EVALUATION

Pre-placement/admission evaluation has several components. The AL nurse is often the first face of care that the resident meets. Communication and language are critically important at this time. The ALC is the person's home, not a unit; the people who live there are residents (in some states, tenants), not patients. The AL nurse should describe possible challenges the resident will likely face upon moving to the ALC from his or her home. Potential residents and their families will quickly sense a nurse who is feeling rushed and oblivious to the challenges and angst of leaving a known domicile for an ALC. They will see the dichotomy between what marketing described and what the reality seems to be. The pre-admission evaluation does not have to be conducted at the ALC; it can be in another long-term care setting, hospital, or the person's home (recommended for a person with dementia who would be discomfited or challenged by having the assessment conducted outside his or her known surroundings). Entering assessment data during the interview on a computer might be off-putting and seem cold or officious; transfer the data later. Pre-admission assessments should not be delayed, however, even if there are no vacancies; prospective residents need to feel valued.

As the complexity of health care needs increases among older adults wanting to live in an ALC, marketing the nursing care has an ethical dimension. The foundation for competent care in an ALC must consider:

■ *Allowable conditions:* Described in the state's regulations as stable and predictable health care needs, with few clarifying descriptors. In some states, a resident

with a specific condition or diagnosis might not be admitted. For example, most states allow admission of an older adult with diabetes mellitus, but those with a recent history of so-called metabolic instability can be admitted only if there is on-site nursing supervision. On the other hand, if an ALC has no licensed professional nurses who can administer insulin (and administration by an unlicensed person or even a certified med tech is not permitted), a diabetic resident might not be admitted. Competent pre-admission assessment requires knowledge of state-specific admission guidelines. In some states, when a resident has become physiologically unstable or exceeds the state's standards for allowable conditions or care, the AL nurse or administrator can contact the area surveyor/health department agency and request permission to retain the resident. However, this kind of arrangement should not be promised to a prospective resident or family in advance of such a condition change.

■ *Safety needs*, especially for the resident who is cognitively impaired, can be physically, emotionally, and ethically challenging for all parties. Previous elopements (or attempts) need to be truthfully reported and carefully evaluated. What is the nature of the person's wandering? Is it loss of way-finding and inability to use cues (e.g., signage, arrows, colors)? Is it purposeful walking toward some goal but the goal was forgotten in the very act of getting there?

■ ALC size and layout can be physically and/or cognitively overwhelming for some older adults. The likelihood of having a room (with or without a roommate) near the shared/common living center (for meals, diversionary activities, etc.) can influence an admission decision.

■ Trajectory of the potential resident's known illnesses. AIP and access to or availability of hospice services (and any additional costs) must be disclosed and discussed.

■ Short-term supportive services that might be needed at the time of admission and then gradually reduced as the older adult settles in to his/her new home in the AL residence.

NURSING'S MARKET IMAGE: ASSESSMENT

Consider asking all the ALC staff, not just nursing, to complete a brief questionnaire about the ALC's health care/supportive services—that is, its nursing service component. Among the yes/no questions, ask:

- Is nursing easy to deal with/approach/responsive/well-informed?
- Does nursing deliver what it promises?
- Does nursing encourage resident autonomy and decision making?
- Does nursing do better with one kind of resident rather than others?

DEFINING QUALITY

Family members think about an ALC's quality in terms of *staffing, environment, services,* and *operations.* As might be expected, staffing type, numbers, and training are important in ALCs caring for persons with dementia. Interpersonal relationships are highly valued, particularly with regard to communication, attitude, caregiving, and a sense of joint accountability among the staff for each resident. Studies indicate that as a resident's condition worsens, more and better trained staff and health care services are more valued than the ALC's activities, ambience, or social program. Continuity of caregivers, achieved by low turnover, is a quality indicator, but absent staff continuity, a well-documented resident profile and record is necessary in order to overcome (new) staff unfamiliarity with residents. A cohesive, social, warm, and homelike environment, established by staff spending time with each resident to explain and discuss things, speaks to quality of life. Before undergoing significant architectural and/or programmatic changes, it might be instructive to query residents about what *homelike* means to them; how do you know when you have it? Make few assumptions about the meaning of this critical factor in quality of life. Every few years, as resident demographics change, it might be worthwhile to do this kind of analysis (see Chapter 1, "The Assisted Living Setting of Nursing Practice," Experience of Home Scale).

In thinking about the key principles of AL, specific quality measures can be articulated and evaluated. Consider, for example, the principle of resident choice and independence: Are bathrooms shared or private? Can the resident bring his or her own furniture? Can the resident keep a pet? Can the resident lock his or her door? With regard to AIP: What are the ALC's retention and discharge policies? Do they have policies about a resident's employing private caregivers? With regard to outcomes: Are staff able to recognize a resident's change in condition? What kinds of medication errors occur? What are the unmet care needs described by residents, families, and staff?

CONSUMER CHOICE AND QUALITY ACCREDITATION

Slightly over half of State Units on Aging (SUA) have information about AL on their Web sites; some Web sites have links to other sources of information. Data about ALCs comes from consumer advocacy organizations, private accrediting agencies (e.g., Commission on Accreditation of Rehabilitation Facilities [CARF], the Joint Commission on Accreditation of Healthcare Organizations [JCAHO]), providers and provider associations (e.g., National Center for Assisted Living, Assisted Living Federation of America, American Association of Homes and Services for the Aging, Agency for Health Care Administration), and federal and state government agencies. However, there is no standardized assessment for AL quality. Many states express interest in developing a rating system for ALCs and in obtaining uniform data across states. Given that every state has different reporting requirements, however, this is a significant roadblock.

Mechanisms to inform consumers about AL options, operations, and quality monitoring occurs via three pathways: state licensing and inspections, complaint monitoring and investigations by ombudsman programs in each state, and voluntary accreditation. The Older Americans Act (2000) requires all states to have an ombudsman program in long-term care, including ALCs. The most frequent complaints about AL to ombudspersons relate to resident rights (dignity, respect), medication management, food choices, and notice of discharge or eviction. Whether there is an ombudsperson in every ALC is unknown.

The two federal and state-approved accrediting bodies for assisted living are CARF and the Joint Commission (JC, formerly JCAHO). Participation is voluntary, however, and is not required as a condition of initial or continuing AL licensure/certification. Both bodies survey similar domains and care processes (e.g., coordination and continuity of care, resident rights, health promotion) and show survey results on their respective Web sites. The CARF standards are organized in three domains: business practices, direct care (including assessment), and instrumental activities of daily living (IADLs, including medication management). The JC has 12 standards including infection control, safety, leadership, and human resource and information management.

The JC's *Assisted Living National Patient Safety Goals* (2006) include guidelines for hand-off communications that are so critical during transitions from one level of care to another (see Chapter 17, "The Continuum of Care" for transitions information). They also recommend development of a standard medication reconciliation form and falls assessment program, a protocol for flu vaccine administration, and a system to address and manage look-alike medications. Among the safety goals, ALCs (and nursing homes) are required to use at least *two resident identifiers* when drawing blood or obtaining other samples and when administering medications and treatments. Identifiers include name band, photo ID, chart number, or other specific marker but cannot be the resident's room number. Although the JC Web site provides comparative data about ALCs via its Quality Check search engine, the data refer only to those ALCs that have been surveyed or accredited by the JCAHO.

Multiple studies describe what is important to consumers: facility characteristics (e.g., cleanliness, space, ambience), staff (e.g., number, type, interaction with resident), food variety and quality, emergency service access, opportunity for choices and choosing (i.e., independence), social factors, and characteristics of the other residents. In addition, architecture, private room and bath, security and safety, staff attitude, and services that contribute to an independent, autonomous lifestyle are major considerations. However, what is not known and what warrants inquiry and understanding, even by a free-standing ALC, is the meaning of these factors for each resident, given the resident diversity. It is folly to assume that every older adult wants to participate in care planning and decision making, or that every resident has the same perception and appreciation of what constitutes a homelike environment, or how each resident (and family) calculates the risk(s) associated with self-determination.

SATISFACTION

Satisfaction feedback draws on resident and family feedback. Interestingly, staff satisfaction appears to be related to the services that may or may not be provided by the ALC. Family satisfaction tends to focus on staff responsiveness, transportation, activities, the family member's impact, and on the interesting notion of resident responsibilities. Many families feel that it is their relative's responsibility to find things he or she likes to do, administer their medications appropriately, and eat enough to preserve his or her health. For residents, satisfaction resides in a felt sense of safety and peace of mind, personal attention, independent decision making and choices, privacy, activities, and staff availability and

knowledge. Using measures of organizational culture, commitment, and job satisfaction, the data indicate a positive relationship between resident satisfaction and staff job satisfaction. For staff, those ALCs that promote and support teamwork and participatory decision making are positively associated with job satisfaction. Data indicate that residents with higher educational levels tended to be less satisfied with AL.

ADMISSION AGREEMENTS

Three *business models* appear to describe AL residences: (a) those that admit residents with high acuity and service needs and are more concerned with meeting their needs than with the impact on resident mix, costs, and reimbursement; (b) those that admit low- to moderate-acuity residents and retain them even as their care and service needs increase (note: acuity levels rise but tend to be cyclical as these residents leave/die and new low-acuity residents are admitted); and (c) those that admit low- to moderate-acuity residents but rather than discharge them as their acuity/needs rise have the residents meet their needs privately. It is important for an AL nurse—as well as prospective ALC residents—to be aware of the business model of the facility and how it affects, for example, move-in/move-out decisions.

Most states require ALCs to give (i.e., disclose) specific information prior to admission, and in the admission or residency agreement as well, about the services included in the basic rate or the cost of the service package. However, only about half of the states require ALCs to disclose their admission, retention, and discharge policy, the services that can be provided beyond the basic package and their respective cost(s), payment and billing practices, resident rights, and grievance procedures. Fewer than 10 states require disclosure of ALCs' staffing practices, medication management, or services that are simply not available. Several states require that the disclosure and resident rights document be written in plain language, not legalese. Resident rights information can be provided in a specific resident rights document rather than in a residency or admission disclosure document. The extent to which individual ALCs disclose over and above what the state requires is unknown. The AL nurse needs to be aware of what state regulations require and what the ALC chooses to disclose.

Admission and Retention Criteria

Virtually all states take into consideration the (potential) resident's functionality with regard to activities of daily living (ADL) assistance, need for health-related services such as nursing supervision or monitoring, cognitive status, health status stability, and cognition. Three categories of admission and retention policies have been identified: *full continuum, discharge triggers,* and *level of licensure.* Facilities in states that permit a full continuum approach can establish their own criteria, albeit within state regulations. In advocating for a resident's right to remain in an ALC, an AL nurse should be aware of the state's regulations regarding, for example, a resident's options when his or her needs exceed what the ALC can safely provide (or what the resident/family can purchase through supplementary services). For example, some states permit ALCs to admit and retain residents who require nursing supervision or are bedridden for more than 14 days, but treatment complexity (e.g., mechanical ventilation, Stage III or IV pressure ulcer care) may be cause to recommend transfer to a higher level of care, such as a skilled nursing facility. Discharge triggers with regard to certain conditions or needs can be similar to criteria forbidding admission or retention beyond a certain amount of time. In general, these conditions refer to treatments that cannot be safely administered in an ALC, such as IV fluids administration, or sterile dressings.

It is important to know that, within each state, several approaches to admission, retention, and discharge can be in effect at the same time. Some states grant waivers for ALCs to retain residents whose care needs exceed what is permitted by regulation. If the ALC, resident, and family arrange a (service) plan of care that safely meets the resident's needs, and the costs are identified and agreed to by all parties, the resident can remain in the ALC—given physician approval of the plan. Of those states that have levels of licensure, an ALC can pick and choose what kinds of services it will and will not provide. There is no question that this mix-and-match approach can facilitate AIP, but it can also be very confusing to the consumer/prospective resident (see Chapter 14, "Resident Assessment and Service Plan Construction").

Aging-in-Place and Negotiated Risk Agreements

AIP is a major tenet of AL philosophy and service. Whether specifically described or alluded to in state or facility-specific retention language, AIP requires that an ALC respond to a resident's changing needs and adjust its services and level of care criteria. When this happens, a resident is presumably less likely to be discharged to a higher level of care, that is, to a nursing home or skilled nursing facility. AIP means not having to move from a current residence to one that can provide support services needed to maintain comfort and well-being. A managed negotiated risk agreement (NRA) can be a record of the recognition and accommodation of the resident's risks of remaining in the ALC. As such, an NRA can facilitate AIP; but it bears noting that AIP has positive and negative outcomes for residents and the facility.

While more than half the states address AIP in their AL regulations, far fewer provide guidelines for negotiated risk discussion and service plans. An increasing number of states permit ALCs to offer additional (or skilled nursing) health services for an intermittent or limited time; this facilitates AIP. Retention or discharge (e.g., to a nursing home) is dependent on state regulations about specific resident characteristics and the services that may or may not be provided. However, individual ALCs have the right to be more restrictive. Most states do not permit retention of residents on continuous bed rest or requiring two-person transfer. The exception to all of this is that virtually all states permit hospice services/care in ALCs, in which case the additional services needed would be provided via hospice; the ALC is not liable for failure to provide care or neglect of obvious needs.

Administration of injectables, including insulin, is a major issue for AIP. Nurse practice acts and state regulations vary across all states in this regard and should be closely read. For example, the New Jersey Health Department agreed in 2008 that medication aides/techs in ALCs can administer insulin using insulin pens. This single factor can be very important in selection of an ALC that meets an older adult's continuing needs.

Managing the decline associated with chronic disease is a cornerstone of AIP service plans. The notion of resident–facility fit to manage decline resides in two strategies: one, preventing decline with health promotion and maintaining therapeutic regimens; two, responding to decline by attempting to balance needs with an ALC's resources. The second strategy is met, wholly or partially, by increasing fees to hire additional staff, and/or bringing in additional equipment (e.g., mechanical lifter), and/or increasing the family's financial or physical support for increased care. Both strategies pose a risk for the resident and the ALC. The resident might choose to refuse the additional care/services needed for a variety of reasons including increased costs. The ALC's risk might be failure in their genuine attempt to provide the care needed and subsequent accusation of neglect.

An NRA is a way to manage the risk(s) associated with a resident's choice(s). However, few states have provisions and/or statutes regarding NRAs. Almost all states regard the NRA (concept or practice) as an expression of resident choice when that choice might be in conflict with medical advice or ALC norms, but some states restrict their use. The resident's service plan should reflect the situation, contingencies, and constraints that are discussed in the NRA.

Some states require a negotiation process when a resident's behavior is placing him/herself or others in harms way. Fewer than 10 states have specific guidelines that address the resident's capacity to understand the provisions in his or her NRA. Some states prohibit an ALC from attempting to use the NRA to avoid liability.

RESOURCES

Agency for Healthcare Quality and Research. (2006). *Environmental scan to inform consumer choice in assisted living facilities* (Pub. No. 07-0032-EF). Rockville, MD: Author.

Ball, M. M., Perkins, M. M., Whittington, F. J., Connell, B. R., Hollingsworth, C., King, S. V., et al. (2004). Managing decline in assisted living: The key to aging in place. *Journal of Gerontology: Social Sciences, 59B*(4), S202–S212.

Chapin, R., & Dobbs-Kepper, D. (2001). Aging in place in assisted living: Philosophy versus policy. *The Gerontologist 41*(1), 43–50.

Edelman, P., Guihan, M., Bryant, F. B., & Munroe, D. J. (2006). Measuring resident and family member determinants of satisfaction with assisted living. *The Gerontologist, 46*(5), 599–608.

Hawes, C., & Phillips, C. D. (2007). Defining quality in assisted living: Comparing apples, oranges, and broccoli. *The Gerontologist, 47*(special issue), 40–50.

Jenkens, R., O'Keefe, J., Carder, P., & Wilson, K. B. (2006). *A study of negotiated risk agreements in assisted living: Final report.* Retrieved December 1, 2008, from http://aspe.hhs.gov/_topic/topic.cfm?topic = Long-Term%20Care

Joint Commission. (2006). *Assisted living national patient safety goals.* Retrieved April 24, 2008, from http://www.jointcommission.org/PatientSafety/NationalPatientSafetyGoals/06_npsg_asl.htm

Joint Commission for Accreditation of Healthcare Organizations. (2006). *Accreditation programs assisted living.* Retrieved December 1, 2008, from http://jointcommission.org/AccreditationPrograms/AssistedLiving/06_npsg_asl.htm

Mitty, E., & Flores, S. (2008). Aging in place and negotiated risk agreements. *Geriatric Nursing, 29*(2), 94–101.

Mollica, R. (2004). *Residential care and assisted living policy: 2004. Section 1.* Retrieved December 13, 2007, from http://aspe.hhs.gov.daltcp/reports/04alcom1.htm

Mollica, R. (2006). *Residential care and assisted living: State oversight practices and state information available to consumers* (AHRQ Publication No. 06-MO51-EF). Washington DC: National Academy for State Health Policy.

Mollica, R., & Jenkins, R. (2001). *State assisted living practices and options: A guide for state policy makers.* Portland ME: National Academy for State Health Policy.

Nursing and Organizational Theory, Practice, and Culture

Ethel Mitty

There is no one nursing theory that perfectly captures what nursing is or does, can prescribe what nursing should do, or predict what will happen as a result of nursing acts. Two nursing theorists looking at the same activity, for example, ambulation assistance, will attribute different meaning to that assistance and its basic elements. This chapter briefly describes two nursing theories that can guide practice in assisted living (AL), the manual of nursing practice, and the various terms that guide nursing, such as, protocols, procedures, policies, and nursing orders. Knowledge of the concepts and language of organizational and management theory are vital for nursing effectiveness in meeting resident goals. This chapter describes autonomy and empowerment, characteristics of participatory management and shared governance, and offers some criteria for assessment of organizational culture and climate.

NURSING MODELS

The two most relevant theories or models for AL nursing practice are Roy's (1989) adaptation model and Orem's (1991) self-care model.

- *Adaptation model*: This model holds that the individual is a biopsychosocial being who must cope with internal and external environmental stressors; coping is either adaptive or it is ineffective. Illness is a manifestation of a problem coping with stressors. Adaptation is a kind of equilibrium that is needed to free energy for healing and reach a level of wellness. Nursing's role is to promote adaptive responses.

- *Self-care model*: Widely used in nursing homes, this model holds that people want to understand their health care needs and make choices about (and participate in) their care. Also known as the self-care deficit theory, this model states that a patient is someone who needs assistance in meeting his or her health care *demands*. The notion of self-care is that it is a *universal requirement* needed to maintain and improve life and health status. The nurse assists the individual in achieving his or her maximum self-care competence.

The *nursing diagnosis model*, used in some nursing homes, is a typology of health patterns (not a nursing theory) that guides data collection, assessment, and nursing intervention. This model can be useful in structuring the resident's service plan. A health problem is either actual or potential and is expressed by the problem statement (e.g., falls risk), the likely etiology or cause (e.g., postural hypotension), and the presenting signs and symptoms (e.g., unstable gait, low blood pressure). Terms such as "impairment of," "limitation in," and "alteration of," refer to both cause and effect of the problem. Currently, there are more than 100 nursing diagnoses distributed in 12 categories: activity/rest, circulation, ego-integrity, elimination, food/fluid, hygiene, neurosensory, pain/discomfort, respiratory, safety, sexuality, social interaction, and teaching/learning. Assessment instruments, care plans, and guides are available.

Manual of Nursing Practice

Many health care publishers have nursing practice manuals; it is important to select the manual that has the best fit with the AL resident population *and* the staff who will be providing the assistive care. The manual should be a reflection of both the nursing theory and standards of practice that are guiding nursing care delivery in the AL community (ALC). It describes the objectives of care and the nursing acts to achieve them. The manual should be reviewed annually and at such times as the mission of the ALC has changed. A manual contains policies, protocols, procedures, and nursing orders.

- *Standard*: a competency for which a nurse (or personal care assistant) is accountable; directs practice; is evidence-based.
- *Policy*: a kind of standard; a strict rule or regulation that must be followed because of regulation, facility policy, scientific evidence, or professional standards; an outline of actions that must be taken.
- *Protocol*: a kind of standard; a guideline to manage a specific problem, diagnosis, or syndrome (e.g., pain, confusion).
- *Procedure*: a road map or sequence of steps to conduct a specific activity; a standard for delivery. This is a detailed formal model that *assumes limited knowledge or skill.*
- *Guideline*: a less authoritative type of standard that suggests flexibility in decision making about care or treatment decisions given patient-specific attributes. Based on evidence and expert opinion, they guide procedures and approaches to care.
- *Nursing order*: a specific evidence-based (if available) intervention that does not require a physician's order (e.g., measures to prevent skin breakdown, oral hygiene, reminiscence).

ORGANIZATIONAL THEORY, PRACTICE, AND CULTURE IN ASSISTED LIVING

Regardless of size, and whether free-standing or part of a corporate or network group, the nursing service in an

ALC is an organization consisting of people and with *formal* and *informal* structures. Mission, goals, policies, procedures, and the table of organization constitute the formal structure. The human element—management/ leadership style, interpersonal relationships, communication style, personal beliefs and values, and group history and norms—constitute the informal structure. The informal structure (re)interprets nursing's (i.e., the organization's) values and is critical to goal achievement.

Managerial beliefs about workers (i.e., staff) influence how staff will be perceived, appreciated, and given decision-making power over their work. This is as true in AL as it is in any white- or blue-collar work setting. Given the extensive and costly turnover of personal assistive staff (e.g., nurse assistants) in long-term care— including AL—these constructs about workers can be useful with regard to retention efforts.

Two managerial beliefs about workers prevailed during the 20th century: *theory X* and *theory Y.* Theory X holds that workers, in general, are not really interested in their work or in problem solving, are motivated only by salary and benefits, need constant monitoring and threats to be productive, avoid responsibility, have little loyalty to their work unit, and entertain few expectations about their management or leaders; management style is therefore autocratic. Theory Y holds that workers have a good attitude toward their work, are interested in problem solving, and are motivated because of the respect between management and workers. Management style is supportive, humanistic, and based on the belief that workers are self-directed, have little need for monitoring, seek and enjoy responsibility, feel that their personal goals are achievable through organizational goals, and feel that management values them. *Theory Z* emerged in the 1980s, is similar to Theory Y, and holds that workers seek responsibility and are the key to productivity. A theory Z management technique, *quality circles,* involves workers from all levels in problem-solving discussion and empowers them to make recommendations; data show that it raises morale, productivity, and quality.

Autonomy and Empowerment

The social architecture of a nursing service (i.e., organization) consists of the interaction between the formal and informal structures, the way in which roles are enacted by all members (i.e., the staff, the workers), and the degree of autonomy and empowerment given to them. Roles are defined by job descriptions, but how they are enacted depends on the workers' personalities and willingness to adhere to the organization's rules (i.e., policies), norms, and their understanding of what is expected of them.

As a nurse manager, it is important to know whether and to what extent the values of nursing and staff/worker are similar. For example, is there a match between residents' rights, such as respect and choices, and staff rights, such as input into the construction of a performance evaluation tool, or opportunity for career growth? To what extent do values differ among different staff classifications (within nursing and with other ALC staff)?

Autonomy

Autonomy means the right to be self-determining and to at least participate in decisions that affect one's work and well-being. To a considerable extent, autonomy is a cornerstone of the *culture change* movement that seeks to empower nursing home residents so that they receive self-directed care and to empower caregivers who are closest to the bedside (that is, the nurse assistant or personal care assistant). Empowered staff must be able as well as willing to assume responsibility and accountability for their actions as well as their attitude. This can happen only if management commits time and resources for education and training in problem-solving and decision making.

Participatory Management Theory

This theory holds that those who will be affected by a decision should be involved in making it. These staff will be more committed to organizational goals than those who were not involved. Empowerment and the shift from a *centralized* to a *decentralized* social architecture moves the span of control from being embedded solely in the chief executive (and supervisors) to placing authority and accountability at the lowest possible level of the organization; staff will make decisions that directly affect their work.

Shared Governance

Shared governance is a key element of participatory management and empowerment. It is an opportunity for creativity and development of staff problem-identification and decision-making skills. An ALC nurse manager should be able to answer the following questions.

- How ready (and willing) are staff for decision-making accountability?
- What are staff members' decision-making skills?
- What will happen to the decision makers if they make a poor or wrong decision?

- What decisions should and will continue to be made by the nurse manager? The main office? (In general, decisions that affect the entire service or facility, such as sick time policies, should be centralized.)
- What decisions should be made by the frontline staff? At the unit level?
- If decision making is resident-centered, what skills do staff have in recognizing and managing poor or faulty resident-made decisions?

A participatory management style and decision-making process is inappropriate when staff lack knowledge, skills, or expertise about the issue; when a decision is needed quickly; and/or when the issue is minor and/or affects very few staff. It is very appropriate when staff really have something to say about the issue and when they have experience, knowledge, skills, and expertise—perhaps even more than upper management! Participatory management decision making is also very useful because it can draw in diverse and sometimes highly ingenious ideas, can help a group reach consensus around controversial issues, and can facilitate collaboration across services or disciplines if that is needed for program or goal achievement.

Staff unaccustomed to give-and-take discussion need encouragement and support to engage. Use open-ended questions; follow up a "yes" or "no" (or "I don't know") response with a probe; ask "what" instead of "why" (asking why something is important or was done or not done can elicit a defensive response). There are no wrong answers. Consider this opener: "That is an interesting point you made. I'd like to hear more about . . ." Then add one of the following questions.

- If you could modify one thing . . .
- What, in your opinion, makes XX important?
- If XX is done, what is likely to happen, in your view?

Table of Organization

A table of organization should reflect the philosophy of the ALC (e.g., resident-centered care) and its management style (e.g., participatory management), especially with regard to reporting lines, communication, and accountability. Most tables of organization are organized by top-down decisional authority. Typically, authority and decision making flow down and accountability flows up. A solid line indicates accountability and reporting relationships; a broken line indicates a communication relationship only. The concept of resident-centered or resident-directed care has influenced revision of tables of organization: circular constructions place the resident in the middle of the decision-making nexus; vertical constructions place the resident at the top of the decisional pyramid, from which all decisions flow.

Culture and Climate

An organization's culture, such as nursing, includes management/leadership style, its values and reward system, and its history. Culture is observed in staff and leadership behavior and in the norms of the organization. The fact that staff fail to call in sick at least 2 hours before start of the shift—a management policy—is a cultural norm.

Climate is a measurement of staff perceptions and attitudes about their work and the workplace. Some writers use the words "climate" and "culture" synonymously. Nursing climate assessment instruments address, to a greater or lesser degree: communication, trust, interpersonal relationships, rewards, status symbols, work norms, autonomy, supervisor support, control, work pressure, conflict management and change, climate, and quality of care. This information (i.e., data) can be important in preparing for change, such as the decision to admit residents needing rehabilitation services or a change in ownership or nursing leadership.

A study conducted in 61 ALCs and with more than 300 staff analyzed the relationship between staff perception of organization culture and their work-related attitudes. Using several different instruments measuring job and coworker (i.e., team) satisfaction, organizational commitment or loyalty, morale, communication, supervision, and other aspects of an organization's structure and style, the findings clearly indicated that organizational culture is associated with, and even a predictor of, job satisfaction and work-related attitudes. Perceptions of the work environment, specifically teamwork, strongly influenced satisfaction with coworkers. There was a strong relationship between staff feeling that they were treated with respect and their commitment to the ALC.

To estimate staff receptivity to change, for example, or to policies associated with new ownership or new direction (mission) of the ALC, a questionnaire addressing the following factors, can be useful. Staff would be instructed to respond (anonymously) yes-or-no or to a Likert-type graded scale. What is the . . .

- Degree of adherence to the *chain of command* for all issues and decisions?
- *Distribution of information method:* verbal, written, rumor?

- Staff's *participation in decisions* that affect their work?
- Sense or evidence of *teamwork?*
- Formal or informal *terms of address* among staff, including administration?
- Adherence to *dress policy?*
- Maintenance of *confidentiality* of resident and staff personal and health issues?
- Culture of *safety:* reporting errors and near misses?
- Extent to which *deadlines* are met or ignored or to which promises are kept?
- Core of *resistance* to any change or innovation?
- Opportunity for staff to *celebrate* a special moment (e.g., birthday, baby, etc.) while on duty.

Staff's likely response to change can be assessed using maturity models, some of which draw on Maslow's hierarchy of need satisfaction and motivation, or on a continuum of immature to mature. For example, a personal care assistant (PCA) who is dependent on supervision to prioritize her residents' care needs and has no interest in problem solving (i.e., theory X) is immature in contrast with a self-directed PCA who likes to engage in creative problem solving (i.e., theory Y). Another maturity model characterizes workers as: unwilling and unable to engage in decision making (i.e., immature); being willing but unable; being able but unwilling; or being able and willing (mature). ALC nurse managers should think about how their staff currently manage change and are likely to do so given future contingencies.

Trust is a special component of manager and worker relationships. Two positions on trust reflect different (and almost opposite) management styles: you trust a person until proven otherwise; you cannot trust a person until proven otherwise.

RESOURCES

Eaton, S. (2000). Beyond "unloving care": Linking human resources management and patient care quality in nursing homes. *International Journal of Human Resources Management, 11,* 591–616.

Gordon, M. (1982). *Nursing diagnosis: Process and application.* New York: McGraw-Hill.

Mitty, E. (1998). *Handbook for directors of nursing in long-term care.* Albany, NY: Delmar Publishers.

Orem, D. (1991). *Nursing: Concepts of practice* (4th ed.). St Louis, MO: Mosby Year Book.

Roy, C. (1989). The Roy adaptation model. In J. Riehl-Sisca (Ed.), *Conceptual models for nursing practice* (3rd ed., pp. 105–114). Norwalk, CT: Appleton & Lange.

Sikorska-Simmons, E. (2006). Organizational culture and work-related attitudes among staff in assisted living. *Journal of Gerontological Nursing, 32*(2), 19–27.

Leadership/ Management Style and Assessment

Ethel Mitty

An assisted living (AL) nurse functions within several role constructs: leader/manager, clinician, and educator/ resource person. For purposes of this book, the terms "leader" and "manager" are treated as if they are the same thing, unless otherwise stated. This chapter describes several leader/manager styles and how to assess them from several perspectives: decision making, trust, and so forth. Assessment is a nonthreatening way to indicate areas of strength and those areas in which some tweaking, development, or maturity is needed. These assessments might be applicable, as well, in organizational climate, job satisfaction, and retention analyses. All the tools described in this chapter are publicly available.

Also discussed in this chapter is transformational leadership, communication and feedback, the one-minute manager, assertiveness, components of an employment interview, and characteristics of an ethical nursing practice model and a professional nursing practice model.

LEADERSHIP/MANAGER STYLE

Leadership is shaped by multiple factors: the leader's intellect and interests, abilities and attitudes, staff trust and maturity, the internal and external environment, and the organization's work ethic. Roles have elasticity; a leader can be a role taker (i.e., business as usual perspective) or a role maker (i.e., responding to the situation; a force for change). Three leadership role-categories exemplify the range and depth of leadership: *interpersonal, informational,* and *decisional* roles.

Management or leadership style involves the distribution of decision-making between leaders and followers (i.e., workers) and reflects the leader/manager's beliefs about the staff's right to participate in decision making. The seven leadership styles described in the following list refer to manager–worker decision making and can be useful in framing problems and discussing solutions in nursing management in AL.

- *Autocratic/authoritarian.* The manager's focus is on task completion and goal achievement; only the manager makes decisions; there is no input from staff. Trust between managers and staff is minimal; individuals and groups/teams (within nursing or between departments in the AL community [ALC]) compete rather than collaborate. Rewards (e.g., promotions, going to a conference) and punishments are based on outcomes and are the exclusive right of the manager to bestow. It bears noting that this leadership style is highly valued and very effective during times of crisis (e.g., power outage, strike).
- *Paternalistic.* Staff are completely dependant on the manager, who not only makes all decisions but

assumes responsibility and accountability for the staff's activities and the outcomes of their efforts. This kind of leader might be just as overbearing as an autocratic leader but tries to protect workers by preventing their mistakes or preventing them from making poor judgments. During a survey, this kind of manager can reassure staff that they will not be taken to task by negative survey findings.

- *Participatory.* While the manager only has decision-making power, the staff provide input. This concept of leadership is not the same as shared governance.
- *Democratic.* Sometimes confused or used synonymously with participatory leadership, this style more closely resembles shared governance—which is not a leadership style, per se. Staff set policy, establish goals and plans, make decisions, describe and detail tasks, and determine when goals have been achieved.
- *Laissez-faire.* Some management theorists do not consider laissez-faire a leadership style; rather, they feel it is a complete absence or abdication of leadership. This type of leader/manager gives advice and offers guidance only when asked, provides the resources needed, and is not invested in outcomes evaluation. Given the total freedom—and responsibility and accountability—of the group, it could be argued that this type of leadership requires the highest level of worker maturity.
- *Bureaucratic.* This manager enforces organizational policies so that staff have little opportunity for creative initiatives, that is, other ways of doing things. Staff participation in decision making lacks authority and meaningfulness. Nursing middle managers can fall into this role when their domain of practice or responsibility is unclear.
- *Technocratic.* This manager relates to the group as an expert consultant. With a mature, self-directed work group, this can be an effective leadership role but it lacks visioning and motivation. It is not a recommended role model in AL, where nursing is more than a skill set.

Transformational nursing leadership is a leadership style that epitomizes engagement in which leaders and followers, through mutual trust and respect, motivate and raise each other to higher levels of aspiration and achievement. This kind of nursing leader is inspiring/visioning, ethical, and provides a practice environment that supports trust, creativity, and caring. In management terms, a transformational nursing leader is both people and production oriented and incorporates shared governance and collaborative practice.

What Is Your Leadership Style?

It is important to understand one's management style and assist staff in working (and thriving) with it or, alternatively, moderating your style to match the contingencies in the situation, including staff maturity, threats in the environment, and so forth. Four behavioral styles with respect to interpersonal relationships have been articulated in the following list. Know that a manager is not exclusively of one type with no other characteristics; you are likely a composite. The question before you is whether you are too much of one and scarcely enough of another.

- *Controlling leader/manager.* Staff know that you are not going to waste time with niceties but will get to the point quickly and remain focused on it. You are likely to offer options from which followers/staff may choose. This style can be very effective and desirable in a crisis situation, especially during a tough state survey.
- *Supporting leader/manager.* Your focus is on relationships, cooperation, eliciting staff ideas and avoidance of conflict. Perceived as nondemanding and loath to engage in major conflicts, you might be unwilling or unable to engage in difficult change or conflict situations or to recognize poor performance or productivity.
- *Promoting leader/managers.* You are rather like an entrepreneur: you have lots of ideas, you bore easily, and you change your mind with stunning rapidity if something does not work out. It is fruitless to challenge you. Sometimes, you rely on scanty evidence, settle for second-best or so-called satisficing (although you refuse to recognize that), and jump to the next step.
- *Analyzing leaders/managers.* You are supremely comfortable with structure, orderly process, data, and substantive feedback. Characteristically, you are an information gatherer, maintainer of standards, and are risk averse. As such, you may have been described (perhaps unfairly) as a procrastinator, unable to make a decision. You hate surprises and prefer logical, organized, referenced reports.

Extensive research on various leadership/management styles in nursing homes consistently finds that a combined leadership style of consideration/relations-oriented and structure is more likely to achieve quality resident care than is either leadership style alone. Successful leadership respects and meets staff needs *at the time* and considers *all* the factors in the situation.

Consider a collaboration with nursing faculty at a local school of nursing to conduct modest studies to evaluate leadership/management style in the ALC and its effect on resident outcomes and on staff.

COMMUNICATION

Communication is interpersonal, by definition. It is also affected (and arguably, effected) by trust between senders and receivers, whether the message/information is lateral, upward, or downward. Senders and receivers interpret the information, much like a translator does from one language to another. This process may be like the old telephone game: what was the message that came out at the end compared to the message that went in? The fact that all staff initial that they read a memo in no way ensures—nor should it be assumed—that the information or guidance was applied correctly.

Leaders/managers communicate in order to *tell* or to *sell*. A tell communication brooks no discussion; the intent is to inform, direct, and clarify (e.g., "Attached please find the changed policy on vacation benefits"). A sell communication seeks to persuade and solicit feedback—up to a point (e.g., "Attached please find the feedback from staff on all shifts with regard to vacation policy. It appears that most staff want xyz"). Effective leaders/managers are good sellers; they invite discussion but also know when to end the debate, usually at the time the feedback is repetitive.

Memos, in organizational parlance, are a mediated communication. A memo is desirable as a mode of communication because everybody gets the same information. However, a memo that is more than one page long is not a memo; it is a report. Be cautious, also, of so-called memo blitz (i.e., too many memos arriving at the same time). The assumption that message distortion is reduced because there are no intermediaries to (re)interpret the message is a happy delusion. Personal, socioeconomic, educational, and cultural factors influence how a memo is decoded. Talk with staff about how they prefer to receive information. Should the type of content (e.g., vacation policy, birth announcement) determine whether the message will be verbal or written? Decide with staff how to check that the information was accurately received. It may be that some staff (or managers) will always prefer one communication style, whereas others are willing to trust/risk other ways of being informed. Continue to check back with regard to accuracy of the message received.

Feedback can be positive or negative, verbal or written, a message to "go" or to "stop," and can be disas-trously ineffective if not timely or sensitive. Negative feedback is a "no" or "stop" message; it should not be about a worker's personal characteristics. Comments should be framed around the value or lack of value of the activity—not the value of the person; it should be about the performance behavior. Positive feedback says "continue this valued activity/behavior"; negative feedback says "stop it; it has no value." Negative feedback requires that the sender and receiver formulate a mutually agreed-to plan of correction (utilizing principles of adult learning) with targeted performance goals and timelines.

One-Minute Management

Countless nurse managers in long-term and acute care have received as well as given copies of *The One Minute Manager* (Blanchard & Johnson, 1982) to their staff. It is a remarkably thin (available in paperback) guide for effective management. Three core ideas constitute the successful one-minute manager: *one-minute goals, one-minute praisings,* and *one-minute reprimands.* When managers and staff agree on goals, there has to be open discussion regarding whether or not resources (i.e., time, equipment, support services) are available and sufficient for goal achievement. Absent this discussion, goal achievement is unlikely, for either party. Goals, whether individual or group, have to be recognizable: "How will I know it when I have it?" The gap between what was achieved and what is still desirable is the area for improvement.

Catch your staff doing something right instead of doing something wrong. That is the essence of one-minute praisings, and it means recognition and praise at the time that something specific is observed, not several months later as part of the performance evaluation. "Well done!" is nice to hear, but it lacks specificity; well done for doing what? The praiser could also say how good it made him or her feel about what the worker did, then and there.

The third secret, the one-minute reprimand, is exactly what its name implies and is based on prior agreed-to performance standards. Staff need to know that they are accountable for their actions. A reprimand should not be delivered to someone who is learning a new skill, nor should it wait until the annual performance evaluation. A reprimand is negative feedback, but it can also lead to a root cause analysis of an error, a revisitation of the goal(s), or an indication that additional education/training is needed. The reprimand (delivered in private) should also speak to how much the person and his/her efforts are valued.

Assertiveness

Acting assertively does not mean acting aggressively; those styles have different strategies, expression, and goals. The benefits of acting assertively include increased self-respect and self-confidence, reduced feelings of incompetence and of being poorly treated, and, interestingly, the desire to be held accountable for one's actions. Just as leaders are made, not born, assertiveness has to be learned. In some cultures, particularly for women, this is a major undertaking and carries emotional if not physical risk. Assertiveness competency appears in many leadership roles and domains. For example, giving negative feedback is an aspect of the monitoring role; expressing an opinion is an aspect of ethical and decision-making skills; saying "no" is a time management skill. The process and skills of problem solving/decision making, advocacy, and assertiveness are similar in that all require problem identification and data collection, evaluating alternative actions and their consequences, and outcome analysis.

How can you assess your (or others') assertiveness skills? Do you always say "yes" to a request, legitimate or not—rather than risk feeling guilty if you say "no"? Are you generally silent at meetings, ask no questions, or make no comments? Do you feel others think you are uninformed or not too bright? How do you feel about accepting compliments? How do the people you work with feel about and describe assertive people? Do they view them as cold, aggressive, or power-hungry? A heated discussion is not necessarily a power struggle. These openers are examples of healthy and respectful assertiveness and still get at the issue:

- "Tell me what I did/said that set you off; this is really important to me."
- "Help me understand . . ."
- "I rely on your feedback; you have to let me know when, in your view, I am off track."

Practice being assertive and making your case. Test out how wording and intonation might affect the listener/receiver; written and verbal assertiveness will likely have totally different receptions. Know in advance whether body language and touching (e.g., reaching out to give a back pat or stroke the person's arm) is permissible or offensive. Is eye contact an absolutely necessary part of the conversation or is it to be avoided (as in some cultures)? It is very important to consider the likely risks and consequences of the assertive act: social, professional, resource access. As an exercise, move the emphasis on each word of the following statement: "*When* can I expect the repair to be done?" "When *can* I expect the repair . . ." "When can *I* expect the repair . . ."

Employment Interview

An employment interview is somewhat like a commercial exchange of selling and buying; investment (i.e., cost) in a new employee is high (estimated at $2,500/per person). Items on a standard application form generally request information about the applicant's education (licensure, certification) and past employment history; some ask how the applicant learned about the position. Federal regulations prohibit asking about marital status, children and family planning intentions, race, religion, age (i.e., date of birth), arrest and civic violation history, and financial status. Questions that can be asked speak to citizenship verification, English and foreign-language proficiency, and person(s) to notify in an emergency. It is acceptable to administer a skills inventory and medication administration quiz at this time, if only to introduce them into discussion during the interview. Most states have established a registry of certified nurse assistants that contains information about criminal violation.

An interview with a licensed nurse applying for a staff or leadership position (e.g., unit/nurse manager) should cover the position's role and responsibilities in AL nursing practice. Questions one might ask would address the following:

- Role and responsibilities: the applicant's perception of the role/position's opportunities and constraints, risks, and benefits; clinical and managerial responsibilities; experience in teaching and learning evaluation; research experience; understanding of the rules, regulations, and reimbursement of AL; and current activities with regard to professional growth.
- Nursing theory and practice: the nursing theory/model that has guided the applicant's practice and care planning for older adults; concepts of interdisciplinary care; indicator(s) of quality of care; notion of a culture of safety; and evolution and evaluation of resident/person-centered care.
- Interpersonal relations: thoughts about performance evaluation; understanding of delegation and accountability; and feedback and progressive discipline.

Interviewing an applicant for a personal care assistant position might begin by asking what the person knows about AL (mission, facility, residents). It might help establish trust between the potential employee and the ALC by asking him what frustrated or disappointed him in his last position/job. This speaks to motivation and job satisfaction, which, in turn, is seen in resident care outcomes. It is fair to ask the applicant what kind of resident they do not want to work with or are most comfortable with. In closing out the interview, after talking about the salary and benefits the applicant is seeking, ask her what kind of supervision and leadership she likes, how she feels about being part of a decision-making group, and how she wants to be told if she is (or is not) doing a good job.

Ethical Nursing Practice Model

An ethical nursing practice model takes the four major ethical principles and puts them into practice in clinical and management nursing acts.

(1) *Beneficence and nonmaleficence*—to do good and prevent or reduce harm—is seen in nursing practice as assistance with personal hygiene, pain management, and informed observation regarding change in condition. In nursing management, it is seen in job descriptions and performance evaluations and in employee health programs.

(2) *Respect for persons* resides, for ALC residents, in confidentiality of the medical record (particularly with electronically recorded and transmitted resident data); for staff, it involves negative feedback and grievance processes.

(3) *Autonomy and informed consent* (i.e., self-determination) for residents is their (or their surrogate's) participation in service plan construction and in negotiated risk agreements (NRAs); for staff, it entails their participation in shared governance and participatory decision making.

(4) *Distributive justice* means the fair distribution of goods and services. Care assistance should be based on assessed need and not on ability to pay. In the management domain, this principle is seen in resource allocation. Using resident/family satisfaction survey findings, determine if food and dining room service are more valued than personal care assistance. How are the needs of those who value and/or need personal care assistance to be balanced by the interests of those who value an aesthetic dining experience? Or a robust activity program?

Professional Nursing Practice (PNP) Model

This model is a relatively recent (re)construction of what nursing practice is all about; the patient and family are central, and care is patient/resident-centered. The core of this approach is that care is guided, coordinated, and provided by clinically competent and caring professional nurses. The requisite structures and processes in the PNP model include leadership, research/evidence-based practice, support systems, collaboration within and across disciplines, standards of practice, self-governance, and continuing professional development. A growing body of research demonstrates the interrelationship of these factors in providing quality of care and, as well, a nurse's intention to remain in the nursing profession.

RESOURCES

Anderson, R.A., & McDaniel, R.R. (2003). Nursing homes as complex adaptive systems: Relationship between management practice and resident outcomes. *Nursing Research, 52*(1), 12–21.

Blanchard, K., & Johnson, S. (1982). *The one minute manager: The quickest way to increase your prosperity.* New York: Wm. Morrow and Company.

Scott-Cawiezell, J., Main, D.S., Vojir, C.P., Jones, K., Moore, L., Nutting, P.A., et al. (2005). Linking nursing home working conditions to organizational performance. *Health Care Manager Review, 30*(4), 372–380.

Sullivan-Marx, E.M., & Gray-Micelli, D. (2008). *Leadership and management skills for long-term care.* New York: Springer Publishing Company.

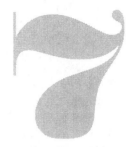

Problem Management, Change, and Team Building

Ethel Mitty

For an organization to persist and grow, change, conflict resolution, and continuity are all inherent components; an assisted living community (ALC) is no exception. This chapter describes critical thinking, problem identification, decision making, strategies of change, conflict resolution, and principled negotiation. Voting methods and team process assessment are also described.

PROBLEM MANAGEMENT

Problems are best analyzed by critical thinking: a combination of insight, maturity, education, experience, and reasoning skills. It requires recognition of the *aspects* of an issue or problem between staff, residents, departments, or various other parties and combinations. Think of a teaching session where the purpose is to draw out the students to think analytically by asking probing questions.

Alternatives refers to the degree of fit between a proposed or likely outcome and the interests of the parties involved. An alternative that will have an impact on the ALC's mission, organization, resources, structures, and processes needs close scrutiny with regard to resources (e.g., staff classification and numbers, skills, and equipment), costs, burdens, benefits, risks, *and* likely consequences of each alternative. For example, if the ALC decides to admit persons with severe cognitive impairment or dementia, what impact will this have on the current residents, programming, and skills needed? Sometimes the most challenging aspect is the evaluation criteria with regard to each alternative.

The terms *problem identification* and *decision making* are sometimes used synonymously; problem identification is sometimes called *problem solving*. A decision can be *optimizing*: there is sufficient time and information to think about each alternative and its consequences. Or it can be *sufficing*: the information at hand is sufficient—or has to be—to make a decision. Decision making begins with identification of a problem and ends with choosing among alternatives; it has six essential steps:

(1) Collect and analyze relevant data, then ask if any data/information is missing. If so, will it be difficult or easy to collect and/or analyze?
(2) Differentiate between fact and myth or rumor; estimate the likely power of each of these sources to influence the decision.
(3) Estimate the type or nature and the degree of conflict about each alternative and the staff (and/or residents) whom the decision will affect.
(4) Identify the values—cultural, ethical, spiritual—that may be embedded in the problem.
(5) Classify the problem using Donabedian's structure-process-outcome model of quality (Donabedian,

1988), if possible. Is the problem more associated with overall organization? Is it a process issue, such as communication between shifts? Is it a resources issue: budget and finances (internal) or reimbursement (external)?

(6) Is the problem the tip of an iceberg? And if so, how can it be chipped away?

When a problem fails to generate several alternatives, the wrong staff may be working on the problem—or the staff who are working on the problem don't have the expertise to generate solutions, or the time and interest to work on it. It might be that the problem was inadequately described or presented. Staff have to be not just empowered to make decisions but educated/trained in the decision-making process. Similarly, AL residents might need clarification or assistance in making decisions and choosing among the options that affect their lives.

CHANGE AND CONFLICT RESOLUTION

Change means both the means to an end and the end in and of itself. In the face of an impending survey, it might be better to continue a policy or practice. Staff, out of anxiety, might respond with misinformation when asked a question by a regulator and thus undermine the good intentions of the change. Stay with the tried-and-true in the face of two competing pressures: impending survey versus the need to change practice for quality of care/safety reasons. Explain or describe to the regulators/surveyors the planned change; if available, give them copies of new/revised practice guidelines. In the event that a new practice has to be implemented and the survey is very soon, then plan a response to surveyors' likely identification of deficiencies: explain that the protocol/procedure is new and was implemented because of the ALC's quality improvement plan feedback. Assure staff, in advance, that their anxieties are recognized.

In the face of change, staff as well as managers are likely thinking about their preparation and readiness for the change, performance evaluation, and job security; they need information. It is difficult to change behavior and even more difficult to change attitude. Cognitive science suggests that if the behavior is changed first (and the rewards are meaningful), then attitude change will follow. For example, personal care assistants (PCA) might resist having their assignment become fixed instead of the usual practice of rotating every few days. It has been repeatedly demonstrated that, after a few

days, the PCAs are likely to value not having to learn about new residents every few days. They also become invested in the goals of care for their permanent group of residents and become their advocates!

To implement change:

- *Sell or tell* (verbally or in writing) the advantages or values of the change in comparison to the status quo and how it fits with staff self-interest and/or resident well-being.
- Identify the person in charge who has the authority to modify or discontinue the change plan or the planned change.
- Those who will be affected by the change should be decision-making partners in how the change will be implemented *and* evaluated (this can include residents).
- Identify the barriers and likely sources of resistance *as well as* the supporters.
- Identify the data needed before and after the change and how the change will be evaluated.
- As with any structural or process change, anticipate likely consequences of the change process and the change itself. For example, if you intend to change shift hours, medication administration schedule, or meal times, then think about the unanticipated consequences.

If a change process or outcome is worse than the problem itself that precipitated the change, abandon it and evaluate what might have gone wrong in the problem analysis and resolution. What facts were at hand and what facts were missing? How was goal achievement going to be recognized?

Conflict can be healthy or destructive, it invites creativity regarding goals and process, it improves productivity or diminishes it, it encourages cohesion among staff and groups, or it ushers in divisive partisan loyalties. There are a variety of approaches to *conflict resolution*, some more satisfying than others and some more appropriate for the transformational leadership associated with effective nurse managers. Think about the history of conflict in the ALC, approach(es) that were used to resolve them, and the outcomes. In selecting a conflict resolution approach (see the following list), it might be helpful to have a desirable outcome in mind when going into the discussion.

- *Confrontation*: In this approach, each party presents their case with no guarantee of an outcome satisfying to all parties. This approach implies that there are winners and losers.

■ *Suppression and smoothing*: This approach tries to downplay differences and look for similar opinions and interests between parties. Dangers with this approach include misrepresentation or failure to present relevant information; it can also be perceived as patronizing or paternalistic.

■ *Accommodation*: This approach entails a willingness to please the other party and could be called appeasement. This is not a "you win, I lose" settlement, although it frequently is felt as such. It might be more useful to construe this strategy as one that is mindful of the contingencies in the situation.

■ *Blaming*: This approach attributes the situation to an external force, such as the surveyors/the state. This has a lovely feel-good quality and rationalizes why some policies simply had to be written, but it generally makes staff feel disempowered and impotent. Even though staff feel good about each other—they bonded against a common enemy—this approach is useful but only for the short run.

■ *Compromise*: In this approach, neither party gets what they want ("I lose, you lose").

■ *Collaboration*: The approach entails mutual interest in conflict resolution; both parties give up something they wanted yet both feel they got what they wanted ("I win, you win").

■ *Principled negotiation*: This approach tries to get to a middle ground through tradeoffs that get each party a little of what they each want.

Described in *Getting to Yes* (Fisher & Ury, 1992), principled negotiation tries to avoid the ad hominem (i.e., personal) attack among parties in conflict. This approach wants to put each party in the other person's shoes in order to at least appreciate the values contained in the other's argument. Scenario: conflict between two roommates, each of whom wants the bed by the window; one resident has been there longer; one was private pay longer; and so forth. Another scenario: both PCAs want every Sunday off. The maxims of principled negotiation are quite simple but are not simpleminded:

■ Separate the people from the problem,
■ Focus on interests not on positions, and
■ Think about options for mutual gain by both parties.

Committee and team effectiveness

Depends on role taking by the members in the group, the decision-making processes, and conflict management. A committee charged with making recommen-

dations should not be made too large in an attempt to have all perspectives represented or too small, with the consequence that members are assuming multiple roles and start to wear thin. A committee, group, or team may be dysfunctional because members are ill-prepared for the group's purpose and/or group process, because they do not feel that the issue is important, because there are role (power) battles within the group, because decision-making processes and/or authority are unclear, and/or because members are unsure about the reception to and/or consequences of their actions.

Not every decision requires a committee; think about the individuals or groups who will be affected by a decision. For example, changing a vendor who supplies food staples differs from changing the ALC's menu. If a committee is formed, different *roles* are needed at different times in committee/group/team processes: task roles (e.g., information seeker or provider, coordinator, summarizer, recorder); building and maintenance roles (e.g., monitor and expediter, soother and compromiser, interpreter, standard setter); and individual roles.

Voting

When a committee is formed, members need to know whether their decisions are simply recommendations, that is, advisory, or have authority (i.e., the decisions must be carried out). The three generally accepted voting methods are by *majority, unanimous vote,* or *consensus*. Select a voting method with due regard to who and how many staff will be affected by the decision, scope and intensity of change, and ambiguities and unknowns in the issue that needs to be decided.

■ *Majority vote or two-thirds rule:* This means that up to one-third of the members may not support the decision (and, likely, are uncommitted).

■ *Unanimous vote* (100% pro, in favor, supportive): This is very time consuming to achieve. If the likelihood of acceptance is high and rejection is projected to be low, *but* nevertheless possible, this voting method should not be used.

■ *Consensus voting:* In this method, members recognize that a decision is needed; all agree to support the decision in spite of disagreement; and those who disagree (but vote to support the decision) reserve the right to evaluate the decision at some future date. Consensus voting is a characteristic of team/group/committee maturity.

Assessment of Team/Group/Committee Effectiveness

Given the time involved in team, committee, or group work—and time is money—it might be necessary to look at the team process if outcomes are unacceptable, not timely, and so forth. Regardless of ALC size and organizational or corporate structure, the way(s) in which teams/groups/committees advance the mission and goals of the ALC can be evaluated—as can a resident/tenant council. Assessment methods include:

(1) Role-taking analysis: Write the roles or functions (as described earlier) across the top of a sheet of paper and the names of all members of the group/team/committee on the left. (The rows and columns form boxes.) During a meeting, a neutral observer checks off each time one of the members assumes a particular role/function. Discuss the observations of group dynamics and next step(s) for role development.

(2) Power relationships analysis: Draw a circle, then write the name of each group member on the circumference. A neutral observer draws a directional arrow every time a member speaks, indicating if it was to the group at large or to an individual member(s). The lines drawn can indicate not only who did most of the talking but to whom the talking was directed. The observations are discussed.

RESOURCES

Donabedian, A. (1988). The quality of care. How can it be assessed? *Journal of the American Medical Association, 260,* 1743–1748.

Fisher, R., & Ury, W. (1992). *Getting to yes. Negotiating agreement without giving in.* New York: Penguin Books.

Mitty, E. (1998). *Handbook for directors of nursing in long-term care.* Albany, NY: Delmar.

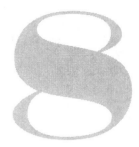

Staff Development and Training

Ethel Mitty

This chapter discusses key responsibilities of a nurse manager/leader in an assisted living community (ALC): job descriptions (JDs) and the performance evaluations that are based on them, and staff development. Providing education and the information needed to perform well is but a small fraction of staff development. This chapter describes many aspects of staff development, including concepts of competency, principles of adult learning, lesson plans and case-based learning, role models and mentors, feedback, and discipline. Suggestions for education in assisted living (AL) nursing practice are also provided.

JOB DESCRIPTIONS

Every organization/department must have job descriptions for its staff, including administration/management staff. Key components of a JD are:

- Job title
- Accountability or reporting relationships (who the position reports to and who reports to the position)
- Position summary (general description of the scope of practice of this role)
- Responsibilities and tasks (an *overall* listing of the daily duties but not necessarily including everything; the last item should be "All other duties as assigned")
- Qualifications or requirements (experience, education, personal attributes, physical capability)

- Optional: whether it is a management or supervisory position (Note: if the ALC has a collective bargaining unit [CBU], this position might be included or exempt)
- Optional: occupational safety issues and potential hazards, including Occupational Safety and Health Agency (OSHA) regulations

Some JDs are quite explicit with regard to the physical requirements of the position, as might be expected for personal care assistants (PCAs). In some JDs, the lifting and physical exertion of the job are described in terms of the percent of time the activity (e.g., one-person lift assist) is required: rarely (> 1%), sometimes, frequently (30%–65% of the time), or continuously. Physical activity can also be differentiated by percent of time the employee would be sitting, standing, walking, pushing or pulling, and so forth.

The JD should be the basis for evaluation but is sometimes fraught with fuzzy wording, for example, terms like "attitude," or "caring." What do those attributes look like? How do you know that a PCA is caring or attentive or respectful? By what a resident says? When a resident says that a PCA is very kind to her, and she gives specifics, does that mean that the PCA is unkind to a different resident who says nothing? A JD should contain behavioral terms and activities that are observable and, ideally, measurable. It is the basis of the performance evaluation. Job descriptions should be reviewed annually and/or when there is a change in the organization's mission, structure, or services. Each state's Nurse Practice Act (NPA) frames the job description of registered nurses (RNs) and licensed practical/vocational nurses (LPN/LVNs), respectively, with regard to scope of practice.

Competency, in a nursing job description, has two meanings: (a) readiness to perform a nursing act and (b) quality of the conduct or performance of the act. Some nursing services use Benner's *novice-to-expert* construct (Benner, 1984) to delineate expected competencies in nursing staff JDs, performance evaluation tools, and career ladders. Benner distributes competencies in seven domains of practice: helping, teaching/coaching, diagnosing and monitoring, managing unstable situations, therapeutic interventions, quality, and work role. Research evidence for this construct is strong; it is a useful model to establish and maintain standards of practice. The novice-to-expert continuum is as follows:

- *Novice*: task performance is rule (i.e., procedure) driven because this practitioner has very limited experience with the work to be done as well as the decision-making skills needed to change any aspect of the procedure/activity. For example, a new RN or LPN, hired shortly after graduation and licensure, makes several basic treatment errors or goes off duty without turning in assessment data: competency level in this case is poor. However, in all fairness, review the nurse's orientation to the ALC, the policies and standards of practice, and the monitoring that was provided; they may have been inadequate.
- *Advanced beginner* (approximately 9–12 months into practice): this practitioner is beginning to understand the context of a health care event or situation, recognize the cues, and develop a plan, but he or she still needs assistance and guidance to make sense of the information/data.
- *Competent*: after several years in the same or similar position, this practitioner has evident mastery over most situations, is an independent decision maker who is knowledgeable about goals and how to achieve them, and is a full participant at interdisciplinary team meetings.
- *Proficient*: this practitioner has the skills to rapidly and correctly appreciate a problem from diverse perspectives, construct an approach with several options and consequences about which all parties (including the resident) need to weigh in, and move forward effectively and efficiently.
- *Expert*: given years of experience with successes (and failures), this practitioner is a problem solver with

the knowledge and skills to both guide as well as share and instruct.

The task performance of an RN and LPN/LVN might look exactly the same, but the difference resides in the analysis and approach to problem solving. Informed by a more extensive knowledge base, this is what differentiates an RN from an LPN/LVN. The American Association of Colleges of Nursing (AACN, 2000) and the John A. Hartford Institute for Geriatric Nursing described the core competencies, knowledge base, and role requisites of a nurse who could (and should) provide quality care to older adults. Although based on the expected competencies of a nurse graduating from a baccalaureate program (i.e., BSN), it would not be unreasonable to expect the competencies in the following list of an AL registered nurse—or, in many cases, an experienced LPN/LVN. (These competencies relate to the professional nursing practice model described in Chapter 6, "Leadership/Management Style and Assessment.")

- Critical thinking with regard to attitudes about aging and person-centered care;
- Communication that recognizes the influence of age, gender, culture, and cognitive and physical changes of aging;
- Assessment of risk factors using validated tools;
- Illness and disease management of geriatric syndromes common to older adults and the interaction of acute and chronic (i.e., comorbid) conditions as well as the altered presentation of illness;
- Information and technology for monitoring and communication;
- Ethics, particularly with regard to the parameters of autonomous decision making;
- Cultural competence;
- Health care systems knowledge regarding provider systems and reimbursement for care; and
- Care at the end of life.

PERFORMANCE EVALUATION

Performance evaluation (PE) is a type of feedback based on standards of practice and descriptions of activities in the JD. A properly administered PE—it is a process as well as a document—is a "go" message that can improve the work of satisfactory staff and is a "no" message to those who are performing unsatisfactorily. There should be no surprises; a performance expectation that was not described in the JD should not be a PE criterion. Domains of PE generally include

- Care outcomes with regard to the resident and the unit/facility;
- Evidence of knowledge and skills and their application in practice; and
- Varying with the job level: communication, interpersonal relations, decision making, and conflict resolution.

Rating scales are somewhat arbitrary and perhaps could be left to staff to choose which kind of rating scale they prefer and for which aspects of their work. Failure to provide performance feedback—N/O (not observed) or N/A (not applicable)—about critical aspects of the job is disrespectful to the worker and does not build organizational trust or loyalty. Rating scales can use Benner's novice-to-expert construct, but the performance or activity has to be specifically described. Commonly accepted descriptive terms for a performance scale are:

- O = Outstanding: the very best that can be expected; a role model.
- G = Good: performance is above required standard of practice.
- S = Satisfactory: performance meets expected/required standards of knowledge and skill.
- U = Unsatisfactory: required standards have not been met. A remediation/education plan using principles of adult learning must be implemented (including the support that will be available and what the worker will independently do to improve performance). A specific date or length of time until performance re-evaluation should be agreed to and documented.

Performance evaluation criteria will differ across job classifications. For example, the specifics of the criteria of evaluation will be different for the nurse manager than for the PCA—and such criteria should be spelled out.

The PE tool or measure should be discussed at the time of employment. Feedback has no value if it is not specific to the action(s) that met or failed to meet a standard. An employee has the right to refuse to sign the PE; this should be noted on the document as well as the reason(s) for refusal (by the employee or by the person who administered the evaluation). A *self-evaluation tool* can be used for all levels of staff, in all disciplines. Easily constructed, it should be based on what the employee *and* their supervisor/manager think is important. In fact, importance could be drawn from the job description! A self-assessment tool for ALC nursing staff could consist of these items:

- My outstanding abilities are . . .
- My performance on the actions listed below is: Good, Could be better, or Could use some education about . . .
- *Perhaps most importantly:* What the ALC can do to help me reach my goals . . .

STAFF DEVELOPMENT

Orientation for new staff should include a walkabout and introductions, general policies of the ALC (possibly in an employee handbook) and those specific to the nursing service. Policies and protocols applicable for all employees include the ALC's mission, values, and goals; table of organization; fire safety and disaster preparedness plan; tipping and gifts; smoking; visiting hours, including pets; complaint and grievance process (for residents, family, staff); and sick, lateness, and vacation accrual guidelines. More specific policies and protocols for nursing staff only are:

- The nursing model that guides ALC nursing practice
- Hazardous substance management (also for housekeeping/environmental services)
- Infection control plan (a variation would be applicable for the preceding services as well as dietary services)
- Resident rights (specifically confidentiality, privacy, and access to records)
- Medication management system and the culture of safety in the ALC
- Dress code
- Abuse, mistreatment, and neglect reporting
- JD and PE criteria
- Ombudsman access to resident records

The ALC, and hence the nursing service/department, is morally obligated to describe and discuss with every (new) employee the relationship between the JD, PE, and the benefits or rewards that can be achieved. It is recommended that new staff complete a *skills inventory* relevant to the work they will be expected to do. This helps develop the education/training plan that will bring the employee up to a level of acceptable practice.

In-service education is the maintenance of existing—and the introduction of new—knowledge and skills. Topics should be relevant to AL nursing practice, not just what is hot in the marketplace or a freebee from a drug rep. *Principles of adult learning* recognize that an adult's motivation and receptivity to new knowledge is borne of personal history of achievement in something that mattered, and the person's needs, values, and aspirations. An adult learner is someone who is in control of what and when new information will be accepted or learned. The notion of a *learning contract* is built on mutual respect between teacher and learner, agreed-upon goals or outcomes by both parties, an honest appraisal of the learner's strengths and weaknesses, and the learner's felt need to learn. In cases where a disciplinary action has been invoked, either by continuous errors in practice or infraction of facility policy (e.g., sick calls), the learning contract should have specific measurable outcomes. Any on-site teaching or in-service referrals should also be documented and include a description of the reason for the teaching (e.g., procedural update, safety/medication management, infection control, etc.).

Lesson plans are similar to an application for continuing education units (CEU) or contact hours (CH). In general, a lesson plan has a title and states the purpose or goals/objectives of the program in behavioral terms, such as, "At the end of this program, the learner will be able to . . . describe, discuss, demonstrate . . ." Avoid attitude outcomes, as they are notoriously difficult to measure although seemingly easy to describe. Three to four objectives are sufficient. Each objective should have one to three statements describing the relevant content that will be provided. A lesson plan includes the name and title of the instructor (including department), teaching method(s) (e.g., lecture, Q and A, pre- and posttest, role play, etc.), required reading or viewing (including Web sites), and method and criteria of evaluation.

Case-based learning, also known as the case study method or problem-based learning, is extensively used in medical, nursing, and business education. This method is an opportunity to explore a complex situation from different perspectives and requires critical thinking and decision making. The case can contain both the problem and the solution(s). The purpose is to teach, not to test, like a tutorial. Participants debate the merits of each solution, its risks, benefits, burdens, and consequences for the person(s) involved. Role playing can also be used to add drama as well as ambiguity.

Ideally, the case should be only a few paragraphs long but should be authentic to the ALC *and* to the role and responsibilities of the likely players (e.g., resident, family, nursing staff, administrator). In ALCs, what situations lend themselves to case-based learning? Examples: a diabetic resident who finds various ways to eat cake and candy; a resident who refuses to bathe;

a family who constantly complains about the services; the need to protect the resident with impaired decision making from the consequences of poor judgment regarding, for example, leaving the ALC unattended; a life-long smoker, fully capacitated, forbidden by ALC policy to personally keep his or her smoking materials and needing permission to go to the smoking area(s).

The *SOAP (subjective-observation-assessment-plan) format* can also be used to structure the case format.

S: What is the issue or problem from the resident's (family) perspective? What values, interests, or preferences are embedded in the issue? What actions has the resident taken, to date, to further his or her interests, albeit riskily?

O: What is known about the issue? What are the risks and dangers: resident/family perception? Staff perception? What is ALC policy? What information is missing from our analysis/discussion of the problem?

A: What is (are) the likely outcome(s) if nothing is done? If the ALC does XYZ? What are the risks, benefits, and burdens for the resident, and the staff, with each option?

P: What is the rationale/justification for the plan that has been agreed to by all parties? If the resident does not agree, is it still a viable plan?

Role Models, Mentors, and Preceptors

A *role model* teaches by example; nothing special is demonstrated specifically for the new employee; there is no show and tell. A *mentor* or *preceptor* (the terms are often used synonymously) is more actively engaged: guiding, teaching, counseling, coaching, correcting. A mentor is recognized for his or her competence, knowledge, and human relations and communication skills, as well as being a role model. Mentors should be volunteers with a passion for teaching who believe that, because of their efforts, the likelihood of retaining a new employee increases (and the odds of resignation or termination decrease). Mentors are not replacements for in-service staff, they are adjuncts, and they should be on staff for at least 1 year before becoming a mentor. It should not be assumed that a mentor knows how to teach or to coach; this should be evaluated and discussed with the prospective mentor. It is important to teach the mentor to recognize when their mentee requires more direction and training than they (the mentor) can provide. Having a mentor when someone is promoted in-house, for example, from a staff to a nurse manager position, can enrich and smooth the transition. Having an experienced buddy for a new personal care staff member is like a combined role model and mentor. This has significant benefits for new staff who are trying to learn the work and the norms (culture) of the PCA position at the same time. There are no guidelines about specially compensating a mentor, preceptor, or buddy.

Discipline and Negative Feedback

Discipline is a kind of negative feedback, a stop sign that is meant to correct behavior or change unsatisfactory performance. For negative feedback and discipline to be effective in an organization that respects its staff, *progressive discipline* relies on the existence of clear policies, complete JDs, known standards of performance, PE instruments that contain measurable criteria, and a learning contract. A referral to in-service education can be an appropriate first step prior to initiating a disciplinary action or notice. It can be argued that recourse to disciplinary action (up to and including termination) is as much a failure of leadership as it is of the worker. Employees are entitled to protest or grieve a warning or disciplinary action.

A written warning, with relevant attachments, generally consists of:

(1) The policy, procedure or standard that was violated (or ignored).
(2) Evidence of the violation (e.g., medication record, time card). Avoid hearsay.
(3) The employee's version of the situation. Note: The employee is entitled to have someone with him/her, either as a witness, for friendly support, for union representation, and so forth.
(4) Record of previous situations that are identical or closely similar to the current situation (e.g., medication error, lateness pattern, failure to respond to a call bell).
(5) Record of interventions taken to correct the previous *and* current situation (e.g., in-service referral, coaching).
(6) The next step(s) to be taken in the course of modifying/correcting performance.

(7) The next step in progressive discipline should the employee be unable to do his or her work satisfactorily (and safely).
(8) Name(s) and title(s) of other persons present during this discussion.
(9) Employee's signature that the disciplinary statement has been seen *and* discussed. (As with PE, the employee can refuse to sign.)

Education for Assisted Living Practice

A national survey revealed that most direct care (personal/assistive) staff have no knowledge about normal aging; 80% feel that urinary incontinence and confusion are normal age-related changes. Many staff have scant information about antipsychotic medications and the manifestations of dementia yet feel that they know how to manage such behavior. States vary with regard to the required hours of training and content (e.g., age-related changes, psychosocial needs of the older adult, dementia, death and dying).

Recommended education for all ALC staff based on reports and suggestions from multiple sources, including expert clinicians, includes the following: normal aging and age-related changes, cultural aspects of care, person-centered care, communication, depression, pain assessment, relationship with families, holistic assessment, manifestation of dementia, models of dementia care, and death and dying care.

RESOURCES

American Association of Colleges of Nursing. (2000). *Older adults: Recommended baccalaureate competencies and curricular guidelines for geriatric nurse care.* Washington, DC: American Association of Colleges of Nursing and the John A. Hartford Institute for Geriatric Nursing.

Benner, P. (1984). *From novice to expert. Excellence and power in clinical nursing practice.* Menlo Park, CA: Addison-Wesley.

Hawes, C., Phillips, C. D., & Rose, M. (2000). *High service or high privacy assisted living facilities, their residents and staff: Results from a national survey.* Washington, DC: U.S. Department of Health and Human Services.

National League for Nursing. (1983). *Competencies of graduates of nursing programs* (Pub. No. 14-1905). New York: Author.

Waters, V., & Limon, S. (1987). *Competencies of the associated degree nurse: Valid definers of entry-level nursing practice* (Pub. No. 23-2172). New York: National League for Nursing.

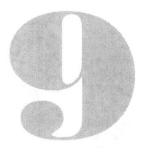

Staffing, Assignments, Delegation, and Time Management

Ethel Mitty

This chapter provides a brief overview of the recommendations proffered by the Assisted Living Workforce (ALW), convened by the U.S. Senate Special Subcommittee on Aging in 2001, regarding assisted living (AL) nursing responsibilities. Given that delegation (of nursing acts) is such an inherent part of AL—and nursing responsibilities—the principles and rules of delegation are discussed in some detail. Types of time use are described, as is a time waste assessment that might be helpful in guiding a fledgling nurse manager toward a more mature managerial style.

STAFFING, ASSIGNMENTS, AND DELEGATION

Nursing staff, both licensed and unlicensed, provide *direct care* (e.g., personal hygiene care/assistance, medication administration, treatments), *indirect care* (i.e., things done on behalf of the resident but not at the bedside), perform *management activities* (e.g., report writing, meetings, scheduling, resolving conflicts), and engage in *personal activities* (i.e., meal and break), all of which are budgeted. An *assignment* transfers the responsibility for an activity to another person(s), but it is not the same as *delegation,* which is an action that *empowers someone to act on another's behalf.* In both cases, however, accountability has to be identified.

The ALW, by a two-thirds majority, recommended the following: criminal background checks of personal care staff, establishment of a federal abuse registry, compliance with federal employment statutes, 24-hour awake staff, discussion of the job description with a future employee, administrator qualifications, recruitment and retention practices, orientation and performance evaluation. A recommendation that an AL community (ALC) should ensure the right number of staff 24/7 to meet residents' predictable and unpredictable needs, and fire safety needs, was not adopted. The ALW members disagreed about the staffing requirement; many felt that staffing should be at the discretion of individual providers, albeit in keeping with state guidelines. Most ALW members agreed, however, that dementia unit staffing should be at least two staff members per five or more residents.

The ALW recommendation for a registered nurse (RN) presence in the ALC was not adopted even though research indicated that residents in an ALC with an RN who was involved in care plan development and monitoring were less likely to be transferred to a nursing home. Similarly, the ALW did not adopt a recommendation regarding personal care assistant (PCA) training performance objectives and workload. Nursing staffing standards suggested by the Consumer Consortium in Assisted Living (CCAL) were based on resident acuity and a resident-centered/directed philosophy of care;

staffing varied by shift and by the number of residents with dementia. The CCAL recommendations included having a licensed nurse, as well as a direct care supervisor, on call 24/7. Another staffing recommendation specified RN staffing as *hours per week per number of residents* and suggested that on-site nursing managers should have some gerontological nursing education. In this model, ALCs with 10 or fewer residents would require an RN only 10 hours per week, whereas ALCs with 21 to 30 residents would need an RN at least 30 hours per week, increasing by 10 hours per week for every 10 residents greater than 30. This recommendation did not pass. Many ALW members felt that each state should determine staffing needs or adequacy based on an instrument that assessed resident needs.

Most states' regulations regarding staffing are couched in terms such as "sufficient," "adequate," or "awake" staff to meet residents scheduled and unscheduled needs. Some states specify having sufficient staff in the event of evacuation or having at least one staff person who is CPR trained on duty 24/7. There is no staffing model or ratio of resident acuity-to-staff-needed for ALCs such as is used to guide staffing classifications and numbers in skilled nursing homes. Corporations that manage and are invested in ALCs (philosophically and financially) have staffing models but have not made them available to the public, nor has any data been published with regard to outcomes, such as satisfaction, aging-in-place/nursing home transfer, hospitalization, medication error, turnover, and so forth.

Delegation

Delegation is key to effective human resources management and service delivery. In a sense, the table of organization is an outline of delegation: authority and responsibility are hierarchically arrayed from the top down. Some Nurse Practice Acts (NPAs) differentiate between *assigning* and *delegating*. Delegation refers to a skilled task/nursing act administered or provided to a particular resident by someone other than a licensed nurse. The National Council of State Boards of Nursing (NCSBN, 1997) defines it as "the act of transferring to a competent individual the authority to perform a selected nursing task in a selected situation." In some states, by virtue of the NPA, an RN can delegate to a licensed practical nurse/licensed vocational nurse (LPN/LVN) the authority to delegate a nursing task/activity to unlicensed assistive personnel (UAP). *Accountability* for the outcome of the task (activity) resides with the person who delegated it. Most NPAs have guidelines

for assigning and delegating, including legal restrictions on what level of licensed nurse can delegate, what can and cannot be delegated—and to whom—but there is no uniform NPA that applies in all states. In general, *only those health-related activities that do not require professional nursing knowledge, skill, or judgment can be delegated—and then only by an RN.*

Nursing assessment cannot be delegated, nor can the formulation of nursing diagnoses or care/service plan development. However, LPNs/LVNs and PCAs can collect data and participate in care/service plan development. In those states where UAPs are trained in medication administration (a skilled nursing activity), and may administer meds (including injectables), this is often by authority of the state's AL regulations rather than by the NPA of the state, which might, in fact, not permit such delegation!

The *Five Rights of Delegation* (NCSBN, 1997) delineate the accountability, critical thinking, communication, and decision making associated with safe delegation.

(1) *Right task:* A specific task is matched with a specific caregiver who is capable of performing the activity safely. Tasks appropriate for delegation are routine activities, rely on a standard procedure, are low risk, have predictable results, and do not require the caregiver to make a nursing judgment or decision. Inasmuch as medical technicians (med techs) take vital signs and decide whether or not to administer a particular medication based on those data, the concept of right task has been considerably broadened for medication management or administration by UAPs (who are then known as med techs or by similar titles).

(2) *Right circumstances:* This refers to the best fit between task complexity, the caregiver's competency, and available supervision. With regard to medical administration by UAPs, this step implies, at the very least, that the resident's medical status and nursing needs have been evaluated. Common situations in ALCs include the following: lab reports with regard to administration of anticoagulant therapy, blood glucose measurement, and insulin dosage.

(3) *Right person:* This refers to assessment of the delegatee's knowledge and skills and the degree of monitoring that will be necessary.

(4) *Right direction/communication:* Specific instructions or directions (written or verbal) have been given, including the expected outcomes of the activity. For med techs, communication should

include education about the expected/desirable effects of specific medications and observation for adverse reactions. The ALC should have clearly written policies regarding resident refusal of medication, situations requiring nurse and/or physician notification, out of stock medications, borrowing, and *pro re nata* (PRN) medications. Some states have specific rules about PRNs: the resident must have the capacity to describe and communicate his symptoms or his need for the PRN medication. For some medications, such as pain meds, an RN must be contacted prior to administration. These policies (steps) should be periodically reviewed.

(5) *Right supervision/evaluation:* This connects the dots by documenting structure, process, and outcome. Simply put: How is a UAP/med tech judged capable to assist with or administer medications? Who made this determination? How often is the activity monitored? How are gaps in knowledge or skill identified and how are they rectified?

A *delegation decision-making grid* can be used in conjunction with the *Five Rights of Delegation*. It combines assessment of the patient's stability (and potential needs), readiness and competence of the UAP to perform the delegated act, the number of times the UAP has previously performed the act or task, the licensed nurse's competence in delegating a nursing act (that includes the nurse's knowledge base about the patient's condition), the potential for harm associated with the nursing act, the patient's ability for self-care, and the level of decision making associated with the nursing act. This tool can assist the nurse in determining whether or not to delegate a specific nursing act (or task) to a specific person (e.g., UAP or other licensed nurse). Novice nurses might be unprepared for delegation of some skilled nursing acts that require a certain level of knowledge, experience and judgment (the grid is available at https://www.ncsbn.org/delegation_grid_NEW.pdf).

Delegation of medication administration to UAPs who are variously trained and supervised is of considerable concern, especially in that most boards of nursing are not familiar with the context or practice of nursing in AL.

TIME MANAGEMENT

Time is an expensive resource that can and should be (re)allocated, as other resources are, depending on the situation. An AL nurse manager needs to be aware of how time is (mis)spent by self and staff; this has important budget considerations. The three *sources of time use* are: boss-imposed (e.g., meetings, special events, data collection); system-imposed (goes with the job title/responsibilities of, for example, nurse manager, and includes managing, monitoring, and communicating); and self-imposed (or discretionary). Some boss-imposed tasks can be delegated. Differentiating how time is spent on various tasks uses the notions of *urgency* and *importance*:

- Type A tasks are important, urgent, and cannot be delayed.
- Type B tasks are important but not urgent. These tasks need to be done and are worth the effort.
- Type C tasks are urgent but not important and tend to be a result of a hasty decision, like agreeing to chair a meeting that is of no value to nursing. Learn how to say "no."
- Type D is busy work and is neither urgent nor important. Such forms of work are diversions and share characteristics of procrastination, the art of putting things off.

Prioritizing means deciding if a task or activity will lead to goal achievement. Priorities can be set according to urgency and importance. Slice a task into smaller, manageable segments; do nothing else until one segment has been completed. Table 9.1 is a personal assessment of one's attitude and actions in managing time.

The Pareto principle or the 80/20 rule of the vital few and the trivial many holds that very few of all the items on a to-do list are really important. If the important things were attended to, then prioritizing was done well. Check your daily calendar of things to do in terms of their urgency and importance. Work smarter, not harder; develop habits of self-preservation *and* effective managing.

- Information processing includes sorting written material (e.g., reports, memos) into those needing a callback, immediate action, filing, or reading and those that are low-priority. Use the vertical file (i.e., trash basket); do not save or file what can easily be retrieved if needed or is simply not necessary to retain.
- File or save a meeting announcement only if it has the agenda on it.
- Create a stamp for incoming mail or documents that need to be routed to others.

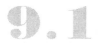

Time Waste Assessment: A Personal Inventory

1. I generally do not have a plan in writing when initiating a change.

2. It is difficult for me to say "no" when someone asks me a favor.

3. I can get hung up on details; I need *all* the facts when I have to make a decision.

4. It is difficult for me to prioritize what I have to do.

5. I am frequently asked to put out the fire.

6. I prefer to communicate by phone rather than by memo.

7. My desk (briefcase) is not large enough to hold all the things I need to be monitoring or doing.

8. I wait for latecomers rather than start a meeting on time.

9. I am not that good at differentiating between what is urgent and what is not urgent.

10. I tend to make too many commitments, such as giving a talk or holding a meeting.

11. I don't think it is a good idea to delegate data collection to someone else.

12. I am not a procrastinator, but I tend to put off things that I am uncomfortable with.

13. I am unable to describe what I want from a data set or report, so I get reams of paper instead of a summary.

Note: Scoring: If 10 or more items were answered "yes," then you have a time management problem.
From *Handbook for Directors of Nursing in Long-Term Care* (p. 79), by E.L. Mitty, 1998, Belmont, CA: Delmar Learning. Adapted with permission.

- Using a personal, desk, or electronic calendar, note due dates of reports and so forth. Remind staff about reports due (e.g., evaluations) until such time as they submit them on time.
- Ask for an executive summary if scrupulous reading of a report is not necessary.
- Your open-door policy that closes the door on occasion is a sign of time management and prioritization.
- Say "no" and control interruptions. Teach telephone manners by asking "Is this a good time to talk?" so that you can one day be on the receiving end of such a courtesy. Saying "no" is not indicative of avoidance of responsibilities—it is essential time management.
- Learn about nursing informatics and information technology (IT): what is out there and suitable for your size ALC, staff, and residents?

RESOURCES

Assisted Living Workgroup. (2003). *Final report. Assuring quality in assisted living: Guidelines for federal and state policy, state regulations, and operations.* Retrieved April 24, 2009, from http://www.fhca.org/fcal/news/wkintro.pdf

National Council of State Boards of Nursing. (1997). *The five rights of delegation.* Retrieved February 16, 2007, from http://www.ncsbn.org/fiverights.pdf

Mitty, E., & Flores, S. (2007). Medication management: Part 2. Supervision and monitoring of medication administration by unlicensed assistive personnel. *Geriatric Nursing, 28*(3), 153–160.

Reinhard, S.C., Young, H.M., Kane, R.A., & Quinn, W.V. (2006). Nurse delegation of medication administration for older adults in assisted living. *Nursing Outlook, 54*(2), 74–80.

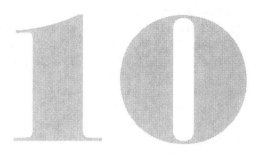

Medication Management

Ethel Mitty and Sandi Flores

An assisted living community's (ALC's) *medication management system* consists of policies and procedures for ordering (and delivering), administering, documenting, storing, and disposing of prescription, over-the-counter (OTC), and herbal or alternative remedies. These directives should be reviewed at least annually and whenever the ALC changes its mission, the population it wishes to serve (e.g., those with dementia, hospice, short-term rehabilitation, etc.), its drug provider, or those authorized by law to administer medications. It is estimated that 50%–75% of assisted living (AL) residents need assistance with medication management.

This chapter describes several approaches for assessment of a resident's ability to self-administer medications, addresses unlicensed personnel administration of (or assistance with) medication and their performance evaluation, states the six standards of medication administration, and discusses management of a medication/treatment error and the ALC's culture of safety.

Options with regard to stabilizing, normalizing, and creating a medication management system that is sensitive to resident wishes, staff workload, and safety concerns can emerge from discussion with the resident's primary health care provider, ALC nurse, and the consultant pharmacist. These might include:

■ Can a three-times-a-day med be given twice a day?
■ Can a long-acting medication replace a shorter-acting medication and thus be given once a day?

■ What medication(s) are really no longer indicated?
■ What other time(s) of day can a med be given? For example, if not at mealtime, can the med be given at night?
■ In keeping with resident-directed care, are the meds being given when residents prefer?

RESIDENT SELF-ADMINISTRATION OF MEDICATION

Some states require assessment and documentation of a resident's ability to self-administer medications by a licensed health professional (i.e., physician, nurse practitioner [NP], registered nurse [RN], pharmacist). Even though it is documented that the resident is able to self-administer medications, this does not preclude staff from assisting the resident with her or his medications. There are at least 17 different regulatory definitions of assistance, ranging from retrieving the drug, opening the container, verifying that the correct pill is being taken, to placing the medication in the resident's mouth. In terms of safe practice within the limits of the state law and delegation of nursing acts, it is critically important to know your state's definition of assistance with meds.

In some states, self-medication ability is not an issue of functional ability but, rather, of awareness: the resident has to be able to direct the person (e.g., the personal care assistant [PCA]) assisting them, understand the drug instructions (including the unit-dose packaging), and store their medications safely. State-specific definitions can make the difference in whether or not a resident will be permitted to self-administer and addresses the need to have an assessment tool that reflects local conditions. It is pointless to assess self-administration ability if it is not permitted by regulation. If awareness is a key criterion of self-medication ability, then behavioral descriptors and measures of awareness must be part of the assessment tool. A score below 23 on the Mini-Mental Status Examination (MMSE) can be used to exclude residents from self-administration of medications (see the section "Assessment Tools for Self-Administration" later in this chapter).

The following are factors that vary across states and are addressed in some states' AL regulations:

- *Risk* is defined as an insecure location, in which access to medications by a cognitively impaired resident is possible. Failure to identify a resident at risk of harm from an unsecured drug location can incur a deficiency citation.
- The ALC must document whether the resident or the ALC will be responsible for *drug storage*.
- Some states require evaluation of a resident's ability to recognize the drug label and accurately remove the medication from a *pre-filled medication box*.
- *Reminding* can include handing the appropriate pre-filled medication reminder box to the resident and opening the box if the resident is unable to do so. Some states prohibit staff from taking the medication itself out of the box; other states permit this if the resident is aware of the reason for the particular medication.
- Having the *cognitive capacity* to decide whether or not to take a medication, and the ability to recognize and take appropriate action regarding side effects, can be built into a self-medication assessment instrument that contains generic questions about the specific medication(s) for the specific resident.
- In some states, a resident assessed as *unable to self-administer medications* is at risk for discharge or for added personal costs to pay for staff assistance with medication.
- ALCs in some states must advise the resident and/or responsible party that the ALC is not required to have a licensed nurse on staff and that the resident may be receiving assistance with his/her self-administration from unlicensed assistive staff (who may or not be a medical technician).
- Self-administration of *pro re nata (PRN) medications* might require a written statement by a physician (MD) or NP that the resident is able to determine and communicate need for a prescription or non-prescription PRN medication. In some states, assistance with self-administration of a PRN medication can be given to a resident who can communicate his/her symptoms but is unable to decide the need for a PRN medication (e.g., a resident with a diagnosis of osteoarthritis who complains of pain). In some states, if the resident is unable to determine or communicate need for a PRN medication—but the need exists in staff judgment (e.g., body language indicates that resident is in pain)—the MD or NP must be contacted before the PRN drug can be administered. Assessment of a resident's ability to describe his or her need for a PRN medication—and know what and how much to take—should be part of a self-administration assessment tool.

A resident might be unaware that he or she lacks the cognitive and/or functional abilities related to timing, retrieving, pouring, and self-administering medications. Family members might discourage the ALC from medication assistance or administration because they do not want to incur the (likely) additional cost *and* because they are unaware of the risks associated with unsafe medication self-administration. A formal assessment using a standardized instrument makes the determination of the need for medication assistance less haphazard, more reality-based, and less likely to be a source of contention between the ALC and the family.

ASSESSMENT TOOLS FOR SELF-ADMINISTRATION

Self-medication assessment tools usually ask the resident about each drug that she or he is taking. The resident must identify the prescribed medication, state the dosage and when the medication is taken, the reason for the medication, and how it is stored. Additional probes might ask the resident about drug-specific adverse reactions (e.g., sleep disturbances, vision changes, alterations in mobility, dizziness) to assess the resident's ability to detect and report changes possibly associated with the medications. If staff are noticing changes that the resident is not noticing or reporting, this might be an indicator that the resident is no longer able to safely self-administer his or her medications. Described in the following list are two assessment instruments, either of which can be useful in assessing a resident's ability to self-administer medications. Select the instrument that contains the criteria of interest—and safety—for the resident and the ALC.

(1) The Medication Self-Administration Assessment Form (from the American Society of Consultant Pharmacists [ASCP]) assesses a resident's ability to read the instructions on the medication container (i.e., literacy); to state what each drug is for, its common side effects, correct time, and dose (i.e., number of tablets); to open and remove the correct amount of medication from the container; to place the container in a secure place; and to document self-administration. This instrument also assesses the resident's awareness of indications or need for a PRN med and documentation of self-administration. An observation component assesses self-administration of drops, patches, inhalants, suppositories, inhalants, and subcutaneous (sub-q) injected medications. Additional items may be needed with regard to the resident's ability to negotiate Medicare Plan D options, particularly after hospitalization, when a resident's medications might have been changed or dosages adjusted. (See Chapter 1, "The Assisted Living Setting of Nursing Practice," regarding health literacy, and Chapter 17, "The Continuum of Care," regarding medication reconciliation between care settings.)

(2) The Medication Management Instrument for Deficiencies in the Elderly (MedMaIDE) tool assesses (a) knowledge (about the medication being taken), (b) administration (how to take the drug), and (c) procurement (how to reorder the drug and/or get it from a pharmacy and check that the correct medication was refilled). Among the eight knowledge questions are reason for the drug, dosage, time of day instructions, and side effects. The resident's functional ability to manipulate the container and ingest the medication is observed. This assessment can be completed in 30 minutes (Brandt, et al., 2006).

UNLICENSED ASSISTIVE PERSONNEL ADMINISTRATION OF MEDICATION

Accountability for medication management resides with a licensed nurse (RN or licensed practical nurse/licensed vocational nurse [LPN/LVN]) even if delegated to unlicensed assistive personnel (UAP) who are trained and monitored in a variety of ways. Tasks and responsibilities for medication assistance and administration should be part of the job description of staff providing this service. The ALC's policy should address continuing education, monitoring and performance evaluation of these staff, and the medication error reporting system. An AL nurse is at some degree of risk with regard to a state's requirement of nursing supervision and monitoring of UAP/med tech activities, but there is little case law that addresses this. A UAP/med tech who is making repeated errors, even after retraining, should be removed from medication assistance/administration. Justification for this prudent action is a valid and reliable performance evaluation tool.

Performance evaluation of medication assistance/administration competency can be constructed around the six rights of medication administration. These are generic standards of practice that apply across settings. Observable and measurable competencies for each practice standard are as follows:

(1) *Right medication:* multiple medications for the same resident are crushed in separate medication cups (particularly important for vital-sign dependent drugs or anticoagulants); med container labels are read and compared to the order or medication administration record (MAR), three times. The med tech/aide can also be asked to explain the hold policy or order.

(2) *Right dose:* order is rechecked if more or less than one tablet is required; medication cup (not a spoon) is used to measure liquid medication; wait 3–5 minutes between administration of different eye meds to the same eye (e.g., glaucoma meds).

(3) *Right time:* administered in the correct window of time, that is, 1 hour before or 1 hour after the stated time.

(4) *Right route:* checked placement of gastrostomy tube before administering medications via tube; site rotation (e.g., Fentanyl patch, insulin injection); instructed resident where to look while administering eye drops.

(5) *Right resident:* carried out ALC policy regarding resident identification.

(6) *Right documentation:* site of application/administration; relevant vital signs (e.g., blood pressure) or lab data (e.g., international normalized level or prothrombin time); annotation of refusal of medication and a written note; medication that is out of stock (OOS) and action(s) taken; medication missed and given at a later time.

MEDICATION/TREATMENT ERRORS

Several studies report that most medication errors in ALCs are related to the 1-hour time window and had no statistically significant relationship to whether the medications were administered by a licensed nurse or a UAP/med tech. Other errors, ranging from 1%–13% of all errors, were wrong dose, omitted dose, extra dose, unauthorized medication, and incorrect medication (least frequent). Few medication errors are clinically significant, with the exception of insulin, furosemide, and warfarin sodium. However, this does not excuse or rationalize the med errors.

A culture of safety in health care organizations is slowly changing how a medication (or treatment) error is handled. Organizations are moving away from name and blame approaches toward a systems-oriented cognitive science approach that seeks to understand why an error occurred. An organization interested in safety has as much interest in actual errors as in potential errors—the near misses. Respect for persons, a fundamental ethical principle, requires that the resident and/or significant other be told that an error has occurred. This has not engendered more lawsuits, as was originally feared among providers. In addition to being told that a medication error has occurred, residents are also told what to expect as a result of the wrong med (or dose, or treatment), what will be given to them to mitigate the effect of the error, how they will be monitored for any adverse effect, and the likelihood of certain outcomes. Genuine apology for an error maintains the resident's sense of self-esteem. It is important that the individual(s) most associated with the error speak to the resident; this is not the time for a messenger. Some apologies include what was learned from the error and what the organization (i.e., ALC) will be doing to prevent such an error from happening again.

All staff involved in the medication management system should participate in developing a (medication) error reporting system. Basic elements of an error report include the type of error, related facts associated with the error, notification, actions taken, and relevant attachments (e.g., the medication order, MAR, relevant nurses and/or physician notes). Types of errors include the following:

- Wrong resident, wrong dose, wrong route or site
- Wrong day, wrong time, wrong med
- Med given despite vital sign or lab result hold order
- Expired order, med not ordered, order not transcribed correctly
- Med not charted, vital signs or lab data not charted
- Med given yet resident has known allergy to that med

- Failure to document refusal, omission, held med, OOS med
- Med given beyond auto stop date
- Ordered but not given
- Given but not ordered
- Related facts: order not written clearly, order written incorrectly

If not on the error report itself, the continuing care/progress notes should describe the effect of the error on the resident, how the resident was advised of the error and by whom, what the resident was told, and follow-up. An ALC's culture of safety should include systematic or root cause analysis of the error, an educational approach to preventing future errors rather than the traditional name and blame method, and an attitude about safety that incorporates recognition and reporting of the near miss error.

RESOURCES

American Society of Consultant Pharmacists. (2006). *Consultant pharmacist requirements for assisted living facilities.* Alexandria, VA: Author.

Brandt, N., Orwig, D., & Spellbring, A.M. (2002, November). *Evaluation of the MedMaIDE to assess medication management deficiencies in the elderly living in the community.* Poster presentation at the Annual Meeting of the American Society of Consultant Pharmacists, Orlando, FL.

Hawes, C., Phillips, C.D., & Rose, M. (2000). *High service or high privacy. Assisted living facilities, their residents and staff: Results from a national survey.* Washington, DC: Office of the Assistant Secretary for Planning and Evaluation, Department of Health and Human Services.

Liebel, D.V., & Watson, N. (2005). Consolidating medication passes. *American Journal of Nursing, 105*(12), 63–64.

Maddigan, S.L., Farris, K.B., Keating, N., Wiens, C.A., & Johnson, J.A. (2003). Predictors of older adults' capacity for medication management in a self-medication program. *Journal of Aging and Health, 15,* 332–352.

Meade, V. (2001). A new comprehensive model for assisted living medication management and wellness care. *The Consultant Pharmacist, 16,* 9–18.

Mitty, E., & Clark, T. (2003). Assisted living: Safety vs. autonomy. In M.B. Kapp (Ed.), *Ethics, law, and aging review* (vol. 9, pp. 61–76). New York: Springer Publishing Company.

Mitty, E., & Flores, S. (2007). Medication management: Part 2. Supervision and monitoring of medication administration by unlicensed assistive personnel. *Geriatric Nursing, 28,* 153–160.

Young, H., Gray, S.L., McCormack, W.C., Sikma, S.K., Reinhard, S., Trippet, L.J., et al. (2008). Types, prevalence, and potential clinical significance of medication administration errors in Assisted Living. *Journal of the American Geriatrics Society 56*(7), 1199–1205.

11

Finance and Budget

Ethel Mitty

This chapter describes the processes that pertain to financial management including budget preparation, a description of a patient classification system (PCS), master staffing formulae, computing full time equivalence (FTE), and materials management.

A *budget plan* draws on forecasts about the services that the assisted living (AL) residents (i.e., population mix) will seek or require, the projected costs and the AL community's (ALC's) likely reimbursement. The notion of *opportunity costs* speaks to the tradeoff between the costs (and anticipated revenue) of one service (e.g., rehab) compared to another (e.g., dementia care). Health care institutions' financial planning draws on PCSs that use acuity measures and severity of illness indices of one kind or another, such as diagnostic related groups (DRGs), time spent per DRG or relative intensity measures (RIM), or resource utilization groups (RUGs) that cost out the care required by different classifications of residents.

The Balanced Budget Act (1997) changed skilled nursing home reimbursement from a cost-based retrospective payment system to a prospective payment system (PPS) (i.e., predetermined fixed payment for an episode of care for a specific group or set of resident characteristics/needs). The nursing home RUGs system is a PPS consisting of seven categories of characteristics: special rehabilitation, extensive care, special care, clinically complex, cognitively impaired, behavior problems, and reduced physical functions—all of which produce 44 different resident classifications (or RUG groups). Nursing homes must use a standardized assessment tool called the Minimum Data Set (MDS), which contains clinical and functional items and measures, to place each resident in one (and one only) of the 44 RUG groups—each of which has a specific payment rate. To date, there are no staffing recommendations based on RUG levels or the aggregated *case mix index* (CMI). There has been some discussion and testing of a RUGs-like tool for AL.

PCSs use terms such as *work analysis, direct and indirect care,* and *workload index.* Although PCSs for reimbursement purposes to ALCs do not exist, some states (and some ALCs) use PCSs to address regulatory requirements for types and numbers of staff. Relevant terms for PCSs are:

- *Work analysis:* the time taken to provide a specific kind of care, or administer a treatment/procedure, or the nursing care hours (NCH) needed by the average resident.
- *Direct care:* usually means hands-on care. *Indirect care* includes unit management activities, such as staff meetings. Some nurse managers feel that writing a service plan is indirect care, whereas others feel that it is direct care. Both are measured in units of time.
- *Workload index:* a simple mathematical calculation: divide the NCH required by the NCH provided.

The PCS selected should reflect the realities of the ALC's resident population and nursing practice. Time norms of another ALC should not be used unless there is comparability with regard to type of residents, support services (including information technology), and care equipment (e.g., mechanical lifters). Nurse (or nursing-staff led) small group sessions (e.g., memory training) should be included. Items that do not represent actual nursing practice at the ALC, such as catheterization or sterile dressing change, should not be used; otherwise, the real work of nursing will not be captured.

When acuity appears to be rising, it is prudent to check if documentation of resident characteristics and service needs is also rising to meet the needs of the resident assessment or PCS system. Known as "acuity creep," such increases have been used to demand higher reimbursement or even resident relocation. Rising acuity data is highly suspect unless there is a demonstrable change in the resident population as would happen, for example, with admission of persons with moderate to severe dementia or retention of residents with (temporary) need for skilled nursing.

A *cost center* is a resident community/neighborhood/unit. Cost center reports can include supplies as well as staff overtime data. Supplies costs, however, can be distributed among all units or based on unit bed size or on some kind of resident descriptor (e.g., incontinence). Overtime (OT) costs generated by staff call-ins need to be differentiated from OT costs associated with time-and-one-half compensation for work on a legal holiday and so forth. A nurse manager should be aware if responsibility for cost-containment or fiscal accountability is part of the job description and performance evaluation.

BUDGET PROCESSES

The most commonly used budget processes are:

■ *Historical or line-item budgeting*: based on assumptions that resident characteristics and needs, programs and services, and staff and equipment costs will remain essentially unchanged in the coming year. Relatively easy to prepare. Salary increases and anticipated inflation are factored in, as are the likely costs of a new program or service. Monthly expenditure reports are a way to track glitches in the budget.
■ *Appropriations or fixed budget*: line-by-line fixed spending that cannot be exceeded without administrative approval.
■ *Zero-based budget*: used at times of significant inflation and/or cost-containment or cost-reduction demands. All budget requests and expenses have to be justified; data with regard to program effectiveness or efficiency must be presented. Very time-consuming to

prepare, this sort of budget is essentially a prediction about resident acuity and needs, and nursing activities and programs, for the coming year.
■ *Planned program budget*: a specific program allocation; outcome measures are required. A program that fails to deliver on the promised (clinical) outcomes or a program that is costing more than projected (even with acceptable outcomes) could be eliminated in resource-strained times.

CAPITAL AND OPERATING BUDGET

Every organization, including a free-standing or corporate ALC, will have a capital, operating (revenue and expenses), and cash budget. The *balance sheet* identifies the organization's assets (e.g., land and buildings owned, investments, etc.) and liabilities (e.g., mortgage, debt). The *cash budget* identifies money received and distributed over a specific time period. A nurse manager can be required to prepare the nursing-related sections of the capital budget and the operating budget.

A *capital budget* is a written plan and projection for additional or replacement equipment over the next 5 (or 10) years. Each organization sets its own criteria for what constitutes a capital item; this usually includes equipment that cost $100 (or more) and that must endure at least 5 years. The preparation and approval process can take several months because several layers of management and ownership (or the board) have to weigh in on the allocation of resources. Vendors can be asked to prepare a proposal in which there is interest. All requested items need to be justified (with data) and accompanied by a method to evaluate outcome(s).

■ Is the item needed to replace outdated or worn equipment? (e.g., attach repair record or staff injury data associated with equipment)
■ Is the item needed to provide a service that is not currently provided by nursing? (e.g., aroma therapy)
■ In what way will the item improve existing nursing service? (e.g., clinical outcomes, satisfaction data)
■ Is the item needed to improve safety? To decrease the number of complaints?
■ What are the installment costs? The staff education costs?

The *operating budget* consists of a salary budget and other than personnel salary (OTPS) budget.

■ *Salaries* are a fixed cost. Staff receive the same pay regardless of occupancy or resident acuity. The computation of cost-per-unit-of-activity changes, for example, with the number of residents for whom a personal care assistant (PCA) is responsible. The more residents assigned, the lower the fixed cost: a PCA assigned 10 residents and who earns $80 per day generates a cost per resident day of $8. With only 6 residents, the cost per resident day is approximately $13.30.

☐ Salary increases based on some kind of merit-based or performance evaluation system are very difficult to carry out—and defend.

☐ Organizations vary as to how salary increases will be distributed, by percent of the total salary budget or by a specific dollar amount.

☐ In-service education can be its own cost center, or these staff can be included in nursing's salary budget, as can their teaching supplies.

■ The OTPS or nonsalary budget includes minor non-medical and medical equipment (e.g., glucometer) that are not part of the capital budget, professional organization dues, conference costs, stationery and office supplies, and recruitment costs. It can include service contract and repair costs.

☐ Laundry, housekeeping, and utilities costs can be allocated to individual departments, such as nursing, or covered by the organization's total budget.

☐ If residents bring their own furniture and other belongings (e.g., rug, TV), the ALC should have a policy with regard to upkeep and repair of these items.

Budget preparation of the salary and nonsalary (OTPS) budgets commonly occurs in October and generally includes an *inflation factor* used for the OTPS budget. Each organization has its own budget presentation format that might require, also, comparison between current and projected expenses (or costs). The budget can be a combination of narrative and flow sheets (e.g., Excel document) with regard to PCS data and the relationship to staff needed; recruitment and orientation costs (including overlap salary cost for incoming and departing employees); various insurance costs (e.g., malpractice, unemployment, and disability); a cost-benefit or cost-effective analysis (CBA/CEA) about a new program; summer relief staff needed; and overtime and tuition reimbursement projection.

Any *monthly expenditure report* issued after June is used to prepare the OTPS budget. This report generally shows—for each item purchased and provided by the ALC (that is, not by the resident or family), such as food supplements (liquid or pudding)—the following:

■ Budgeted amount for the year (i.e., the annual budget)
■ Year-to-date (YTD) budgeted amount for the item (i.e., amount budgeted or allocated for the particular item since the start of the year up to and including the current month)
■ Budgeted amount for the current month
■ Total expenses YTD and for the current month (compare to second and third bullets)
■ Also shown, per item, are dollars spent above the budgeted amount (in parentheses) or below it for the month and the YTD. This report can also indicate the percent of variance above (in parentheses) or below the budget allocated for the item.

An item can be above budget allowance in one month and below it in another month. This might be attributed to a temporary change in resident acuity (e.g., an infectious outbreak that generated supplies costs). As per ALC financial policy, a greater than $1,500 variance above or below budget might have to be explained.

MASTER STAFFING

There is no prescribed formula for master staffing, by type/classification or number, 24/7, in long-term nursing home care, or in ALCs (except as developed by individual ALCs). States determine staffing numbers and classifications in myriad ways: by facility bed capacity, by whether or not there is a dementia care unit, by fire evacuation procedures, by level of care, licensure, or certification, or not at all. A typical master staffing model is described below.

■ 4-2-1 PCS:
☐ 4 = 4 hours of care needed (i.e., totally dependent, nonmobile, incontinent); 2 = 2 hours (i.e., significant assistance needed; self-feeding but needing tray prep; might be incontinent); 1 = 1 hour (i.e., independent; needs some cueing; requires medication administration).
☐ Every resident is assessed as being at level 4 or 2 or 1.
☐ Establish the nursing care hours per resident day (NCHPRD) needed: multiply the number of residents at each level by the hours of care needed (i.e., 4-2-1).
☐ Add all levels together to reach the *total NCHPRD*.
☐ Divide this figure by the number of total residents to arrive at the NCHPRD needed per resident, on

average. This is a very basic schema, but it gets at resident acuity and service needs.

■ Staffing needed—by number, not by type or classification: divide the total NCHPRD needed by the hours worked by a single staff person in one day (i.e., shift). The resulting figure represents total staffing needed for 24/7 coverage.

To compute NCH provided:

(1) Multiply the number of staff on duty per shift by the number of hours of the shift (e.g., 7.5) to obtain the NCH provided on a particular shift.
(2) Total the three shifts to obtain the NCH provided over 24 hours.
(3) Divide that sum by the number of residents (census) to arrive at the average NCHPRD provided per resident in 24 hours.

Each type or classification of staff should be handled separately. Consistent over- or understaffing must be justified. Some ALCs require a monthly report showing budgeted NCHPRD compared to NCHPRD provided daily.

Full-Time Equivalence (FTE)

The FTE is computed to determine how many of each job type/classification are needed to meet the master staffing plan 24/7. It includes productive and nonproductive time. Steps in computing the FTE are as follows:

(1) Assume that 2.2 NCHPRD are needed for a 30-resident ALC. Calculate the projected annual units (PAU) of service:
    (a) Multiply the ALC's bed capacity by its percentage average occupancy (e.g., 100%) to ascertain the average daily census (ADC).
    (b) Multiply this figure by 365 to derive the PAU: 30 × 100% = 30 ADC × 365 = 10,950 PAU. (If the community has a lower census, use the percent figure that best represents actual census.)
(2) Multiply the PAU by the needed NCHPRD: 10,950 × 2.2 = 24,090.
(3) Using a staffing model wherein every staff person works 5 days or shifts per week: each employee works 231 days × 7.5 hours, which equals 1,732.5

hours worked per year per employee. Explanation: if every employee has two days off per week, 52 weeks per year equals 104 days not on duty. On average, every employee has 2 weeks vacation per year, which equals an additional 10 days not on duty. On average, every employee has 10 paid holidays and is entitled to 10 sick days per year, an additional 20 days the employee will not be on duty. Added together, this makes 134 nonproductive days. With 134 nonproductive days a year, that means there are 231 productive days per year. (For staff with longer vacation benefits, the FTE overall will be larger.)

(4) Divide the annual NCHPRD needed by the hours worked annually per employee: 24,090/1,732.5 = 13.9 employees needed per 24 hours (i.e., almost 14 full-time shifts need to be worked).
(5) Determine the nonproductive shifts per employee per week: multiply the number of employees needed per day by an industry average of 15% of nonproductive time: 13.9 × 0.15 = 2.08 nonproductive shifts per employee per week.
(6) Total FTE for the 30-resident ALC: add the productive and nonproductive factors: 13.9 employees needed per 24 hours + 2.08 nonproductive time = 15.98 full-time *budgeted* positions are needed to staff the ALC/unit/community 24/7 needing 2.2 NCHPRD. (Practice doing these computations; it gets easier each time.)

MATERIAL MANAGEMENT

Material management is a feedback system that includes contracts, vendor screening, and visits, and various purchasing approaches. Many product representatives offer in-service education about their line of products that could be useful for residents as well as ALC nursing. Material management includes *inventory control:* every item has a reorder point (ROP) and a reorder quantity (ROQ) based on ease of getting the item, past usage, and budget. *Par levels* are the minimum and maximum levels that an item should be available in the ALC.

RESOURCE

Balanced Budget Act of 1997, 105th U.S. Congress (1997).

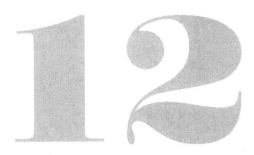

Law, Legal Issues, and Labor Relations

Ethel Mitty

Moving from description of a typical Nurse Practice Act (NPA), this chapter discusses negligence, professional misconduct, and malpractice insurance. The remainder of the chapter addresses workforce issues, such as the rights and protections provided all employees by the National Labor Relations Act, grievance management and work stoppages, Title VII (The Civil Rights Act), employee disability and workman's compensation, and employee satisfaction measures.

LAW AND LEGAL ISSUES IN NURSING PRACTICE

Every state has an NPA for registered nurses (RNs) and licensed practical nurse (LPN). The NPA is based on a deeply embedded societal principle: a social contract exists when society recognizes a specific occupational group. By granting a specific domain and privileges to the group, society has a right to expect that, in return, the group's members will have a special education, special entry (e.g., a test), competency testing of its members, a body of knowledge that is evidence- or research-based, and will hold its members accountable. Many occupational and professional groups have *acta* that address this relationship and rules of practice. The NPA is a law (or statute) that defines what nursing practice *is*, describes licensure requirements and the grounds for license revocation (e.g., professional misconduct), and authorizes a special body—the *state board*—to monitor and process

these responsibilities. Board actions can include reprimand, limiting the license to practice, and sanctions against a nurse who has violated state or federal drug laws. The National Council of State Boards of Nursing (NCSBN) provides information and educational workshops and conducts research with regard to regulations that affect practice. The NCSBN also has a directory of nurse assistant registries that are useful in intake/screening potential new assistant staff (now required by several states).

Negligence is a general term meaning deviation from a standard of care. Nursing *malpractice* is a specific kind of negligence: deviation from a *professional standard* of care. A nurse can be held as having been negligent when a person to whom a nursing act was assigned or delegated by the nurse caused harm to another. *Standards* speak to the necessity of having basic knowledge of the phenomenon or act for which one is responsible. Written in measurable terms, standards reflect the beliefs and values of professional nursing and provide direction for actual practice—and its evaluation. Assisted living (AL) nursing standards are based on gerontological nursing standards and were discussed in Chapter 1 section "The Context of Assisted Living Nursing Practice." The certification exam for AL RNs and LPNs/licensed vocational nurses (LVNs) is based on these standards, as well.

Professional misconduct includes patient abuse, mistreatment or neglect, about which each state has its own regulations and statutes. Most lawsuits against nurses involve medication errors, failure to observe, document, or report changes in resident status, and falls. The notion of *liability* suggests that an undesirable outcome was the result of an incorrect action—or failure to act appropriately.

Four criteria must be met to prove negligence or malpractice:

(1) Duty: that a particular relationship between the resident and the nurse existed;
(2) Breach of duty: that there was a failure to meet an accepted standard of care (usually associated with knowledge and skill or competency; e.g., medication administration);
(3) Causation: proof that the injury (i.e., damage) was caused by breach of duty; and
(4) Damages.

Expert testimony relies on the notion of what a reasonable person (e.g., nurse, personal care assistant) would have done in the same or a similar circumstance. A no-longer-used concept—the locality rule—has been replaced by national standards. An AL nurse will be held to the standard of practice of an average member of that group, regardless of geographic location.

Many AL communities (ALCs) admit residents with dementia; some ALCs have specific units; some ALCs are specific for dementia care. Many states have specific regulations regarding staffing, programs, education, and environment that ALCs must meet if they will be marketing to and admitting these residents. Facilities do not have to retain residents who act aggressively toward other residents or are a risk to themselves. Given that all residents, including those with impaired cognition (e.g., decision-making skills) have the right to refuse treatment, the ALC is obligated to protect these residents from the consequences of their poor judgment. However, determination of the (degree of) risk pursuant to a poor decision is difficult; there are no guidelines other than past history of the resident and health care professionals' experience in managing such behaviors. In some ways similar to a negotiated risk contract (NRA) or even to informed consent for treatment (or the service plan), the notion of *assumption of risk* means that the resident understands the consequences and possibility of risks associated with his/her decision. Faced with a seemingly capacitated (i.e., competent) resident who, in your view, is making an unwise decision, ask the resident to repeat back in his own words his understanding of his decision and risk. If the resident is unable to do this or omits important information or misinterprets what was told him, the primary care provider should be notified as soon as possible. Document the

discussion: what the resident was told, what the resident said (this is similar to what is done in determining capacity to give informed consent for treatment and/or research participation). (See also Chapter 4.)

Malpractice Insurance

Bad things can happen to even the most well-intentioned nurse. The cost of coverage should *not* be a deterrent to playing it safe and having malpractice insurance. Claims and risks in ALCs are predominantly about negligent care practices, resident rights, and elopement. Negligent care is attributed to lack of protocols (i.e., standards of care and procedures). Inadequate staff leads to inadequate supervision and monitoring of residents as well as staff. Although the AL industry has fewer claims, to date, in comparison to the nursing home industry, the average awards per case are higher in AL.

Many ALCs provide liability coverage for their nurses, but the type of coverage can vary. Some ALCs have an *occurrence policy* that only covers incidents that occurred during the policy period without regard to when the claim is reported. Employer liability coverage may be insufficient or not covered at all with regard to defense (or trial) costs. Depending on the claim, bringing to light issues such as inadequate staffing, lack of training, and other issues that seem relevant may not be permitted. *Claims-made coverage* is a type of policy that provides coverage for any suit or incident (i.e., claim) reported in the coverage year. An extended reporting endorsement policy (known as a "tail") can be purchased and will provide coverage for claims reported after the policy was terminated. Inasmuch as nursing malpractice suits can take years to settle, this kind of personal policy might be wise to obtain.

Having malpractice coverage is an important first step in professional protection, but practicing with an overall preventive philosophy and implementing simple preventive techniques is critical. It involves listening to *all* concerns of the resident and/or family and engaging them in the decision-making process. In some situations, this means that the resident and/or family assume not only responsibility for the decision but for their actions to achieve the desired outcomes. For example, the (family of a) resident who wanders might agree to the purchase cost of a wander-guard system or might privately employ an individual to be with the resident during his or her awake hours.

The traditional and commonly used SOAP model—subjective, objective, assessment, plan—is a template for information gathering, but it lacks flexibility and does not encourage a proactive approach to care planning and malpractice risk reduction. The SOOOAAP note (see Table 12.1) is a more comprehensive approach that encourages communication and resident/family/proxy participation in decision making and their responsibility for follow-through with the agreed-upon plan.

In sum, preventive malpractice includes knowledge of the NPA, maintaining and improving practice competencies, discussing an initial or interim assessment with a colleague (even if it means making a phone call to another ALC nurse), clarifying resident and family expectations of care and supervision, and documentation that is descriptive and supported by facts. Charting should be descriptive and objective and respectful. *Chart as if the resident and/or family will read your notes.*

LABOR RELATIONS

The National Labor Relations Act (NLRA) (National Labor Relations Board [NLRB], 1935), also known as the Wagner Act, stipulates the right of employees to organize as well as to grieve or complain about working conditions (including workload). Administered by the NLRB, an independent federal agency, the NLRA is the principal law regarding private-sector employer–employee relations. Under the NLRA, employees have the right, as well, to refrain from involvement in collective bargaining activities. The NLRA does not cover issues or activities that are the responsibility of other government departments. For example, it does not address workers' compensation programs, occupational safety, family medical leave, and other Department of Labor issues, nor does it address issues such as race, gender, and age discrimination in employment, which are instead the purview of the Equal Employment Opportunity Commission (EEOC). The federal Taft-Hartley Act, also known as the Labor-Management Relations Act (1947) made several amendments to the NLRA, among which is the stipulation that employers have the right to oppose unions and cannot threaten or promise rewards to employees who are considering forming a collective bargaining unit (CBU) or joining a union.

Grievances commonly addressed, whether through a CBU or an employee committee (variously named), include wages and benefits, insubordination or refusal (notion of willfulness) to carry out an assignment, erratic disciplinary actions, promotions, and having a say in decisions affecting their work. Supervisors are generally excluded from union membership (or representation) because their activities include hiring and firing, initiating a disciplinary action, and approving

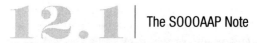

| The SOOOAAP Note |

SOOOAAP	CONTENT
Subjective	Document your attention to the resident; highlight main areas of concern; accurately decribe the resident's mental capacity, physical ability (related to the plan or goal), and mood or affect. Describe the resident's expectations of being successful or achieving the desired goal.
Objective	Each statement should be supported by facts including observation (whether one-time or recurrent), lab data, and/or diagnostic test results. Recheck facts and assessment conclusions.
Opinion	Provide a comprehensive record in support of the assessment; document that this is an initial assessment that will be reviewed and discussed with the caregivers.
Options	Document communication of the assessment with the resident/family/proxy, the available treatment options (as presented to them earlier by the physician or nurse practitioner), and that they can consent or refuse to consent to the treatment plan, in whole or in part. (To confirm understanding, ask the resident to state back in his or her own words what he or she has been told.)
Advice	This section of the documentation reviews the options and consequences of each—given the known research and clinical findings in support of each choice.
Agreed Plan	Describe the agreed-to plan, *including* those options that were rejected (and why) and the reason(s) why an option(s) was agreed to.

overtime. However, given the evolving principles and practices of self-governance, it is somewhat tricky and perhaps arbitrary who or what activities are designated as supervisory and which are part of a professional nursing practice model (see Chapter 6, "Leadership/Management Style and Assessment").

Work stoppages and strikes are forbidden unless the union/CBU has given a 30-day notice to the NLRB Mediation and Conciliation Service followed by a 10-day strike notice. A facility's strike plan generally includes a list of personnel or job classifications that are exempt from a strike call (i.e., cannot go out on strike); how resident care and service needs will be met by the remaining staff; staffing models that will be implemented (including use of contract staff); measures to protect food and fuel delivery, residents, visitors, and staff; communication with residents and families including possible requests to remove the resident to another location during the strike; where the striking workers can meet to express their views; and so forth.

Workplace issues such as age, gender, race, or religious discrimination, sexual harassment, and disabled employee discrimination are addressed in several federal acts.

- Age Discrimination in Employment Act (The U.S. Equal Employment Opportunity Commission, 1967): applies to organizations with 20 or more employees and to adults age 40 and over. An employer may not fire, refuse to hire, or treat the person differently than other employees because of age.
- Title VII of the Civil Rights Act (The U.S. Equal Employment Opportunity Commission, 1964): applicable to all workplaces with 15 or more employees. The act protects individuals against employment discrimination on the basis of sex, race, color, national origin, or religion. Employment discrimination refers to hiring, firing, promotion, wages and benefits, job training, or any other aspect of employment. Importantly, the act prohibits employment discrimination based on stereotypes and assumptions about an individual's ability, traits, or performance on the basis of sex. An employee who requests a specific weekend day off, every week, (e.g., for religious observance reasons or for child care) cannot be dismissed (nor can they be barred from employment) unless it can be shown that meeting this request would create significant hardship on other staff or the facility. Such a request might be accommodated by having the employee work the other weekend day, every weekend.

The act contains rules and prohibitions regarding sexual harassment and pregnancy-based discrimination. The Equal Pay Act of 1963 states that men and women must receive equal pay for equivalent work; the jobs do not have to be identical.

- The Americans With Disabilities Act (ADA, 1992, 1994) is a federal law that provides civil rights protection under the Department of Justice and applies to all employers/organizations with 15 or more employees. From the employment perspective, a *qualified individual* with a disability is "a person who meets legitimate skill, experience, education, or other requirements of an employment position that s/he holds or seeks, and who can perform the essential functions of the position with or without reasonable accommodation" (www.ada.gov). An individual who is unable to perform tasks that are not essential for job performance *cannot* be considered unqualified for a position.
  - ☐ The notion of *reasonable accommodation* to the work or physical environment is based on the so-called but for argument: a physically challenged employee could meet the job requirements but for impediments or lack of accommodation in the physical environment. Physically challenged employees who are unable to meet the job requirements, even after reasonable accommodations have been made in the environment, are subject to the same performance review standards as are non–physically challenged employees. In some cases, a physically challenged person can be hired with the stipulation that they are required to meet all aspects of the job with the exception of a particular activity. This agreement should be witnessed and documented.

Workman's compensation laws, designed by each state, provide a specific payment amount to an employee injured by a job-related event. In contrast, *unemployment compensation* can be paid an employee who was terminated or who resigned voluntarily—and who is able to prove that there was good cause to do so. The need for timely and accurate documentation of progressive discipline, instances of willful refusal to do a job-related task, or attendance or lateness counseling cannot be overstated.

Job Satisfaction

Job satisfaction means different things to different people, both within and between job classifications and levels. Factors in job satisfaction, in addition to the relationship between the job and one's personal goals, include recognition and respect, feedback (communication), policies and promotion systems, job content, resources, and leadership style. There are many job satisfaction instruments; some are combined with or administered at the same time as a climate analysis (see Chapter 5, "Nursing and Organizational Theory, Practice, and Culture"). Job dissatisfaction can be a precursor to workplace unrest. It is important to select an instrument that has a good fit with the job classification or staff from whom you are soliciting feedback and with the residential care setting of an ALC.

A satisfaction survey can be constructed in-house after learning about staff interests and concerns working in the ALC. The tool should include the respondent's job classification, shift, full- or part-time status, and length of time at the ALC, unless it can be used to identify the respondent (e.g., there is only one night staff or only two nurses, etc.). A typical Likert-type scale is: 1 = very satisfied, 2 = somewhat satisfied, 3 = dissatisfied, 4 = no opinion/not applicable. If there are insufficient staff to conduct a meaningful satisfaction survey, slowly and respectfully begin a discussion with the staff and start with the issue that would be easiest to address and/or least likely to explode.

Satisfaction items that can be addressed by survey or in discussion (but not all at one time) include work schedule, responsibilities (and training or preparation for them), decision-making participation, supplies and equipment availability (and in working order), feedback about performance (recognition for work; grievance handling), participation in designing a resident's service plan, salary and promotion opportunities, benefits (e.g., tuition reimbursement, health coverage), sick-time policies (vacation policies), nurse manager support, information sharing (communication processes in the ALC), in-service education and opportunity to attend off-site programs, overall cleanliness of the ALC, and staff amenities (e.g., condition of staff lounge, locker room).

Satisfaction surveys (including climate assessment) should not be conducted during a period of significant change (e.g., change in ownership or top management, new mission, or program) or stress (e.g., survey). Wait at least 6 months after a major change. Some items have more weight or import than others; notice where responses to similar items cluster around a particular level of satisfaction or similar issues (e.g., participation in decisions). After reviewing the data, meet with staff to talk about the findings, what they mean, and what needs to be done. Consider annual satisfaction surveys.

RESOURCES

Equal Employment Opportunities Commission and U.S. Department of Justice Civil Rights Division. (2009). *Americans With Disabilities Act questions and answers*. Retrieved April 25, 2009, from http://www.ada.gov

The Equal Pay Act of 1963. (n.d.). Retrieved April 25, 2009, from http://www.eeoc.gov/policy/epa.html

Fiesta, J. (1988). *The law and liability. A guide for nurses*. New York: John Wiley & Sons.

National Labor Relations Board. (1935). *National Labor Relations Act of 1935*. Retrieved December 1, 2008, from http://www.nlrb.gov/about_us/overview/national_labor_relations_act.aspx

The U.S. Equal Employment Opportunity Commission. (1964). *Title VII of the Civil Rights Act of 1964*. Retrieved April 25, 2009, from http://www.eeoc.gov/policy/vii.html

The U.S. Equal Employment Opportunity Commission. (1967). *The Age Discrimination in Employment Act of 1967*. Retrieved April 25, 2009, from http://www.eeoc.gov/policy/adea.html.

13

Quality Improvement, Research, and Education

Ethel Mitty

This chapter, the last in Section I, "Management and Leadership," places assisted living (AL) nursing on the cutting edge of professional practice in AL: quality improvement (QI), research-based practice, and the AL community (ALC) as a clinical campus. Nursing actions undertaken with regard to quality improvement are a hallmark of nursing's social contract with society: an obligation to continuously assess and improve practice. Key phrases associated with QI are provided, as are descriptions of QI plans or models, characteristics of risk management and infection control programs, and hazardous substance management. Research is discussed from several perspectives: components of a research proposal, levels of research risk, informed consent, levels of research evidence, and institutional review boards (IRBs) for research approval. Community-based participatory research (CBPR) and evidence-based practice/research (EBP/R) are described, as is commonly used research terminology.

QUALITY IMPROVEMENT

Quality assurance (QA), QI, and continuing quality improvement (CQI) mean essentially the same thing and suggest that higher quality through improved (and improving) processes and systems can save money. Few states require ALCs to have a QA plan, or continuous

evaluation, but a growing number of ALCs are choosing to do so. Many QA/QI systems are authorized to implement changes, rely on vertically integrated teams of workers (with mutual interests in resident outcomes) collaborating in quality circles, and use standards or benchmarks by which to measure the quality. Quality improvement is frequently mentioned in ALC mission statements.

The FOCUS-PDCA Model has been implemented in many long-term care facilities both for QA/QI and to process a desired change. FOCUS stands for: Find an issue that needs improvement, Organize a team, Clarify what is known about the issue, Uncover the causes of poor outcomes, and Start the PDCA cycle. As a result of Planning a change, Doing it, Checking the effect of the change, and Acting on what was learned (PDCA), new knowledge is systematically and scientifically generated. Reflecting on Donabedian's (1988) structure-process-outcome model for quality of care, there are three major categories of standards:

- *Structure standards:* the necessary framework to guide, provide and monitor nursing care. This includes the management/leadership and governance model, master staffing model, nursing theory of practice, job descriptions, and policies.
- *Process standards:* the nursing activities necessary for, or associated with, care delivery. These include

performance evaluation (feedback), procedures and care protocols for specific conditions and needs, and best practices guidelines.

■ *Outcome standards:* the results of nursing acts; these standards are (or should be) measurable. They reflect nursing's effectiveness and efficiency and include employee and resident satisfaction, clinical data, and principle-driven outcomes of care such as resident-directed decision making.

Outcomes, Indicators, and Thresholds

Outcomes can be broad (aggregated, descriptive data), generic (i.e., overview of a particular phenomenon but lacking specific descriptive detail; e.g., falls frequency), or focused (i.e., examination of a specific phenomenon; e.g., falls at a particular time of day, resident behavior). Outcome indicators can be measures of residents' physiological status, psychosocial function, pain and symptom control, and quality of life. Focused outcome reporting is associated with a *key indicator* (i.e., a specific measure of quality of life or care or a finding, such as falls) and a *threshold* (i.e., a norm for the resident group, such as falls among older adults living in ALCs). Linking a key indicator and the threshold for the particular phenomenon or group of residents is used to identify areas needing improvement. Examine the number of falls in the ALC over a specific period of time (i.e., the indicator) and compare it to the reported number of falls in similar ALCs with similar residents (i.e., the benchmark). Some outcome indicators are highly subjective perceptions (e.g., quality of life) and should be analyzed cautiously if inferences are to be drawn from the group to an individual resident.

Poor care is an outcome, variously described, and can be attributed to poor structure and/or process standards, including inadequate knowledge and skills to care for the population (i.e., structure). Poor communication is a process standard failure, but it could be one of structure, also. Is all communication verbal? The standard of care to which a nursing service might be held could be unrealistic given the prevailing job market, availability of qualified staff, and resources or time to do the work.

Data collection (retrieval) in QA/QI/CQI can be concurrent (i.e., performance observation, current resident chart audits) or retrospective (i.e., closed record review). *Utilization review* is a kind of QA; it looks at resources used (staffing, supplies, equipment) given the resident characteristics.

Risk management (RM) can be considered an aspect of QA, but its focus and methods are different. Whereas QA/QI seeks the best care possible, RM seeks an accept-able level of care such that substandard care, and with it the risk of lawsuits and a deteriorating image of the ALC in the external community, is avoided. Although both approaches are proactive, RM processes strive to identify high-risk areas (e.g., stairways) in advance of an adverse event, whereas QA/QI processes seek to improve care quality. Both programs seek to identify care delivery associated with high risk, for example, wheelchair use in corridors not designed for that kind of mobility (e.g., an open stairway). *Liability exposure* can be reduced by careful perusal of QA/QI data.

Infection control plans (ICPs) are a kind of RM in that they specifically describe the procedures in place to prevent an infectious outbreak, how it is detected, controlled, monitored, and reported to the appropriate services in the facility as well as to the health department, if required. There are few state guidelines with regard to infection control in ALCs, with the exception of admissions practices. In general, ALCs are not required to have an ICP. However, individual ALCs can have department-specific policies and procedures (e.g., food services) for infection/communicable disease prevention and management, use of universal precautions, education, visitor guidelines, and reporting requirements.

A *hazardous substance management program* is mandated by the federal government office of the Occupational Safety and Health Administration (OSHA), though only a few states require this for ALCs at the present time. The program requires a material data safety sheet (MDSS) for each product used by the ALC to clean the physical environment (e.g., isopropyl alcohol, bleach, mercury, or iodine-based products). The MDSS has to identify other names by which the product is known, the chemicals contained in the product, and the actions to be taken in the event of a hazardous situation; for example, it explains what to do if Clorox (bleach) is splashed into a person's eye. Nursing homes must have a designated safety officer and a readily accessible chemical or mercury spill kit. This is something to consider for an ALC, regardless of size.

RESEARCH

EBP/R is a hallmark of nursing practice in the 21st century. The term "nursing research" implies that nursing conducted the research and/or that nursing is using the research (i.e., research "utilization" or "application"). AL residents and ALCs are an increasingly desirable population and site for researchers. A nurse manager needs to know the purposes of the research, what it wants to demonstrate or prove, and the research methods that will be used in order to meet nursing's core professional obligations to residents and staff.

From the ethical perspectives of respect for persons, avoidance of harm, and informed consent, all research should be approved, either by the owner or administrator and/or by an external (or internal) review board (i.e., an IRB). A research proposal must describe the level of risk for research participants and how informed consent will be obtained from them. Research proposals can use rather arcane/esoteric language; informed consent documents can be pages long. It is important and ethically necessary to clarify that which is unclear, especially when it refers to the research methods. The ethical principle of *distributive justice* means that a research proposal should describe how it will solicit research participants—and why it seeks participation by ALC residents and/or staff, particularly. A properly constituted IRB should include a member of the local (i.e., external) community in order to represent the interests of the typical AL resident. However, most freestanding ALCs do not have an IRB; the presence or use of an IRB-type process in AL corporations is unknown. Nevertheless, that does not remove federal government protections for research participants, no matter where they reside or who is paying their bills (see Chapter 2, "Public Policies, Assisted Living Models, and Regulations," regarding the Health Insurance Portability and Accountability Act's privacy rule).

Components of a Research Proposal

- Purpose of the research: what it wants to demonstrate, assert, or prove; implication(s) or application(s) of the research findings.
- Subject/participant recruitment methods: a resident's direct caregiver (e.g., nurse, personal care assistant) should not ask a resident to participate in research; this can be perceived as coercive. This section should describe the rationale for why ALC residents are being selected (e.g., convenience sample).
- Methodology: interview, focus group, exercise performance, lab test, and so forth.
- Review of the literature: previous research about the phenomenon (issue); why this particular research is needed (e.g., the phenomenon has never been studied before or it has been inadequately studied).
- Risk associated with research participation.
- Informed consent: how it will be obtained.
- Subject/participation protection: procedures to ensure confidentiality or anonymity.
- Limitations of the study: procedural, statistical; potential to generalize the results of the study to other do-

mains and populations. For example, how applicable are the results of a study of a nonrestrictive diet for diabetics in an ALC to community-dwelling older adults who live alone? How applicable are study results on a falls prevention intervention in a small ALC with only 6 residents versus a large ALC with 200 residents?

- Dissemination of the findings: the ethical obligation of the researcher to disseminate or share the findings *whether or not* the results generated new knowledge, best practices, and so forth.

Risk levels in research are as follows: no risk; low or minimal risk (e.g., drawing blood); not greater than minimal risk (i.e., risks associated with daily living activities); greater than minimal risk but only minor (e.g., stress test of an older adult with no history of cardiac disease); or at-risk (an intervention that is not part of an older adult's health care regimen). Psychosocial research can be risky; vulnerable older adults might need special protection (e.g., victims of the Holocaust and other genocidal events).

A *low risk–high burden* ratio assesses the impact of the research methods on the subject/participant. Being interviewed for hours might be delightful and low-risk for a lonely resident. However, the risk for the resident is heightened if the research protocol does not consider how the resident might feel when the interviews are over and perhaps ended too abruptly without proper preparation for leave-taking. Does the methods section address this? Informed consent for participation in research requires attention to the details and cannot usually be done in one session. This is where an AL nurse is a resident advocate!

Informed Consent

The principle of informed consent is based on the ethical principles of *respect for persons* and *autonomy or self-determination*. Among the tenets of informed consent are the following:

- Evidence of capacity: the cognitive capacity to consent or refuse to consent to participate in research, which includes giving a rational, authentic reason(s) for this personal decision.
- Knowledge: the breadth and depth (complexity) of information that a reasonable person needs to make a decision about whether or not to participate in the research.
- Comprehension: evidence of the resident's ability to state (or rephrase) his or her understanding of his or her role and responsibility in the research.

■ Voluntariness: the right to refuse to participate or be a research subject.

Understanding is a key aspect of cognitive capacity. It can be assessed with some degree of assurance by asking the resident to state, in his own words, what he thinks the research is about, his role and responsibility as a research participant or subject, any benefits or risks to him by being a research subject/participant, and his right to withdraw from the research. The notion of understanding is very similar to that required for health care decision making and consent to treatment (see the Chapter 14 section, "Decision-Making Capacity Assessment").

Informed consent documents should be free of legal jargon and use a font size and style that is easy for an older adult to read. Persons with impaired cognition (e.g., dementia) have the capacity to make some decisions (e.g., appoint a health care proxy; consent to a low-risk simple treatment; participate in a survey/interview). However, in comparison to older adults who are not dementia sufferers, those with dementia are unable to describe the consequences of their decisions. The Mini-Mental Status Examination (MMSE), although often used as an indicator of capacity to make a decision, should not be used alone to determine the individual's ability to consent to participate in a study. Other tools, such as the Evaluation to Sign Consent, provide a more accurate accounting of the individual's ability to decide if he or she can participate in a specific study. This tool asks the older adult to recall and rephrase in her own words the information she was given about the study.

Residents should be given every opportunity to participate in a study, as desired. At the same time, it is the responsibility of the ALC to ensure that the investigators and projects that are allowed to come into the ALC and recruit resident participants are ethically sound, safe, and something that the facility feels comfortable supporting. An open discussion with the research team is necessary to determine what will be required on the part of the ALC versus what the research team will provide. Will ALC staff be asked to collect data? Does the ALC have to provide meeting space for the research team? When and what will the research team share with the ALC when the study is completed? The researcher (or team) should meet with ALC staff to describe the purposes of the research, what they will be doing on the premises, and when.

Respect for the resident's dignity is shown by the manner in which she or he is approached to participate in a project or study: Is the resident lying down? Is the person who is seeking his consent standing over him? Or sitting in a chair at the same height as the resident? Is the resident dressed or in night clothes? Is the resident conversing in the language with which she is most adept? Is it a staff person he knows who is asking him to participate?

CBPR, in contrast to classic research, is a research model and process that offers relatively immediate benefit to the population or group being studied. The community is an equal, engaged, and accountable decision-making partner with the researcher (investigator). Community partners (e.g., agencies, schools, ALCs) are involved in the research goals, design, methods, subject recruitment, data analysis, and dissemination of findings (for direct application in the community as well as in scholarly journals). Barriers to CBPR include lack of perceived incentives for communities (such as ALCs) to get involved, limited resources to educate community partners about the research goals and methods, the kind of informed consent needed for subject participation, and IRB concerns about subject protection, especially confidentiality. Nevertheless, CBPR can be an exciting opportunity for ALCs to be involved in a learning experience, research, *and* reap the benefits.

EBP is the use of interventions/practices, supported by sufficient data showing that an approach is effective and efficient. Synonymous terms are research-based practice and evidence-based treatment. In nursing and in medicine, EBP looks at the rationale for using a specific medication, treatment, protocol, or regimen in order to guide decision making for the individual resident.

Research Terminology

■ *Meta-analysis:* A statistical technique that collects and reviews previous research about a particular subject or phenomenon, it seeks to answer the question, "Does XX make a difference?" For example, does using physical restraints alter the frequency and severity of falls-related injuries? Several meta-analyses clearly demonstrated that less use of restraints was associated with fewer falls with significant injury.
■ *Control group:* A control group is used in an interventional study when a treatment (i.e., intervention) is administered to one group of participants but not to another group of participants (i.e., the control) who are identical or matched on several characteristics to the group receiving the intervention (e.g., a treatment ALC vs. a control ALC).
■ *Random design:* This is a selection technique whereby participants are assigned to a control or intervention group. No one group or individual is deliberately sin-

gled out to be in one or the other group. Selection (assignment) is completely up to chance and based, as a rule, on a numerical scheme.

- *Double-blind study:* This is the preferred technique in drug or treatment studies. The intent is to demonstrate that the effect of the drug (or treatment) is produced by the drug itself and not by some other characteristic or variable. Two statistically identical groups or populations are created: one receives the drug or treatment, the other receives a placebo (i.e., a medication with no chemical attributes; a treatment that looks like the real thing but is not). Neither the participants nor the clinician know who got the real thing and who got the placebo. Double-blind random control (DBRC) studies are believed to provide the most accurate results in that not even the researchers know what each participant received—until the study is completed.

Measures of disease frequency:

- Incidence rate: This refers to the rate at which people who are without a disease develop the disease during a set period of time. It focuses on the new cases of a disease.

$$\text{Incidence} = \frac{\text{number of new cases of a disease in a time period}}{\text{total number of people at risk for getting the disease}}$$

- Prevalence: This is a measure of the number of people with a disease at any given point in time.

$$\text{Prevalence} = \frac{\text{total number of individuals with a disease}}{\text{total population}}$$

In considering a *research proposal:*

- What are the goals of the research?
  - What are the best practices for AL?
  - What is the nursing theory development with regard to residential care nursing practice?
- What is the source of the research idea? Academia? Practice? Regulations? Social policy?
- What makes this proposal research rather than a quality improvement study? Is it a CBPR study?
- What are the dissemination plans? Most researchers want to meet the research standard of replicability and generalization of findings, defined as follows: If this research was conducted in another similar setting using the same methodology, it would produce the same findings or outcomes. The researcher might be reluctant to release the findings until the study can be conducted again in another setting.

- What is the imposition on resident and/or staff time in the conduct of this research?
- How and when will the findings be shared with the ALC?

CLINICAL CAMPUS AND SCHOOL AFFILIATIONS

A sustained affiliation with a school of nursing and/or a nurse assistant training center is an opportunity for the school as well as the ALC. Nursing and nurse assistant students can learn about the older adult in a setting that is committed to generative and supportive aging, management of chronic conditions, assessment, and communication skills. The experience can dispel misperceptions about aging and about where and how older adults want to live until they die. A school of nursing affiliation with the ALC is a possible source of future staff as well as access to nursing libraries and teaching materials, the latest information on best practices and on professional issues, and access to continuing education and college courses (at reduced cost, possibly). Affiliation can reduce the felt sense of isolation of many ALC nurses, both registered nurses and licensed practical nurses (LPNs). For the registered nurses and LPNs/licensed vocational nurses (LVNs), it might become a pathway for career growth to become a registered nurse.

A successful affiliation requires thoughtful planning and addresses issues such as:

- Why the school wants to affiliate with the ALC or—at the very least—use it as a clinical campus; what are the learning goals?
- What the ALC has to offer that is desirable to the school. (It could be related to location and students' travel costs.)
- How residents will be selected and the length of the student-resident relationship. Is it a one-time/one-day-only learning experience?
- The benefits that accrue to the ALC in the affiliation *and* any hidden costs.
- The nature of student supervision. What is the ratio of students to faculty for purposes of achieving learning goals as well as with regard to resident safety?

A clinical campus or affiliation agreement can also mean that ALC nurses might be appointed *adjunct teaching faculty* (with appropriate titles on their ID badge) for which they could be compensated financially or by access to courses that advance their career interests.

Student orientation to the ALC should include fire safety measures and resident rights, including the right to refuse to be cared for or interviewed by a student. Approval of students' medication administration, and periodic, scheduled evaluation of the affiliation by ALC staff, residents (families), students, and faculty should be part of the affiliation discussion and agreement.

RESOURCES

Donabedian, A. (1988). The quality of care. How can it be assessed? *Journal of the American Medical Association, 260,* 2743–2748.

Israel, B. A., Eng, E., Schulz, A. J., & Parker, E. A. (2005). *Methods in community-based participatory research for health.* San Francisco, CA: John Wiley & Sons.

Marker, C. G. (1987). The Marker model for nursing standards: Implications for nursing administration. *Nursing Administration Quarterly, 12*(2), 4–12.

Mitty, E., & Post, L. F. (2008). Healthcare decision making. In E. Capezuti, D. Zwicker, M. Mezey, & T. Fulmer (Eds.), *Evidence-based geriatric nursing protocols for best practice* (3rd ed., pp. 521–528). New York: Springer Publishing Company.

Resnick, B., Gruber-Baldini, A., Pretzer-Aboff, I., Galik, E., Custis-Buie, V., Russ, K., & Zimmerman, S. (2007). Reliability and validity of the Evaluation to Sign Consent Measure. *The Gerontologist, 47*(1), 69–77.

Approach to the Resident

The chapters in this section focus on general guidelines and recommendations for approaching residents in assisted living (AL) settings. Specifically, culturally sensitive care, physical activity, and other preventive health recommendations for residents (and methods for engaging them in these activities), and ways to manage prevalent problems such as pain are discussed. In addition, new thoughts and approaches on complementary or integrative medicine and general medical management of residents are described. Each chapter provides not only updated information but also ways to integrate these approaches into AL nursing practice.

14

Resident Assessment and Service Plan Construction

Ethel Mitty, Sandi Flores,
and Thomas M. Gill

The goal of assessment of the AL community (ALC) resident is to promote and maintain wellness, lifestyle preferences, and independent function. This chapter addresses assessment from several perspectives: pre-clinical disability, physical, psychosocial, and mental status, decision-making capacity (including standards of decision making), quality of life, and environment. The section on service plan construction suggests some guidelines to make data into useful information. Guidelines for when to call 911 are discussed in the last section.

Assessment includes the physical, cognitive, emotional, and psychosocial domains and, if at all possible, should be performance based. These data are obtained by observation, interview, and physical examination. Given the high prevalence of sensory deficits among older adults, particular attention should be given to the environment of the assessment (i.e., noise level, lighting). Inexpensive amplification devices, such as lightweight earphones, can be especially useful.

At some point during the assessment, ask an open-ended question, such as, "What would living here (in the ALC) do for you that you would like?" "What is it that you can no longer do that you would like to do again?" Finding out what the older adult wants—in advance of living in the ALC—can identify potential problems, generate trust, and improve satisfaction. Admission data are baseline data; they are the source of

the service plan, goal setting, provision and organization of services, monitoring and supervision needed, and the cost estimate of providing the services.

The nursing assessment tool reflects what nursing thinks is important and can be provided and, by their omission, what is not important or cannot be provided. The focus of the assessment should be on what the resident can and should do for him or herself and the ways in which nursing will optimize that function. Constrained by regulations regarding allowable services as well as retention and discharge criteria, and what an ALC chooses to provide, the pre-admission assessment is a critical professional responsibility bounded by knowledge, skills, and ethics. The fact that some states permit ALCs to admit and retain nursing home level of care residents is confusing to residents and their families and speaks to the need for *disclosure* of the ALC's retention and discharge policies and *transparency* regarding how those kinds of decisions are made. Admission determinations, based in large part on nursing assessment, are shaped by the AL nurse's knowledge of the care capabilities of the ALC staff. A resident with a specific medical condition can be admitted, according to regulation—but will staff need additional training or education to meet this resident's needs? A *holistic nursing assessment* seeks information about residents' preferences and lifestyle habits, what they value and is important to them, and their expectations of living in an ALC.

Assessment tools typically ask about medication usage and the ability to self-medicate, food and drug allergies, functionality, communication, hearing and vision, continence and bowel pattern, mood and behavior, oral/dental status, and chronic or recurrent skin conditions. Some states require the resident's history regarding tuberculosis testing and/or infection. Many states provide a comprehensive assessment tool that the ALC is required to use (see Chapter 2, "Public Policies, Assisted Living Models, and Regulations").

Questions that could be posed to a prospective resident include the following:

- What things that you now do for yourself would you like to continue to be able to do?
- What things that you no longer do would you like to be able to do?
- What things would you *not* mind no longer doing, such as, giving yourself your eye drops? Ordering your meds?
- Who, if anyone, is assisting you with financial decisions, such as bill paying?
- Has your falling made you a little unwilling to go outside or to go on trips? How frightened are you of falling again?
- Tell me how you got through those times when you were sick or something really bad happened?
- What do you regret never having done? What do you want to do next?
- What is in the way of your being as healthy as you want to be?
- What kind of person do you feel most comfortable with? Least comfortable?

The SPICES tool is an efficient and effective way to prevent untoward health events as well as track a health condition that is emerging and signal the need for a more in-depth assessment. It is an acronym for the following common geriatric syndromes:

S: Sleep disorders

P: Problems with eating or feeding

I: Incontinence

C: Confusion

E: Evidence of falls

S: Skin breakdown

Functional status is the ability to perform the tasks required for living safely and for effectively meeting care needs: activities of daily living (ADLs) and instrumental activities of daily living (IADL). The best approach is to ask whether or not the older adult requires (or would like) the help of another person to complete the task(s). Bathing is commonly the basic ADL with the highest prevalence of disability and is often the reason why older adults receive home aide services. To identify *preclinical disability*, that is, personal assistance is not yet needed, ask (a) if the person thinks he or she will have some difficulty with the task(s) at some time in the future, and (b) whether the person has changed the way he or she completes the task because of a health-related problem or condition. Potential residents and/or their families might be reluctant to speculate about these issues out of concern that the ALC costs will increase with additional services, perhaps beyond what they can afford.

It is very important to help residents and families understand that the services provided by the ALC will help optimize their function. This is in contrast to simply completing a task for a resident by having the personal care assistant comb the resident's hair or put on a shirt; it takes away the resident's opportunity to raise his or her arms as much as possible. Assessment means giving the resident time and cues to execute a task (e.g., three attempts to get up from a chair) before helping him or her with the activity. This is an opportunity to see the resident's capability and then build in the necessary assistance.

Ask about use of any assistive device (e.g., cane, walker, weighted utensil) and the circumstances under which it is used. At the time of the pre-admission interview and examination, observe the older adult as he or she completes a simple task, for example, unbuttoning and buttoning a shirt or blouse, picking up a pen and writing a sentence, taking off and putting on shoes, or stair climbing.

Older adults are usually aware of their visual deficits but may not want to talk about them. A brief performance-based screen can ask the older adult to read (wearing his or her glasses, if applicable) a short passage from a newspaper or magazine; however, bear in mind that low literacy is not uncommon among older adults. Likewise, hearing can be evaluated by testing to see if the individual can hear you when you use a whisper, a normal tone of voice, or a loud, low voice. The high prevalence of hearing loss among older adults and its association with depression, dissatisfaction with life, and withdrawal from social activities make it an important assessment. Impaired hearing without appropriate amplification devices can result in a misdiagnosis of impaired understanding attributable to a cognitive cause (e.g., dementia) rather than to a physiological or structural deficit that might be correctible.

COGNITION AND EXECUTIVE FUNCTION

Cognition is a mental function that includes information processing, application of knowledge, reasoning, perception, and changing preferences. Cognitive decline doubles every 5 years after the age of 65 and approaches 40% to 50% at age 90. Even in the absence of dementia, cognitive impairment places the older adult at increased risk for accidents, delirium, noncompliance with the medical regimen, and disability. Most older adults with dementia do not complain of memory loss or even volunteer symptoms of cognitive impairment unless specifically questioned. Short-term memory loss is typically the first sign of dementia: the best single screening question is recall of three words after 1 minute.

Mental status assessment using the Mini-Cog is quick (i.e., 3 minutes to administer) and does not have the same language, literacy, educational level or cultural drawbacks as the Mini-Mental Status Exam (MMSE). The Mini-Cog is a brief screening tool to differentiate those individuals with dementia from those without dementia. It consists of recall of three unrelated words and with the Clock Drawing Test (CDT). If all three words are recalled, the person is not demented. If only one to two words are recalled, the person is classified as demented or not demented based on the CDT (i.e., numbers are placed in correct order on the clock face and clock hands are correctly drawn to a time specified by the examiner).

Executive function is a mental process that is essential for goal-directed behavior. It includes planning, ability to make a selection or choice, decision making, adaptation, self-monitoring, and abstract thinking. Often overlooked in assessment, executive function could be important in an ALC with respect to making safe self-care decisions, particularly self-medication. The test of executive function can be especially useful if the resident's family or direct caregiver feels that the resident is different after an acute episode, illness exacerbation, or hospitalization when other screenings suggest no other cause for cognitive change (e.g., delirium). Three tests recommended for executive function testing are Royall's CLOX (i.e., clock drawing), an oral word association test, and a trail making test that links, for example, the letters of the alphabet with a numerical sequence. Limitations of executive function tests are

related to language proficiency, educational level, and, possibly, depressed mood.

Psychosocial assessment in AL consists of several elements: ethnic, spiritual and cultural background, the older adult's personal support system and economic well-being, possibility of elder mistreatment, and advance directives. *Quality of life* is a convenient catch phrase but there is no standard measurement of it; most instruments include various aspects of physical, cognitive, psychological and social function, and satisfaction. The Short Form-36 Health Survey (SF-36) is the most commonly used instrument to measure quality of life; it includes 36 items organized into eight domains—physical function, role limitations due to physical health, role limitations due to emotional health, bodily pain, social functioning, mental health, vitality, and general health perceptions. It has been tested extensively among community-dwelling and hospitalized older adults, but its value for use among the oldest-old (i.e., those over 85 years of age) has not been established. In addition, the SF-36 is more a measure of health status rather than quality of life; therefore, other ways of identifying or measuring quality of life should be sought. Quality of life assessment should ask about the *effect of living with a chronic illness or condition* on the older adult's desire or ability to do what he or she wants to do. It means having meaningful choices. Service plans that include individual preferences increase satisfaction, improve adherence to medical regimens, and have the potential to improve outcomes.

Decision-Making Capacity Assessment

Capacity and competency are different, but the terms are often used synonymously, albeit incorrectly. *Capacity* is a clinical issue and is clinically determined. *Competency* is determination of the ability to make financial or contractual decisions (e.g., legal tasks) and is decided in a court of law. Honoring the decision of an individual with capacity speaks to the ethical principle of *respect for persons*. Honoring (and moving forward with) the decision of an individual who lacks capacity can be construed as an act of abandonment. The fact that an individual makes a decision that is not aligned with a medical recommendation does *not* mean that the person lacks decisional capacity. Health care decisions are framed by culture, beliefs, meaning of life and death, perceptions of pain, socioeconomics, education, language, and advance care planning.

Decisional capacity is the ability to understand the facts, appreciate their implications, *and* assume responsibility for the decision and its consequences. The *elements of decisional capacity* include the following:

- Ability to understand and process information
- Weighing the relative benefits, burdens, and risk of each option
- Applying personal values to the analysis (and ability to describe or explain what those values are)
- Arriving at a decision that is consistent over time (i.e., over 24 hours. Go through the process again; look for consistency: the person made the same decision)
- Communicating the decision

There is no gold standard tool to assess decisional capacity. Determination of capacity should occur over time. The MMSE and Mini-Cog are not tests of decisional capacity. Capacity is not an on-off switch; it exists to some extent even for those afflicted with dementia. Low-risk, safe, appropriate, and uncomplicated decisions can be made by those with early/mild stage dementia and by individuals with mild-to-moderate mental retardation. Understanding the consequences of a decision is one of the most important indicators of decisional capacity and the test that is failed by virtually all individuals with moderate to severe dementia.

Observe and document the resident's ability to express his/her needs and preferences, follow directions, make simple choices and decisions (e.g., "Would you like ice cream or sherbet?" "The TV or the radio?"), and communicate his or her care needs (e.g., that he or she is in pain). Observe *periods of lucidity*, those times of day (or night) when the resident is particularly clear-headed. The statements in the following list can be helpful in assessing whether or not the resident has the skills necessary to make a health care decision. They are similar to the probes used in ascertaining understanding sufficient for informed consent to participate (or refuse to participate) in research.

- Tell me in your own words what I (or the physician, nurse, etc.) explained to you.
- Tell me which parts, if any, were confusing to you.
- Tell me what you feel you have to gain (or to lose) by agreeing (or not agreeing) to the proposed treatment.
- Tell me why this decision is difficult (important, frightening, etc.) to you.

There are three standards of decision making:

(1) Prior expression of wishes, orally or with a written document/instructions such as an advance directive (see the Chapter 2 section "Public Policies").

(2) Substituted judgment: based on the expressed wishes, previous decisions or behaviors of a *formerly capacitated* person; a decision is made by others for that person.
(3) Best-interest standards: a decision is made by others on behalf of an individual whose health care wishes or preferences had never been expressed and cannot be inferred.

If the resident does not appear to have the capacity for health care decision making, help her identify whom she would want to assist her and speak on her behalf in discussion and decisions about treatments and care.

Environmental Assessment

Assessment based on the concept of *environmental affordances* evaluates the opportunities, actions, and behaviors supported by a given environment. The concept is based on the known psychosocial needs of older adults. There are seven principles of ideal environmental affordance.

(1) Contact with the outside world is assured and available, if desired.
(2) Indoor/outdoor connections and transition zones (doorways) are easily accessible.
(3) Comfort and accessibility with as few navigational barriers as possible—given the functional and cognitive challenges to many residents.
(4) Freedom, choice, and variety are achieved with a variety of locations, observation points, seating, and so forth.
(5) Relationship with nature to the extent desired affords the opportunity to smell, touch, observe, and listen.
(6) Activity and movement, as desired (walkways, exercise stations, etc.), is available.
(7) Safety and security (e.g., minimize risk of falling) is assured.

An in-house survey constructed around these principles could yield some practical information with regard to quality of life, desirable architectural and ambient changes, and marketing.

SERVICE PLAN CONSTRUCTION

The *service plan* is the AL industry-wide term for what, in other domains of health care, is called a *care plan*. Most states require creation of a service plan at the time of admission that is to be updated annually and upon change of resident condition. Most service plans hold to the format of identified needs, goals, and interventions for goal achievement. A function-focused care approach is recommended as the underlying philosophy for the service plan. This approach focuses on what the resident can do for him or herself and how to optimize that ability and function, rather than focusing on the task to be completed by the caregiver. For example, the service plan should indicate that the resident will walk halfway from his or her room to the dining room daily and then will be assisted in the wheelchair the remaining distance or that the resident will receive the verbal cues needed to bathe and dress. This is in contrast to having the caregiver simply take the individual to the dining room or perform all bathing and dressing.

Service planning must be culture sensitive and address, as well, the resident's interest in or need for intimacy and sexual expression, spirituality, activity preferences, and wellness planning. Needs typically addressed in a service plan include the following:

- ADLs: required assistance to optimize the individual's underlying function
- Use of mobility devices
- Continence care and toileting schedules
- Pain management
- Dietary requirements and preferences
- Diagnosis-specific care (and monitoring) needs (e.g., diabetes management)
- Sensory care needs (e.g., glasses, hearing aids)
- Special care such as ostomy or catheter care, oxygen or other gases
- Escort needs (e.g., assistance to dining room, activities)
- Behavioral needs (e.g., resident-specific interventions for catastrophic reaction, wandering, inappropriate sexual activity)
- Psychosocial needs
- Requirement for therapies (e.g., physical therapy)
- Medication management

In most AL organizations, a licensed nurse conducts the assessment, but not all states require this. Assessment is more than data collection. Because it includes interpretation and meaning of the data, it is commonly associated with a registered nurse (RN). Some ALCs use terms such as "appraisal," "evaluation," or "review of care needs" because an RN is not doing the data collection or assessment; however, the hope is that those phrases connote RN involvement in the assessment.

Rushed or inadequate assessments typically yield an inadequate service plan that does not properly coordinate all of the resident's care needs.

Ideally, the service plan is a *collaborative process*. Information is gathered from a variety of resources, including the resident's physician, outside providers such as therapists and home health nurses, family, care staff, and of course the resident whenever possible. In keeping with AL philosophy, the service plan should allow for the necessary care to be delivered with resident preference being uppermost. It is not unusual to arrange for bathing in the afternoon rather than the morning or to schedule care for the early riser as well as the resident who does not want to be awakened before 10:00 A.M. Typically, signatures are required of the resident, nurse, executive director, and responsible party who collaborated on the service plan. Many ALCs tie the service plan to the level of care assessment that drives the billing for care, as such requiring a quarterly update of the assessment and service plan.

Staff introduction to a new resident's service plan should be done on each shift. Many ALCs place the original service plan in the individual resident's chart and a copy of all residents' service plans in a large binder, easily accessible by all care staff. Realizing that most staff do not sit and read every service plan before each shift, it is common to see a resident summary of some type given to staff on each shift, noting key points of the service plan in an abbreviated fashion.

The challenge for the AL nurse is to feel confident that all planned care is carried out. This can be done in a variety of ways, including an end-of-shift report where the care provided is verbalized and noted in a variety of documents. Simply walking about and chatting with the residents can elicit information as to whether or not the necessary (and desired) care was provided. In addition, there are a growing number of electronic information technology (IT) systems to record this information.

As a practical matter, a service plan is a functional tool to meet a resident's care needs. Created and used appropriately, it is also a tool to *control risk;* improperly developed, it can significantly increase an ALC's exposure to risk. Key points in service plan development include the following:

- The assessment on which the service plan is based should be complete (i.e., holistic) and accurate.
- Do not require more interventions than ALC staff can realistically provide.
- Update the plan whenever there is a change in resident condition or ALC service capacity.

- Do not require interventions that are contrary to state regulation (or ALC capacity).
- Do not write improper or unrealistic interventions just because the resident, family, or responsible party requests them.
- Verify that staff know how to perform all interventions appropriately, including the use of equipment and assistive devices.

Some ALCs use a point of care system whereby personal assistive staff record, via hand-held computers, whenever care assigned on the service plan has been provided. Some ALCs routinely create all service plans using a computer-based program that also guides the assessment.

Calling 911 for Condition Change

Condition change and acute illness are often difficult to determine in older adults because the signs and symptoms of diseases are not typical. For example, an older adult can have acute appendicitis and not even have any abdominal pain. Whether or not to call 911 should be based on a systematic assessment and communication protocol that can guide decisions. The SPICES tool can be used to identify and monitor change and alert professional caregivers that the resident may be experiencing an acute medical problem. The FANCAPES assessment tool (see the following list) might also be useful to guide the caregiving staff when it is noted that there may be a change in the resident's condition. The acronym identifier is only the starting point of data collection and leads to a fuller, more relevant communication with the primary health care provider.

- F: Fluids: is there any reason to believe that the resident has too much or too little fluid? Consider oral intake and whether or not that is being maintained. Is there a reason to believe that excessive fluids have been lost (e.g., bleeding, diarrhea) or that kidney failure or an acute coronary syndrome (ACS) that might cause a back up of fluid (e.g., congestive heart failure) is present? (See Chapter 42, "Cardiovascular Diseases and Disorders," regarding atypical presentation in older adults.)
- A: Aeration: evaluate the resident for changes from his or her baseline breathing: count the respirations and determine if these are slower or faster than baseline, listen to breathing for wheezing, observe if the individual is able to take a deep breath in comfortably, and observe for the use of neck and stomach muscles to breath.

- N: Nutrition: evaluate if there is any change in oral food intake from baseline, check for mouth pain that could impair eating, and evaluate for changes in ability to swallow (see Chapter 25, "Maintenance of Nutritional Status").
- C: Cognition and communication. The *delirium mnemonic* can help determine possible causes of changes in the baseline cognition and communication abilities of the resident and can guide assessment:

  - ☐ D = drug use, recent meds
  - ☐ E = electrolytes imbalance
  - ☐ L = lack of drugs, missed medication
  - ☐ I = infection
  - ☐ R = reduced sensory input
  - ☐ I = intracranial problems (e.g., stroke, post-ictal state)
  - ☐ U = urinary retention, fecal impaction
  - ☐ M = myocardium problems (see also, Chapter 31, "Delirium")

- A: Activities (ADL changes, recent fall with or without overt signs of injury)
- P: Pain: A helpful mnemonic to differentiate chronic from acute pain—PQRST—has been effectively used with cognitively impaired patients versus those without evidence of impairment. As with the other assessment tools, it guides data collection, analysis/interpretation, documentation, and communication.

  - ☐ Provokes or Palliates: what makes the pain worse? Better? And for how long? Is there recent trauma?
  - ☐ Quality and Quantity of the pain. Is it consistent? Sharp? Tolerable?
  - ☐ Region/radiation: what is the location of the pain? does it move about? Does the pain affect other functions, such as vision or the ability to ambulate, transfer, or self-propel?
  - ☐ Severity: what does the pain prevent the resident from doing? What is the range of motion tolerance?
  - ☐ Timing: when is the pain worst? Is there any association with activities? (See also, Chapter 21, "Chronic Pain and Persistent Pain").

- E: Elimination: Mental status change is associated with constipation and obstruction (see also, Chapter 45, "Gastrointestinal Diseases and Disorders").
- S: Skin and Socialization: a variety of scenarios, from pressure ulcers to suicide (see also Chapter 33, "Pres-

sure Ulcers," and Chapter 34, "Depression and Other Mood Disorders").

When communicating with the primary health care provider, the AL nurse is as responsible for providing relevant information as is the physician or geriatric nurse practitioner for asking relevant questions. The SBAR Guidelines for Communication Content (see the following list) is a structured communication policy and is in keeping with the culture of safety. It includes respect between parties and the right of the AL nurse to ask questions and make suggestions based on expertise, knowledge of the resident, and informed data collection and assessment.

- S: Situation: what is going on? what are the data, the facts?
- B: Background: what is the resident's clinical history/background, including current diagnoses, context (any advance directives), and medications?
- A: Assessment: the AL nurse states what she or he thinks is the problem.
- R: Recommendation: the AL nurse states what she or he thinks is best for the resident and would like to do to manage the condition (including hospital transfer).

The American Medical Directors Association (n.d.) has a useful *Protocols for Physician Notification: Assessing and Collecting Data on Nursing Facility Patients—A Guide for Nurses on Effective Communication with Physicians* that can be used to further aid nurses in gathering and reporting information to health care providers. (See also, Chapter 17, "The Continuum of Care," regarding transitions between settings.)

RESOURCES

American Medical Association. (n.d.). *Physician's guide to assessing and counseling older drivers.* Retrieved April 25, 2009, from http://www.ama-assn.org/ama/pub/physician- resources/public-health/promoting-healthy-lifestyles/geriatric-health/older-driver- safety/assessing-counseling-older-drivers.shtml

The American Medical Directors Association. (n.d.) *Protocols for physician notification: Assessing and collecting data on nursing facility patients—A guide for nurses on effective communication with physicians.* Retrieved April 25, 2009, from http://www.amda.com/resources/index.cfm.

Doerflinger, D.M.C. (2007). *Mental status assessment of older adults: The Mini-Cog.* Retrieved April 25, 2009, from http://www.consultgerirn.org/uploads/File/trythis/issue03.pdf

Haig, K. M., Sutton, S., & Whittington, J. (2006). SBAR: A shared mental model for improving communications between clinicians. *Journal of Quality and Patient Safety, 32,* 167–175.

Kennedy, G.J. (2007). *Brief evaluation of executive dysfunction: An essential refinement in the assessment of cognitive impairment.* New York: The Hartford Institute for Geriatric Nursing.

Mitty, E., & Post, L. F. (2008). Healthcare decision making. In E. Capezuti, D. Zwicker, M. Mezey, and T. Fulmer (Eds.), *Evidence-based geriatric nursing protocols for best practice* (3rd ed., pp. 521–528). New York: Springer Publishing Company.

Montgomery, J., & Mitty, E. (2008). Resident condition change: Should I call 911? *Geriatric Nursing, 29*(1), 15–26.

Rodiek, S. (2008). A new tool for evaluating senior living environments. *Senior Housing and Care Journal, 16*(1), 3–9.

Wallace, M., & Fulmer, T. (2007). *Fulmer SPICES: An overall assessment tool for older adults.* New York: The Hartford Institute for Geriatric Nursing.

15

Cultural Aspects of Care

Reva N. Adler

There is no gold standard definition of *cultural competence* (or cultural sensitivity). Most definitions describe health care provider behavior and organizational policies and processes to facilitate mutually dignified and productive interactions between patient and provider (and arguably, among staff). Cultural competence is a respectful approach grounded in ethical principles. It draws on personal attitude and awareness of one's own biases, knowledge, and behavior. It is not a stand-alone communication method nor is it a kind of political correctness but, rather, is an approach that recognizes the significant influence that culture plays in life, health, *and* in seeking health care. It should not be assumed that an individual's cultural background will dictate his or her health choices or behavior. Be sensitive about stereotyping a person simply on the basis of his or her ethnic or cultural (or religious) affiliation. Conversely, it is important to be alert to the notion of *ethnocentrism*, the belief or attitude that one's own culture or cultural view is the best or most correct one. *Race* is a social construct based on physical appearance and parentage; many anthropologists feel that it is an inaccurate differentiation given the widespread genetic diversity among many populations. However, federal government documents and processes, such as the U.S. Census, continue to require this identification.

A doorway thought is what enters the mind, shapes questions, and frames understanding or appreciation of an individual and/or an event. Awareness of this unique, person-specific cognitive process can reduce the possibility of a resident's misunderstanding of health care advice and information, unwillingness to adhere to a medical regimen, and, most importantly, mistrust of a health care professional and system. Sensitivity to cultural mores includes the following:

- Preferred form(s) of address and correct pronunciation of the resident's name
- Disclosure norms (e.g., whether or not the resident is to be told his or her diagnosis)
- Food preferences
- Nonverbal communication (e.g., eye contact; touching; physical space between parties)
- History of traumatic experiences (e.g., warfare, sexual abuse, genocide, etc.)
- Extent of acculturation (e.g., language preference; adoption of the majority culture's common attitudes and values; gradual loss of separate ethnic identification)
- Preferred language when talking about health issues, parts of the body, and bodily functions, even if proficient in English
- Consent norms (i.e., locus of decision making; who participates in the decision and who does not)
- Health beliefs and traditional ways of healing (fear of medications and/or of hospitals, beliefs about cause of illness; healers; alternative therapies)
- Gender issues (influence on decision-making roles, truth telling, consent)
- Culture-specific health risks

■ End-of-life decision making, demand for life-sustaining treatments, advance care planning (advance directives), palliative care, willingness to use hospice services
■ Home care preferences
■ Desired location of death (hospital, at home, hospice, etc.)

Truth telling with regard to diagnosis and prognosis is forbidden or constrained in many cultures; it may be that only certain individuals can be told (e.g., male spouse, religious leader). In some cultures, truth telling is believed to cause harm—if you say it, it will happen—or cause suffering to the patient, thereby violating the ethical principle of nonmaleficence or do no harm. Just this aspect alone, absent knowing anything at all about the cultural beliefs of the older adult, can cause irreparable damage to the relationship between health care provider and patient/resident.

PREFERRED TERMS FOR CULTURE-SENSITIVE COMMUNICATION

It is important to learn, at the outset, the older adult's preferred term for his or her *identity* and use it consistently, including in written documents. Attitudes regarding the degree of formality differ widely among cultural groups and can differ, also, with socioeconomic status. Initially, a more formal approach is likely to be appropriate.

Try to learn, as well, how the person prefers to address the provider (physician, nurse, personal care assistant, etc.). In some cultures, the physician is an authority figure; communicating on a *first-person basis* might undermine a trusting relationship. Accept the person's preferred terms and forms of address; this is not negotiable.

Body position and motion is interpreted differently between and even within cultural groups. Vigorous handshakes, a loud and hearty voice, hand and facial gestures (or grimacing), or, on the other hand, an impassive facial expression, avoidance of eye contact, or standing at a distance might be insensitive (or frightening). Ask the resident or family about appropriate body language and distance between parties. Be cautious about attributing negative (or positive) meaning to gestures, facial expressions, or body language. In India, shaking one's head from side to side means "yes"; shaking one's head up and down means "no."

History tells us that health care providers have participated in torture, genocide, and death by lethal injec-

tion. The methods and tools employed (including human experimentation) can resemble legitimate clinical instruments and procedures. Survivors of such experiences might feel unsafe in a medical clinic; it can call up feelings of vulnerability, fear, panic, or anger.

ACCULTURATION AND NOTIONS OF HEALTH/ILLNESS

The degree to which a person has adapted (i.e., acculturated) to Western customs and attitudes is a result of many factors—not just of the number of years living in the United States. Level of acculturation can influence not only health behavior but also end-of-life planning and decision making. Non-Western cultural groups may not conceive of illness in Western terms. Some cultures have highly developed concepts of the causes of health, illness, and death that are vastly different or even incompatible with the concepts of Western medicine. Among non-Western beliefs are that illness has a spiritual causation or is the result of imbalance among bodily humors, or that it is caused by a person's actions in past lives, or is a retaliation for evildoing. Acculturation can divide family members, engendering shame or guilt in association with a decision made, particularly regarding life-sustaining treatments. Medical terms need to be carefully explained. Verify understanding: ask the person to tell you in his own words what he was told.

MEDICATION AND PAIN MANAGEMENT

Not surprisingly, every culture has beliefs about medications: amount, liquid or solid, route of administration, the obligation to share medications, and the positive additive effect of herbal and other nostrums. In some cases, when the person feels better, he or she either stops taking the medication or increases the amount taken to get better faster. If the medication is not working as quickly as expected or desired, ceasing to take the medication is also possible.

Varying among cultures, pain can have several meanings: punishment for past misdeeds, prelude to a spiritual awakening or the pathway to the next life, character building, readiness for a healing ceremony, or to be tolerated by the male (i.e., demonstration of machismo). *Suffering* is existential discomfort and, perhaps, should not to be treated by the same approach used to relieve the discomfort of physiological pain. In some cases, it may not benefit the sufferer to receive analgesics that mute feelings or awareness because that is precisely what she needs in order to express and work through her angst—and journey. Sit with the resident; ask her what her pain is like. How does it make her feel? Ask how you can help relieve her discomfort.

DEATH, DYING, AND DECISION MAKING

Some cultures (and religions) value life such that, in the face of death, residents and families will demand and expect vigorous life-sustaining interventions. This raises moral distress among clinicians, most often nurses: are we prolonging living or prolonging dying? Other cultures fear direct confrontation with death and dying and defer such decisions to the physician. Still, other cultures will take a direct approach to death and dying and reject aggressive life-sustaining interventions. The role of religion in decisions affecting treatments and interventions at the end of life can be significant.

Advance Directives

Written directives may be more common among older adults in North American and in Western cultures than among older adults in minority cultural groups, who might prefer a verbal directive—that is, discussion with the family. However, others want to avoid any such discussion because of their culture's prohibition about talking about (planning for) death. Whether written or verbal, individuals should be given the opportunity to talk about the interventions they want and do not want, even in the abstract (e.g., a discussion group at the assisted living community using case examples or drawing on literature and poetry).

RESOURCES

American Geriatrics Society. (2004). *Doorway thoughts* (vol. 1). Sudbury, MA: Jones & Bartlett.

American Geriatrics Society. (2006). *Doorway thoughts* (vol. 2). Sudbury, MA: Jones & Bartlett.

Curriculum in ethnogeriatrics. (2001). Retrieved November 23, 2003, from http://www.stanford.edu/group/ethnoger/

16

Psychosocial Aspects of Aging

Kenneth W. Hepburn and Ethel Mitty

Older adults face many stressful issues: dependency and care needs, losses and grief, change in role and social status, and lifestyle changes. This chapter discusses stress—its mediators and moderators, role change, and coping strategies (including locus of control theory and self-efficacy models)—with social involvement issues, from the notion of *successful aging* to civic engagement and creative aging.

A *stressor* is a demand that requires a physiological, behavioral, or emotional response. Sometimes, such demands are perceived as threats to well-being or existence; the ability to continue functioning effectively might become drastically reduced. Stressors can be persistent, such as those associated with chronic illness, or they can be acute, sudden, dramatic, unexpected—as might be associated with an acute health event (e.g., fracture; mammography finding) or with unexpected news of a friend's death. Stressors can be related to changes in role identity (e.g., retirement; relinquishing one's driver's license) or alterations in independent function, like the need for a supportive environment such as an assisted living community (ALC). Losses in physical capacity and reserve are stressors, especially when they are acute rather than insidious. Time can make a stressor less threatening; it becomes familiar. Risk factors are stressors, always (hovering) in the background, like those associated with recurrent/chronic illness. Some risk factors might be modifiable with teaching/health education, but others, such as those associated with gender and race, are not. The increased

presence of chronic illness as a person ages means that the number and frequency of stressors are likely to increase as a person ages.

Mediators frame and influence perception of the stress situation and the responses to it. They can filter, although not completely protect against, the impact of stress. Mediators are the external and internal resources that a person can use to evaluate the stress *and* his or her capacity to respond to it. Receiving information about, for example, osteoporosis, can mediate the impact of the diagnosis—the stressor. *Moderators* act on the stressor to lessen its intensity; they work with the mediator(s). Moderators are things that a person does, that probably existed even before the stressor appeared, and that are part of the individual's *coping mechanism*. For example, a resident who regularly exercised (e.g., robust walking) is likely to have a quicker return to full mobility after surgery than the person who had mostly sedentary habits pre-surgery. This highlights the need for a complete admission history.

Three major activities moderate stress: health-seeking behaviors, such as diet control or smoking cessation (i.e., healthy activities), spiritual or religious activity, and social engagement.

Losses and grief are companions of aging, whether associated with the loss of a loved one, diminished function (e.g., post-cerebral vascular accident), and/or sensory losses. Intense grief generally lasts 6 to 12 months and can be accompanied by social withdrawal and mild clinical depression. Acceptance generally occurs after

12 months and is characterized by reemergence into social activities (although there might be fewer of them in which the older adult is interested). Treatment for depression, whether pharmacological and/or counseling, can help avoid prolonged (pathological) grief.

Role shift is associated with retirement, change in social or family role, and, for many, loss of economic rewards. The average age of retirement is currently 62 years of age—at which point (reduced) Social Security payout can begin. At what age did many of your residents move into the ALC? Roles may change within a marriage where one partner is starting to experience functional (or cognitive) loss and the other partner now must become a caregiver. Moving to an ALC could be transformative for the spouse.

COPING STRATEGIES

Some AL residents need help seeing their stress situation clearly so that they can work toward improving or stabilizing their sense of control and well-being. Three useful theories in this regard are described in the following list.

- *Locus of control* (LoC), a psychological model based on *expectancy theory,* can help an individual recognize his beliefs about what he thinks is the cause of the good and bad things that have happened to him (e.g., health, business, etc.). *Internal* control means that the person feels that he is in control; *external* control means that the person believes that whatever happens to him is outside his control; it is fate and there is nothing he can do about it; other people or the environment determine what happens to him. Research indicates that internal LoC people are more able to cope with physical disability, in the long term, than are external LoC people. In contrast to internals, external LoC people tend to have less lofty goals, take fewer risks, and are unlikely to invest energy into self-improvement. Application of LoC principles in diabetes mellitus and obesity management is reportedly successful. Assessment findings regarding residents' beliefs about their control over their lives can be used for counseling and education to manage stress or a stress-inducing event.
- The *health belief model* (HBM), related to the LoC model, posits four beliefs that a person might have about her health status:
  (1) *Perceived threat:* belief that one is at high *risk* for getting/having the disease

  (2) *Perceived benefit:* belief about the *value* or benefit of having a diagnostic test or medical (nursing) intervention
  (3) *Perceived barriers:* belief that access is limited, that care is costly, or that one is ineligible
  (4) *Perceived self-efficacy:* belief that personal actions make a difference

  Showing an older adult woman that many women her age (and population) have had a bone density test can be reassuring as well as persuasive with regard to her engaging in healthy behaviors (e.g., medication, moderate exercise, diet).
- *Self-efficacy,* a social cognitive theory construct, is related to internal LoC and mastery, resilience, and competence. The theory holds that confidence in one's ability to do something can predict one's willingness to act in a certain way. Strong self-efficacy beliefs are related to overall function as well as physical and mental health. Self-efficacy can be weakened by continuous onslaughts and negative outcomes—and can be strengthened by targeted strategies. The components of self-efficacy theory have a good fit with ALC residents:
  ☐ *Skills mastery* (i.e., performance accomplishment): imagining or actually seeing oneself succeed in progressively difficult tasks (e.g., ambulation, weight loss)
  ☐ *Vicarious learning* (i.e., social modeling): observing or learning that others similar to one's self have been successful in a targeted area; use support groups or link one resident to another (i.e., buddies)
  ☐ *Encouragement* (i.e., persuasion): information (i.e., research data) can support confidence in the person's ability to be successful
  ☐ *Reinforcement:* experiencing anticipated or actual pleasure from success; hold achievement parties; create certificates of achievement

Social cognitive theory is the most effective model with regard to changing behavior among older adults. Interventions based on this theory decreased smoking, facilitated weight loss, improved memory, decreased fear of falling, and increased time spent in physical activity.

Using the resident's history of an effective response to stress, *selection, optimization,* and *compensation* are useful measures to assist the resident in moving forward with his life and are described in the following list.

- Selection: help the resident choose to do those things that the resident knows she does well. This could means honing down the type and number of activities in which the resident is engaged in order to maximize success in the (remaining or new) activities she chooses to engage in.

■ Optimization: reframe performance expectations; help the resident compare her performance with others of similar or older age—not what she could do 40 years ago. By engaging in selected activities, the resident gets optimal credit for performing to her own satisfaction and/or having gained the desired outcome.

■ Compensation: this deals with diminished performance and losses. The resident engages in simple activities that show her at her best.

Social involvement can be viewed as a proactive, problem-focused response to stress by virtue of strengthening connection to the internal and external community; it affirms the older adult's value. *Disengagement* is not a normal response to aging; severing ties and increasing isolation does not contribute to well-being. One of the tasks of old age is *integration*: bringing the pieces of the self together such that life at this point is celebratory and that learning and achievement are still possible. The notion of *involvement* (sometimes called productivity) means taking part, contributing (whether through volunteer or paid work), or participating in a meaningful activity. It is as applicable to older adults as to people in all stages of life, including adolescents— and there is no reason why ALC residents cannot be involved. Find out what is going on in the external community. Bridge club? Social dancing? Local politics?

Successful aging theory is based on studies that found that decline was not necessarily an irreversible component of normal aging. It is a multidimensional construct with physical, emotional, cognitive, and psychosocial aspects. Perceptions of successful aging include living a very long time, continuing to learn new things, feeling satisfied with life overall, having no regrets, having involved family and friends who care, not feeling lonely, remaining involved with the world and with people, having meaningful choices, acting according to one's own standards, and being able to cope with the challenges of aging. What an enlightening discussion this could be in the ALC!

Civic engagement includes volunteering, joining an organization to help with fund-raising, getting involved in electoral campaigns or issues, writing petitions and/ or boycotting, letter writing, and so on. It appears to promote a feeling of belonging, meaningful contribution of experience and/or activities, ownership in the activity, and is recommended as a retirement role for *all* older adults. The Older Americans Act reauthorization of 2006 requires that the Administration on Aging develop and implement civic engagement opportunities for older adults. Living in an ALC does not preclude resident involvement; they may need to be informed about what is available, however.

Creative aging refers to the relationship between healthy aging and creative expression. The Society for Creative Aging holds that creativity is a basic need and that all people are naturally creative; that, regardless of background (e.g., education, culture, etc.), all older adults have wisdom that can stimulate the creative process; and that, using memory and life review methods, creativity can be expressed through various art forms. Older adults, like people of all ages, can experience creativity as a participant or as an observer.

Aging well and sustaining well-being requires mental and physical exercise, challenging leisure activities, sense of mastery, and social connections (for many, but not all, older adults). Even for those suffering with dementia, there are opportunities for creative expression and meaningfulness. Adaptation of Montessori's learning principles have been used for effective engagement by persons with moderate-to-severe dementia. Storytelling workshops have elicited robust conversations with dementia sufferers. The Museum of Modern Art in New York City established the nation's first museum visiting program for people with dementia and created a guide and toolkit.

RESOURCES

Kaskie, B., Imhof, S., Cavanaugh, J., & Culp, K. (2008). Civic engagement as a retirement role for aging Americans. *The Gerontologist, 48*(3), 368–377.

Love, K. (n.d.). *A guide for using therapeutic engagement to enhance function for individuals with dementia*. Washington, DC: Office on Aging.

Meet me at the MOMA. (n.d.). Retrieved April 25, 2009, from http://www.moma.org/education/alzheimers.html

National Center for Creative Aging. (YEAR). *Title*. Retrieved MONTH DAY, YEAR, from http://www.creativeaging.org

Rowe, J. W., & Kahn, R. L. (1998). Successful aging. *Gerontologist, 37*(4), 433–440.

Society for Creative Aging. (YEAR). *Title*. Retrieved MONTH DAY, YEAR, from http://www.s4ca.org

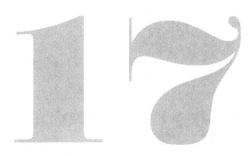

The Continuum of Care

Ethel Mitty and Barbara Resnick

A continuum of care for older adults involves the following: matching their care and service needs with the *least restrictive setting of care* and resources in order to achieve desired health benefit outcomes. Residential care options can be an older adult living in a community-based residence and receiving home care, a continuing care retirement community (CCRC), or an assisted living community (ALC) where most residents *intend* to reside until their death. Nursing homes (NHs) and hospice are not generally considered residential but are instead treatment options. This chapter describes CCRCs, home (health) care, NH care, and hospice services and eligibility, including dying in an ALC. The notion of so-called *slow medicine* nursing style is discussed, as is the need for honest discussion with residents (and their families) regarding their goals of care and advance care planning. The chapter also discusses what is known as *handing off* or transitions between health care settings.

In any one calendar year, an older adult could be in acute care, an NH, an ALC, or his own community-based residence receiving formal or informal home care services. Given these transitions, an AL nurse should be aware of what is available in each care setting in order to provide accurate information to AL residents and/or their families who are contemplating relocating to or from an ALC.

HOME (HEALTH) CARE

The purpose of home health care is to promote, maintain, or restore health and/or functionality by maximiz-

ing independence and minimizing the effects of illness and disability (including terminal illness) on individuals and their families. In 2007, slightly over 7.5 million people received home care services from 83,000 providers. A home care organization can be Medicare certified, providing acute care services as well as end-of-life care (via a hospice agency), or it can be an organization providing domiciliary/nonmedical/custodial care. Home care can be paid for by a managed care organization (including a health maintenance organization or HMO), Medicaid, the Older Americans Act, the Veterans Administration, and private insurance. Of those receiving home care, almost 70% are over 65 years of age and female. The difference between home care and home health services is that the latter is more medically oriented and almost always includes licensed health care professionals who implement and monitor a plan of care; most of these individuals work for licensed home health agencies, hospitals, or health departments. Therapeutic services can include enterostomal and IV therapy, rehab therapies (physical therapy [PT], occupational therapy [OT], speech therapy [ST]) and dietary or nutritional therapy. Psychological and counseling services can also be provided. Home health care services may include some home care (i.e., homemaking) services that typically includes housecleaning and other services, including meal preparation, shopping, and so forth.

Medicare home health care regulations no longer require that the recipient of care is home bound; however, the patient must require medically necessary and reasonable skilled nursing and/or skilled rehab at least intermittently. A physician has to order the home health care services and provide a written plan of care. An ALC resident who is a Medicare beneficiary could receive skilled home care services at the AL residence.

CONTINUING CARE RETIREMENT COMMUNITY

CCRCs range from independent living/housing (in a cottage), to assistance with personal care (such as in AL), to skilled or custodial NH care. Whereas CCRCs originally offered life-care contracts that offered a continuum of care and services to meet the older adult's needs as he or she became more dependent or disabled, this is no longer the case. The scant data that is available suggests that a CCRC resident might transition to a NH or ALC for a short time and then return back to his cottage/apartment once his condition has stabilized. For a growing number of residents, however, AL is the last stop on the continuum; this is especially relevant given that many ALCs bring hospice services into the facility. Given the age at which older adults are coming to a CCRC and the fact that many of the current residents are aging in place, there appears to be a demand in some CCRCs for AL-type services to be brought to the cottage or independent-living apartment.

A variety of payment and service options offer different combinations of access to and provision of supportive, health-related (i.e., AL), and skilled nursing services (i.e., NH) in CCRCs. Medicaid does not reimburse CCRCs or individuals who choose to live in them; it is primarily a private pay arrangement. However, many CCRCs will cross-subsidize residents who have spent down their private funds over time, usually because of deteriorating health status and increasing personal and health care needs.

NURSING HOMES

NHs are federally certified as Medicare skilled nursing facilities (SNFs) and/or as a Medicaid nursing facilities (NFs) or are not federally certified but are licensed by the state. NH resident acuity has increased since the 1990s: many NHs are providing care and services previously only provided in acute care. Most NHs are under 100 beds. Slightly over 67% are for-profit (FP); 27% are not-for-profit (NFP); the remainder are government facilities. In 2007, there were approximately 16,100 nursing homes with almost 1,730,000 Medicare and/

or Medicaid-certified beds occupied by 1,492,000 residents. Despite the rise in the number/percent of the aging population, NHs are reporting vacancies (the 2008 average occupancy rate was 87%) attributed, in part, to the option for formal home care services or to AL. The average length of stay (LOS) is 892 days. However, the average LOS of discharged Medicare-reimbursed residents is 62 days (typically, those admitted for short-term rehab).

Almost two-thirds of NH residents are dual eligible (Medicare and Medicaid beneficiaries). Medicaid is the primary payer for almost 60% of residents; private pay accounts for almost 40%; private insurance accounts for 3%–4%. An NH resident admitted from acute care is likely to be Medicare covered but only for a maximum of 100 days of skilled nursing or skilled rehab.

Just under 6% of the elderly cohort in the United States are in a NH on any given day; 46% are admitted from acute care. Risk factors for NH admission are advanced age, medical diagnosis, living alone, loss of self-care ability, decreased mental status, bed immobility, lack of informal support/caregivers, poverty, hospital admission, and female gender. The fact that NHs cannot admit those who are mentally ill, developmentally disabled, or retarded (without clear evidence that therapeutic services are available—and provided by the NH) might be an opportunity for ALCs to provide these necessary services.

NHs must provide care and services to meet the overall goals of *resident-centered* (or *directed*) care to maintain or improve physical and mental function, reduce or eliminate pain and discomfort, offer a meaningful leisure/recreational program, provide a safe environment, reduce (re)hospitalization, and assure a dignified death. They must also provide dental care, podiatric care, medical specialty consultation, social services, mental health services, and nutrition services. Some NHs have fully equipped clinical laboratories, dental and podiatric suites, radiology equipment, and an on-site pharmacy. All NHs provide care at the end of life—some by formal arrangement with a hospice agency, others by virtue of internal policy and practices. Although all NHs must have a full- or part-time medical director, the physician does not have to be a certified geriatrician; this varies by state. Every resident has a physician of record who is responsible for the plan of care. The physician can be among a panel of physicians caring for the NH residents or an independent outside practitioner. Virtually all NHs provide skilled rehabilitation (OT, PT, ST), but the availability of these services can vary with regard to whether or not the facility is Medicare certified to provide post-acute care.

About 20% of all NHs have a designated *special care unit* (SCU) (approximately 7% of all NH beds). The most common SCUs are dedicated Alzheimer's and related dementias units (5.5% of all beds); only 1% of beds are for skilled rehab. The philosophy and operational principles of SCUs include specific admission, retention, and discharge criteria, specially trained staff, special programs, a distinct space, and program evaluation. There are fewer AIDS and hospice SCU beds in comparison to ventilator-dependent SCU beds. Some NHs might be caring for hospice residents on a regular unit rather than relocating them to a special hospice SCU with unfamiliar staff and routines. The data remain unclear if residents with dementia decline more slowly on a dementia SCU in comparison to a traditional (mixed) unit.

Most NH residents are White; 12% are Black. Among all residents, most are female. Slightly under 50% of all residents are age 85 or older; 12% are under 65 years old. The most common admission diagnoses are hypertension, post-cerebral vascular accident, heart disease, and dementia (see Table 17.1).

The percent of residents receiving a psychoactive medication of some kind (e.g., anxiolytic, antidepressant, antipsychotic) increased from 48.5% in 1998 to 63% in 2004 and is attributed, in part, to better recognition and treatment of depression, sleep disorders, and so forth. Approximately 75% of residents have short- and long-term memory loss, are not oriented to place or season, nor are they able to recognize staff. One-third of cognitively impaired residents have inappropriate or aggressive behavior. Wandering, defined as moving about with no obvious goal or rational purpose and oblivious to safety needs, is a major care (and risk management) issue. Only 7% of NH residents currently need a physical restraint; in some NHs, there is zero tolerance for restraint use.

Some NH residents can be hospitalized as many as four times in 1 year (i.e., the ping-pong phenomenon). Among the many factors—some clinical, some economic—that influence a hospitalization decision are the receiving hospital's vacancy rate and physician practice pattern in the NH, family pressure, staffing contingencies (especially on the weekend), NH resources (e.g., diagnostic services, IV therapy), advanced age, significant activities of daily living (ADL) dependency, chronic obstructive pulmonary disease (COPD), genitourinary or respiratory track infections, congestive heart failure (CHF), and payment source. Having a do-not-hospitalize (DNH) order does not preclude the possibility of hospital admission. Some data indicate a relationship between low NH Medicaid reimbursement rate and the greater likelihood of hospital transfer.

17.1 | Nursing Home Resident Characteristics

ITEM	%
Hearing impaired	21%
Visually impaired	27%
Difficulty understanding or being understood	44–60%
Activities of daily living (ADL) assistance needed	95%
Need help with ≥ three ADLs	75%
Use a walker	25%
Wheelchair dependent	62%
Transfer assistance needed in/out of bed	29%
Bathing assistance needed	94%
Eating assistance needed	47%
Dressing assistance needed	87%
Bowel and bladder incontinent	50%
Dementia: moderate/severe	65%
Clinically depressed[a]	21%
Hospitalized annually	25–50%
Advance directive written	65%
Have a do-not-hospitalize order	4–6%
Expire in the NH	66%

[a]Many clinicians feel that the percent of clinically depressed NH residents is closer to 50% or more.

Staffing is predominantly nursing: registered nurse (RN), licensed practical nurse/licensed vocational nurse (LPN/LVN), and certified nurse assistant (CNA). In many NHs, but by no means all, the CNAs have a consistent assignment. Workload is based on resident acuity, weekday versus weekend, shift, and budget. Typical day shift staffing for a CNA can range from 7 to 10 residents; staffing is reduced on the eve and night shift. An RN must be on duty at least 8 consecutive hours a day; licensed personnel (i.e., LPN/LVN) must be on duty 24/7. An NH can be waivered from meeting the RN requirement if the facility shows that it is unable to do so because of local shortages *and* that resident health and safety are not in jeopardy if there is no RN on the premises. Total nursing care hours per day (NCHPD) vary but typically hover around 3.7 hours per resident (i.e., RN: 0.6 hours; LPN/LVN: 0.7 hours; CNA: 2.3 hours). An Institute of Medicine evaluation of the relationship between quality outcomes and staffing recommended 273 minutes or 4.55 hours of nursing care hours per resident day. Some NHs may be at or near this level, but it can differ between units as well as between residents (i.e., some having more hours of care, some fewer).

Fewer than 5% of NHs have an *advanced practice nurse* (APN) (i.e., clinical nurse specialist [CNS]; gerontological nurse practitioner [GNP], adult nurse practitioner [ANP]) on staff or in collaborative practice with a physician. However, the data are clear that APNs make a significant difference with regard to fewer hospitalizations, less use of indwelling catheters, pressure ulcer prevention and treatment, mobility, incontinence, restorative nursing, mental health, and so forth.

All NHs have an *interdisciplinary team* with joint accountability for the plan of care and outcomes. The team typically consists of the primary nurse and CNA, social worker, nutritionist, rehab therapist, activities therapist, and physician. The resident and family are invited to the resident's quarterly team meeting; it can be more often if the resident's status change warrants.

Regulatory oversight and quality of care monitoring were firmly established with passage of the Omnibus Budget Reconciliation Act of 1987 (OBRA, 1987), also known as the Nursing Home Reform Law. Provisions of this monumental act included resident rights, an interdisciplinary team care planning approach, staffing minimums, creation of a uniform resident assessment instrument (RAI) and a minimum data set (MDS) instrument for comprehensive care planning and data collection, nurse assistant training and certification, justification for use of physical restraints, and a revised quality of care survey that was resident-centered. Every NH has an unannounced survey every 9–15 months that is conducted by the state's health department acting as agents for the federal government (i.e., Center for Medicare and Medicaid Services [CMS]) and state requirements for ongoing NH certification or licensure. In addition, the state surveyors can be accompanied by federal Medicare surveyors conducting a so-called look-behind survey.

The CMS Web site *NHCompare* draws data from the MDS and the Online Survey, Certification and Reporting (OSCAR) databases to provide information on *every* NH in the United States regarding the NH's ownership, bed size, resident characteristics, survey and deficiency information, staffing, and Medicare and Medicaid program participation. The data are NH-specific and can be viewed in comparison with other NHs in the state and nationwide. In addition, data are presented, by NH, with regard to long- and short-term resident quality measures that include pain management, pressure ulcers, use of restraints, and delirium. Deficiencies are classified by *scope* (i.e., number of residents actually or potentially affected) and *severity* (degree or potential for actual harm). All NHs must have an ongoing quality assurance/improvement (QA/QI) plan. The data indicate that pain management has significantly improved in NHs. Review and accreditation by the Joint Commission is not required except for those NHs seeking managed care contracts and/or those that are hospital affiliated.

It is estimated that 46% of older adults will spend some time in a NH. Technological inroads in NHs include electronic charting (especially medication administration), alarm systems, and rehabilitation. Emerging best practices in NHs include mentoring programs (especially for nursing directors), staff empowerment models that facilitate decision making at the bedside, a homelike environment, and meaningful resident choices regarding their preferred lifestyle, such as awakening and bath time, food choices, and engaging in dignified recreational/leisure activities (i.e., the culture change movement).

HOSPICE

Hospice care is compassionate care for a person facing a life-limiting illness or injury and for his or her family/significant others. Provided by an interdisciplinary team that consists of nurses, therapists, physicians, spiritual counselors, home health aides, social workers, volunteers, and bereavement counselors, the principled belief of hospice care is that all people have the right to die with dignity and without pain. The team manages the patient's pain and symptoms, provides needed drugs and medical supplies, helps the patient cope emotionally and psychosocially, delivers special services if needed for symptom relief (e.g., physical therapy), can arrange for inpatient care to improve pain and symptom management, and offers bereavement counseling to family and friends. Signing on to a hospice program and receiving its benefits requires waiver of Medicare benefits, but it does not preclude hospitalization to ameliorate symptoms or manage an incident condition that is causing pain or discomfort (e.g., pathological fracture).

Persons suffering with end-stage dementia are eligible for hospice; it is not limited to those with terminal cancer or other end-stage illness. Studies indicate that an individual with dementia who has progressed to Stage 7c on the Functional Assessment Staging Scale (FAST) is likely to die within 6 months. Stage 7 of the FAST scale is the inability to walk, speak a few or even a single word, smile, hold the head up, or sit; the person is asleep most of the day. Concomitant MDS criteria—significant ADL dependency, bed-bound status, bowel incontinence, co-morbidities (specifically cancer, congestive heart failure, dyspnea), medical instability, weight loss, urinary tract infection, male gender, and age 83 years or older—are prognostic of a life span of 6 months or less.

Just over 5% of ALC residents received hospice care in 2007, a slight increase from 2006. The Alzheimer's Association prepared an evidence-based document, based on interviews with family members of dying nursing home and AL residents, that addresses quality of care at the end of life for residents with dementia. Guidelines for care address communication and decision making with the resident's family about the goals of care, the likely course of the illness and the resident's decline, and the advantages and disadvantages of different interventions. Recommendations regarding symptom management, albeit complicated by the resident's inability to communicate, speak to the need for skilled assessment and monitoring, and recognition that the resident's behavior, even if dying, might be communicating a need.

Families of residents dying in an ALC, while satisfied overall with the care, express concerns similar to those expressed in other settings: that staff do not seem knowledgeable about symptom management and fail to adequately monitor the resident. According to family informants of the decedents, dying ALC residents were in pain and had dry mouths. Interestingly, some of the other reported care inadequacies were that the dying resident was drowsy, had no appetite, and lacked energy—all of which might be what dying *is*, and not a reflection of poor care.

SLOW MEDICINE VERSUS HOSPICE CARE

The notion of slow medicine suggests that some interventions (including invasive diagnostic tests) may have risks that outweigh the benefits. If having a breast biopsy, even if positive, will not lead to a lumpectomy, mastectomy, or a curative intervention, what is the value of the exam? Academic curiosity? Source of metastases? The goal of care and standard of practice should be pain and comfort management—and respecting a patient's preferences. It is critical to be mindful when talking with residents and families that medical and nursing interventions are not withdrawn; rather, they are optimized for the specific clinical conditions and the mutually agreed-to goals of care. As such, health care providers are encouraged to put on the brakes and talk with the patients (family, proxy) about the goals of care—and where they can be met best. Hospital transfer may not be the best thing for the resident. Treatment options, including comfort measures and their consequences, should be discussed.

A resident with an advance directive that addresses wanted and unwanted treatments, including CPR, should be reviewed in a timely way after an acute event or significant change of condition. The resident (and/or family, agent) with COPD or CHF, needs information about the disease's natural history or *trajectory*. With each exacerbation, the decision about whether or not to hospitalize might be made more thoughtfully, given the questionable benefits of hospitalization and the likely adverse effect on the resident (e.g., pressure ulcer, weight loss, disorientation). In some cases, and for a defined set of circumstances, a DNH order might be written. But you should verify whether this is permitted in AL in your state.

In almost all cases, it is an AL nurse who is making the decision to transfer a resident to the hospital. While some cases have a very small therapeutic window (e.g., first occurrence of chest pain)—many situations can afford *slow medicine nursing style*. The nurse's critical role in these cases is to present information to the resident (and family) for their consideration regarding likely tests, interventions, and outcomes of hospitalization. The conversation includes reassurance that slow medicine (like palliative care/medicine) does not mean abandonment; treatment and care continue. In a gentle way, the nurse tries to differentiate between prolonging living and prolonging dying. The principles and actions of palliative care are explained: person-centered goals of care; symptom management and aggressive comfort care; interdisciplinary attention to care needs; and a plan of care.

TRANSITIONS BETWEEN HEALTH CARE SETTINGS: HANDING OFF

Transitions occur at the interfaces of care, that is, between geographically separate settings or in one setting (e.g., discharged from a neurology unit and admitted to a rehab unit in the same hospital), between levels of care, or between practitioners. Transitional care involves a sender and a receiver. The notion of transition has replaced the transfer process and entails a broader appreciation of what is involved in moving between sites of care, providers, and the goals of care. Most transfer/transitional problems occur because of poor communication and lack of coordination, resulting in the loss of continuity of clinical and supportive management and monitoring. The American Geriatrics Society (AGS) position statement, *Improving the Quality of Transitional Care for Persons With Complex Care Needs* (AGS Health Care Systems Committee, 2002), addresses the need for clinicians—and the patient and family—to be completely aware of the treatment and medication plan of care, the patient's treatment preferences, the potential for high-risk events, and the need for patient and family education.

Medication reconciliation, a necessary component of transitional care, consists of five steps.

(1) List the medications that the patient was on prior to admission
(2) List the medications that are to be ordered or prescribed
(3) Compare the two lists
(4) Decide which medication is most appropriate
(5) Communicate the decision to the relevant health care professional(s) *and* to the resident and family

As a practical matter (in case of future events), what is the resident going to do with those no longer necessary medications now sitting on her kitchen table? If the patient educator told her that the new medication was for hypertension, then why can't the old medication prescribed for hypertension (by a doctor she trusted) still be used? On return to the ALC, this has to

be discussed with the resident who was self-medicating prior to hospitalization and retains the stash of formerly used medications. Medication reconciliation is not just a clinical exercise; it has significant economic ramifications for many residents that can, in turn, affect clinical outcomes.

The most common errors in transitioning between care settings are wrong dose (of the same medication that the patient/resident used to take), followed by errors of omission (i.e., failure to prescribe) and commission (i.e., administering the same med twice because of failure to communicate or document that it was given prior to transfer/relocation). Medication reconciliation should occur within 24 hours, sooner for high-risk medications (e.g., Coumadin, insulin), and should be conducted by a knowledgeable practitioner with appropriate resources at hand, including pharmacist assistance, as needed. *Blanket orders* such as "resume pre-op orders" are not permitted by the Joint Commission medication standards of care; they are an obvious source of medication errors. The Institute for Healthcare Improvement (IHI) Web site has a downloadable medication reconciliation review and flow sheet (IHI, n.d.).

RESOURCES

American Geriatrics Society Health Care Systems Committee. (2002). *Improving the quality of transitional care for persons with complex care needs*. Retrieved December 1, 2008, from http://www.americangeriatrics.org/products/positionpapers/complex_care.shtml

Institute for Healthcare Improvement. (n.d.). *Medication reconciliation flowsheet*. Retrieved April 26, 2009, from http://www.ihi.org/IHI/Topics/PatientSafety/MedicationSystems/Tools/Medication + Reconciliation + Flowsheet.htm

National Hospice and Palliative Care Organization. (2008). *Facts and figures. Hospice care in America*. Retrieved November 1, 2008, from http://www.nhpco.org/files/public/Statistics_Research/NHPCO_facts-and-figures_2008.pdf

Resnick, B. (2008). "Slow medicine" nursing style [Editorial]. *Geriatric Nursing, 29*(6), 367–368.

Tilly, J., & Fok, A. (2007). *Quality end-of-life care for individuals with dementia in assisted living and nursing homes and public policy barriers to delivering this care*. Retrieved December 1, 2008, from http://www.alz.org/national/documents/End_interviewpaper_III.pdf

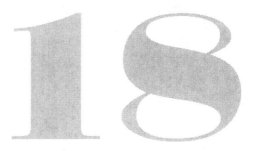

Physical Activity

David M. Buchner
and Barbara Resnick

Physical activity is defined as bodily movement produced by skeletal muscles that expend energy. Exercise is a subset of physical activity that involves a structured program designed to improve one or more components of physical fitness or optimal functional ability. The primary attributes of physical activity are type (mode), frequency, duration, and intensity. Physical activity is one of the most important and effective preventive and therapeutic interventions for older adults. There is conclusive evidence that regular aerobic activity has major health benefits. Resistance training (e.g., weight lifting) and balance training also have important health benefits in older adults. Flexibility training is important for maintaining the range of motion required to do physical activities.

PREVENTIVE HEALTH EFFECTS

Regular physical activity has a beneficial effect on most, if not all, organ systems. Consequently, it prevents a large number of illnesses/diseases. Physical activity reduces the risk and progression of cardiovascular disease, hypertension, cerebral vascular accident, some lipid disorders, non-insulin-dependent diabetes mellitus, obesity, osteoporosis, colon cancer, and breast cancer. There is substantial evidence that physical activity reduces the risk of fall injuries, sarcopenia, depression, and anxiety disorders and some evidence that it reduces sleep problems, cognitive impairment, osteoarthritis, and back pain. The Centers for Disease Control (CDC) reported, in 2008, that physical activities for community-residing older adults reduced the development of two major chronic diseases: hypertension and type 2 diabetes.

Consistent with its broad physiologic effects, regular physical activity decreases both cardiovascular and noncardiovascular mortality in older adults. Observational studies consistently report that regular physical activity substantially delays the onset of functional limitations and loss of independence (disability). Higher levels of physical activity, such as jogging, are associated with fewer years of disability preceding death. The health benefits of physical activity accrue independently of other risk factors. For example, sedentary overweight smokers experience health benefits from increasing physical activity, even if they continue to smoke and do not lose weight.

THERAPEUTIC EFFECTS IN CHRONIC DISEASE MANAGEMENT

Physical activity has therapeutic benefits in the management of a wide variety of chronic conditions. Clinical practice guidelines (prepared by groups such as the American Geriatrics Society and the American Medical Directors Association) identify a role for physical activity in the management of dementia, pain management, heart failure, syncope, reflex sympathetic dystrophy, prophylaxis of venous thromboembolism, back pain, some sleep disorders, and constipation.

It is possible that physical activity will assume a prominent role in the management of mental health conditions in older adults. There is substantial evidence that both aerobic activity and resistance training reduce/modify symptoms of depression. Physical activity should be considered as an adjunct to medication and psychotherapy for older adults with depressive illness, pending more studies clarifying which patients can be prescribed activity as a substitute for medication and psychotherapy. Cognitive ability is positively correlated with higher levels of physical activity and fitness.

The therapeutic use of exercise to reverse low fitness, physical functional limitations, and disability has been carefully studied since the 1990s. Randomized trials of exercise in sedentary older adults show that *aerobic capacity* (defined as the highest amount of oxygen consumed during maximal exercise in activities that use the large muscle groups in the legs or arms), muscle strength, flexibility, and balance can be improved by appropriate forms of exercise.

RECOMMENDED AMOUNTS OF PHYSICAL ACTIVITY

The American College of Sports Medicine and the American Heart Association recommend that all older adults engage in moderately intense aerobic exercise 30 minutes a day, 5 days a week, or that they do vigorously intense aerobic exercise 20 minutes a day, 3 days a week. In addition, it is recommended that older adults do 8 to 10 different strength-training exercises, doing 10–15 repetitions of each of these exercises two to three times per week. Balance exercises are recommended for those at risk of falling. Moderate-intensity aerobic exercise is the most realistic level of activity for the majority of older adults.

Aerobic Activity

Aerobic activity is activity that uses the larger muscle groups over an extended time period where the energy is supplied by the oxygen-utilizing process. Sample activities include walking, jogging, or biking. Physical activity intensity is often expressed in metabolic equivalents (MET) units. Moderate-intensity physical activity is defined as aerobic activities that expend 3.0 to 6.0 METs. One MET is the amount of energy expended sitting quietly at rest adjusted to body weight (1 MET = 3.5 ml oxygen consumed/kg of body weight/minute). This level of activity is a 6 on an intensity scale of 1 to 10; one should still be able to carry on a conversation during exercise. The standard example of a moderate-intensity activity

is brisk walking at 3 to 4 miles per hour. Activity bouts of at least 10-minute duration count toward meeting the requirements of 30 minutes of exercise per day. Further daily physical activity can be accrued during usual activity for residents such as walking to the mailbox, dining room, or a friend's apartment.

The benefits of aerobic activity on cardiovascular health are based on the finding that aerobic activity increases the body's oxygen demand as measured by ventilatory oxygen uptake (Vo_2). A 1-liter increase in Vo_2 produces an approximate 6-liter increase in cardiac output. With regular exercise, there is an increase in $Vo_{2\,max}$ ($Vo_{2\,max}$ is the maximum amount of oxygen in milliliters that one can use in 1 minute per kilogram of body weight). As the $Vo_{2\,max}$ improves, any submaximal physical task (e.g., walking to the bathroom) requires the use of a smaller percent of $Vo_{2\,max}$ and therefore places less stress on the heart muscle.

Resistance Training

Resistance training means increasing muscle strength by moving or lifting some type of resistance, such as weights or elastic bands, at a level that requires some physical effort. Examples of resistance exercise programs can be found in the Exercise Assessment and Screening for You (EASY) tool. The amount of resistance recommended and number of repetitions vary for each individual and muscle group. In general, one to three sets of 10 to 12 repetitions are regarded as optimal for increasing muscle strength. Resistance exercises, or strength training, should not be performed on consecutive days in order to give the muscles time to recover between sessions.

Flexibility Training

Unlike aerobic activities and resistance training, flexibility training by itself does not have substantial health benefits. It is recommended because regular physical activity requires an adequate range of motion, and flexibility training permits and facilitates the types of physical activity that have health benefits. Flexibility-related activity facilitates greater range of motion around the joints. Flexibility training is recommended at least twice weekly.

Balance Training

Balance is the ability to maintain control of the body over the base of support (i.e., the area of the body where most of the weight is supported) in order to avoid falling. Static balance is the ability to maintain balance without moving, while dynamic balance is the ability to move without losing balance or falling. Unlike aerobic exercise, or resistance and flexibility training, balance training is not recommended for all adults. At the present time, balance training is recommended only for adults at increased risk of falls. These exercises should be performed a minimum of 2 days a week. Some balance exercise programs focus on maintaining balance over a narrow base of support, such as a tandem stand (standing heel to toe) or one-leg stand. Other exercises train dynamic balance, such as the ability to do a tandem walk (walking heel to toe). Balance training is typically designed so that exercises are graduated in difficulty, and older adults progress to more difficult exercises as training improves balance. For example, a tandem walk is easiest when holding on to a table and becomes progressively more difficult/challenging/scary with arms in any position, arms close to the body, and arms close to the body while holding a weight.

Tai Chi Chuan is often mentioned as a form of exercise that improves balance and prevents falls. Early studies of Tai Chi reported an almost 50% reduction in falls; a follow-up study reported a (nonsignificant) 25% reduction. Reasonably, Tai Chi remains a promising intervention that is popular, fun, and social and is appropriate for the balance training component of a falls prevention program.

RECOMMENDING PHYSICAL ACTIVITY TO OLDER ADULTS

The EASY tool can be used to guide older adults and nurses as to what exercise is safe and appropriate for the individual to perform. Examples of aerobic, resistance, flexibility, and balance exercises are available in the EASY screening tool. Nonambulatory residents can likewise engage in physical activity. In fact, these individuals are most likely to benefit the most from an exercise program. Muscle weakness and atrophy are probably the most functionally relevant and reversible problems in nonambulatory older adults, and attempting to reverse these deficits through exercise can have a major impact on function and quality of life.

Preference for Moderate Intensity Aerobic Activity

The vast majority of sedentary and insufficiently active older adults should gradually increase their moderate aerobic activity, especially walking, in order to achieve moderate intensity exercise. Moderate exercise is as-sociated with lower cardiovascular risk, lower risk of musculoskeletal injury, and in comparison with vigorous exercise, generates/motivates higher adherence to training. Most older adults prefer moderate intensity activities: 30 to 60 minutes of moderate activity, 5 to 7 days per week, is appropriate for most older adults.

The traditional emphasis on walking is appropriate and is the most common physical activity reported by older adults. The obvious advantages of walking are that it requires no special skills, equipment, or facilities and the risk of injury is relatively low. Greater amounts of walking are not associated with higher injury risk.

Importance of Resistance Training

Age-related decreases in skeletal muscle mass and quality, termed *sarcopenia,* contribute to functional limitations and dependence in older adults. Sarcopenia is more than just disuse atrophy; even highly trained athletes lose muscle mass with age. Epidemiologic studies report that regular physical activity reduces age-related loss of muscle mass. Randomized controlled trials demonstrate that resistance training increases muscle mass and counteracts sarcopenia. Whereas early studies of resistance training prescribed vigorous training similar to that prescribed for young adults, it has subsequently been demonstrated that less training has both physiologic effects on muscle function and on health benefits. Gains in strength are typically reported for those who use weight machines. For older adults with good fitness, weight machines are usually the most feasible and safest training method. Randomized trails have also tested resistance-training programs that use body weight or free weights, such as weight cuffs or dumbbells. These programs are more appropriate for adults with lower fitness levels, where lower amounts of weight will be sufficient for the individual to achieve some gains in strength and function. In theory, resistance exercises in a home-based program can be adjusted on the basis of the ability of the individual. He or she can start by doing the exercises with no resistance (i.e., without using any weights) and then when this is easy can add a 1 pound weight and increase as tolerated.

CONSIDERATIONS IN OLDER ADULTS WITH LOW FITNESS

With regard to aerobic activities, a different definition of intensity is necessary for adults with low fitness. Intensity is defined not as absolute energy expenditure in METS but relative to the person's level of fitness, as judged by the heart rate response to exercise. Moderate intensity activity has a heart rate response in the range of 55% to 69% of maximal heart rate (220 – age for men; 220 – [0.6 × age] for women). An 82-year-old man should try to exercise (e.g., walk) at a speed at which his heart rate ranges from 80 to 95. With this definition of intensity, unfit older adults (i.e., those who are sedentary and do not engage in 30 minutes of moderate physical activity at least 5 days a week) need not do a brisk walk or equivalently intense activity in order to meet the moderate intensity recommendation. Rather, the person should walk at a speed that causes a heart rate response in the range of moderate intensity.

Physical activity should be increased very gradually in adults with low fitness. Initially, short bouts of activity less than 10 minutes are appropriate and should be encouraged at the level in which the individual can tolerate the activity. Older adults in assisted living communities benefit from physical activity. Supervised classes of a few months duration cause improvements in fitness and functional limitations, even in those who are physically frail or have mild or moderate dementia. Physical activity may improve sleep and decrease agitation and other behavioral problems associated with dementia. Exercise programs for assisted living residents should include all of the components previously addressed.

OBESITY

The obesity epidemic in the United States has focused attention on the role of physical activity in maintaining a healthy body (weight). Public health recommendations advise that weight loss should be achieved by both reducing caloric intake and increasing energy expenditure. Regular physical activity during weight loss may be more important for older adults than for younger individuals. Obesity increases the risk of many chronic diseases and of functional limitations in older adults, but it also has the beneficial effects of increasing bone and muscle mass. For older adults advised to lose weight, a reasonable approach is to meet the exercise recommendation of 30 minutes daily at least 5 days a week and to limit caloric intake. Physical activity level can be gradually increased as necessary to achieve and maintain a healthy weight.

OSTEOPOROSIS, FALLS, FRACTURES, AND BALANCE TRAINING

Regular physical activity by older adults has a modest effect in slowing age-related loss of bone mass. Evidence indicates that resistance and high-impact exercises are most beneficial. Weight-bearing aerobic activities can also provide the stimulation to the bone that maintains bone mass (see also Chapter 48, "Musculoskeletal Diseases and Disorders" and Chapter 29, "Osteoporosis").

In older adults at increased risk for falling, randomized trials demonstrate that falls can be prevented by multicomponent interventions targeting factors such as sedative use, environmental hazards, and poor balance. Increasing physical activity is regarded as an effective component of falls prevention programs. A meta-analysis of randomized trials reported that aerobic activity, resistance training, and balance training are all associated with reduced risk of falling in older adults. Balance training is specifically recommended in clinical practice guidelines for falls prevention in adults at increased risk. There is no experimental evidence suggesting that exercise reduces either total fractures or hip fractures. However, a meta-analysis of epidemiologic studies reported that physical activity reduces the risk of hip fracture by up to 50%.

THE RISKS OF PHYSICAL ACTIVITY

Although the benefits of physical activity far outweigh the risks, promoting physical activity should include strategies for minimizing risk. The main risk of physical activity is musculoskeletal injury; some of these risks are modifiable. The risk of injury is higher with vigorous exercise, higher volume of exercise, and with obesity. It is less with higher fitness, supervision, protective equipment such as bike helmets, and in well-designed exercise environments. The principle that physical activity should be increased gradually over time is critical for reducing risk of injury. Generally, it is recommended that older adults begin resistance training with one set of 10 to 15 repetitions of each exercise, rather than the 8 to 12 repetitions for younger adults. That is, for older individuals it is best to do more repetitions of a single exercise but to do this using less resistance (relative to maximal strength). This helps reduce the risk of injury.

The risk of both exercise-related myocardial infarction and sudden death is rare and is greatest in individuals who are the least active. Sedentary adults should avoid isolated bouts of vigorous activity and should increase activity gradually over time.

PROMOTING PHYSICAL ACTIVITY

The causes of inactivity in adults are multifactorial; motivation has a major influence on exercise activity.

In addition, time constraints, environmental barriers and lack of appropriate exercise facilities, unpleasant consequences from exercise, dislike of the activity or boredom, lack of knowledge about the type and amount of exercise to perform, lack of belief in the benefits of exercise at an advanced age, impaired health, and fear of injury contribute to lack of adherence to physical activity by older as well as younger adults.

To maximize adherence to exercise programs, consider a multidimensional framework as afforded by social cognitive theory. This theory is based on a model of reciprocal determinism in which behavior, cognition, and other personal factors, and environmental influences all operate interactively as determinants of each other. According to social cognitive theory, human motivation and action are essentially regulated by forethought. This cognitive control of behavior is based on self-efficacy expectations, that is, an individual's beliefs in his or her capabilities to perform a course of action to attain a desired outcome and his or her beliefs that performing a behavior will result in the specific outcome he or she desires (see Chapter 16, "Psychosocial Aspects of Aging"). Strengthening self-efficacy and outcome expectations can positively influence adherence to an exercise regimen.

Motivating Residents to Exercise: The Seven-Step Approach

Based on self-efficacy theory, a seven-step approach (Table 18.1) was developed to help motivate residents to exercise. Education about the benefits of exercise and delineating the type and amount of exercise to perform are critical first steps for engaging the residents in regular exercise. This can be done formally in classes or informally during care interactions. Education should include families and proxies as well as the resident. Pre-screening using the EASY tool will help establish the optimal exercise program for each resident. Goal development can be incorporated into the resident's service plan and is a helpful reinforcement for the resident as to what he or she *can* do and is *expected* to do with regard to exercise/physical activity throughout the day. Exposing the individual to exercise, particularly to activities that he/she can be successful at, is important to strengthen his or her confidence (i.e., self-efficacy) and help him or her experience the positive benefits of exercise. What is most important is to continue to monitor, ask how the resident is doing in his or her exercise, and provide ongoing encouragement.

18.1 | The Seven-Step Approach

SEVEN STEPS	ACTIVITIES TO FACILITATE IMPLEMENTATION
1. Education	To facilitate learning about the benefits of physical activity and teaching the staff and residents what to do in terms of activity, the information should be given in multiple formats: an interactive lecture, a written handout, or video tape. The information must be repeated and reinforced both informally one-on-one with residents and/or formally in teaching programs.
2. Assessment of needs/ interest in physical activity	Evaluation of the resident (and the ALC[a]) to establish the resident's need to participate in an exercise program and specifically what he or she should do. Activities include: —Physical examination including health history —Exercise screenings —Evaluation of the barriers to engaging in the behavior (fear, no access, too old, etc.)

(continued)

18.1 | The Seven-Step Approach *(continued)*

SEVEN STEPS	ACTIVITIES TO FACILITATE IMPLEMENTATION
3. Goal identification	Set realistic goals with the resident and let him or her know exactly what behavior to engage in, for example: —Walk daily for 30 minutes —Perform resistance exercise two times a week —Walk to the dining room Set realistic goals for the ALC —All residents will be screened for exercise —All residents will be encouraged to walk to the dining room or self propel to the dining room —All residents will be given an exercise program/goals
4. Elimination of barriers	Eliminate the barriers associated with a given activity at the individual level such as: —Pain through medication, ice treatment, and so forth —Facilitate access to information and screening; for example, make exercise opportunities easy to access Eliminate the barriers associated with a given activity at the ALC —Reallocation of resources may be needed to identify and support a resident who will serve as a champion for implementation of the activity —Bring screening to the facility (e.g., a health promotion exercise screening day)
5. Role models	Provide examples of successful residents who have changed health behaviors and noted benefits. ˙ Implement interventions across a neighborhood or floor (or in an ALC); draw on an exemplary neighborhood or ALC that successfully implemented a walk-to-dine program as a role model.
6. Ongoing follow-up and verbal encouragement/ rewards	Ask the resident about his or her health behaviors and provide verbal encouragement toward any positive change. Continue to monitor and support at an administrative level the champion who is working on a health maintenance activity across the facility.
7. Implementation of environmental and policy facilitators for ongoing adherence	Facilitate change in the resident's environment to ensure adherence to health maintenance activities: clear paths to facilitate walking, provide heart healthy foods in the home or at neighborhood stores, remove alcoholic beverages, if possible, from the home setting. Facilitate change at the architectural level: provide access to the outside for exercise opportunities; clear walkways and create pleasant pathways; provide heart healthy food options; provide access to screening (health fairs); promote health education. Establish policies that promote and are consistent with health maintenance recommendations, such as annual screenings, immunizations at the ALC, or transportation to immunizations or screenings.

[a]Comprehensive evaluation of the ALC regarding the exercise and physical activity options available.

RESOURCES

American College of Sports Medicine and the American Heart Association. (2007). *Guidelines for physical activity.* Retrieved August, 2008, from http://www.americanheart.org/presenter. jhtml?identifier = 3049282

Church, T. S., Earnest, C. P., Skinner, J. S., & Blair, S. N. (2007). Effects of different doses of physical activity on cardiorespiratory fitness among sedentary, overweight or obese postmenopausal women with elevated blood pressure: A randomized controlled trial. *Journal of the American Medical Association, 297*(19), 2081–2091.

Cornelissen, V. A., & Fagard, R. H. (2005). Effect of resistance training on resting blood pressure: A meta-analysis of randomized controlled trials. *Journal of Hypertension, 23*(2), 251–259.

Haines, T. P., Hill, K. D., Bennell, K. L., & Osborne, R. H. (2007). Additional exercise for older subacute hospital inpatients to prevent falls: Benefits and barriers to implementation and evaluation. *Clinical Rehabilitation, 21*(8), 742–753.

Neuberger, G. B., Aaronson, L. S., Gajewski, B., Embretson, S. E., Cagle, P. E., Loudon, J. K., et al. (2007). Predictors of exercise and effects of exercise on symptoms, function, aerobic fitness, and disease outcomes of rheumatoid arthritis. *Arthritis Rheumology, 57*(6), 943–952.

Resnick, B., Ory, M., Hora, K., Rogers, M., Page, P., Chodzko-Zajko, W., et al. (2008). A new screening paradigm and tool: The Exercise/Physical Activity Assessment and Screening for You (EASY). *Journal of Aging and Physical Activity, 16*(2), 215–233.

Thompson, P. D. (2005). Exercise prescription and proscription for patients with coronary artery disease. *Circulation, 112*(15), 2354–2363.

Thompson, P. D., Franklin, B., Balady, G. J., Blair, S. N., Corrado, D., Estes, N. A. III, et al. (2007). Exercise and acute cardiovascular events placing the risks into perspective: A scientific statement from the American Heart Association Council on Nutrition, Physical Activity, and Metabolism and the Council on Clinical Cardiology. *Circulation, 115*(7), 2358–2388.

Westhoff, T. H., Franke, N., Schmidt, S., Vallbracht-Israng, K., Meissner, R., Yildirim, H., et al. (2007). Too old to benefit from sports? The cardiovascular effects of exercise training in elderly subjects treated for isolated systolic hypertension. *Kidney Blood Press Research, 30*(4), 240–247.

19

Prevention

Harrison Bloom
and Barbara Resnick

As the population ages and average active life expectancy increases, primary and secondary prevention become increasingly important. The prevalence of *undetected, correctable* conditions and comorbid diseases is high in the older adult population. Fortunately, a growing number of older adults are highly motivated with regard to disease prevention and health promotion. The assisted living (AL) nurse has the unique opportunity to provide AL residents with preventive care information that can help them make decisions about what health promotion activities to perform.

A number of factors, including age, functional status, comorbidity, resident preference, socioeconomic status, and the availability of care, affect health care decisions of older adults. Generally, older individuals will not receive any survival benefit from cancer screening unless their life expectancy exceeds 5 years. Careful consideration must be given, however, to the identification and elimination of cancer at an early stage so that progression does not occur, even among those with limited life expectancy. The risks of screening and its follow-up diagnostics and treatments (e.g., perforation from colonoscopy; impotence or incontinence from prostate surgery) need more emphasis at the time of discussions regarding screening recommendations. For example, finding a preventable cancer that might result in death in 5 to 10 years if not detected early is of no benefit (and can result in actual harm and considerable cost) in an individual whose life expectancy is less than 5 years. It is important, too, that the values, beliefs, and preferences of older adults be factored into discussions, as should issues regarding quality of life.

RECOMMENDED PREVENTIVE SERVICES

A number of preventive services are effective in the care of older adults and are widely endorsed. These include screening, counseling, prevention, immunization, and so forth (See Table 19.1).

Screening

Obesity or Malnutrition

Routine measurement of height and weight is used to calculate body mass index (BMI = kg/m^2). Obesity in men is defined as a BMI $\geq$ 27.8 and in women as a BMI $\geq$ 27.3. Unintentional weight loss of 10 pounds in 6 months can indicate malnutrition or a serious occult illness.

Hypertension

The prevalence of hypertension increases with advancing age. Treatment in older adults is associated with reduction in morbidity and mortality from left ventricular hypertrophy, heart failure, myocardial infarction, and stroke. However, older adults are more susceptible to adverse effects of antihypertensive therapy, such

19.1 | Evidence-Based Preventive Services Recommended for Older Adults

PREVENTIVE ACTIVITY	FREQUENCY	CONDITION TO DETECT OR PREVENT
Screening		
Height and weight	At least annually	Obesity, malnutrition
Blood pressure	At least annually	Hypertension
Vision testing	Annually	Visual deficits
Hearing ability	Annually	Hearing impairment
Depression questionnaire	—[a]	Depression
Alcoholism questionnaire	—[a]	Alcoholism
Serum lipids (with prior MI, angina)	Annually	Recurrent CAD
Abdominal ultrasonography (men aged 65–75 years who have ever smoked)	Once	Abdominal aortic aneurysm
Bone density measurement	—[a]	Osteoporosis
Glucose (with hypertension or hyperlipidemia)	—[a]	Type 2 diabetes mellitus
Mammography	Every 2–3 years	Breast cancer
Pap smear	At least every 3 years[b]	Cervical cancer
Fecal occult blood testing and/or	Annually	Colorectal cancer
flexible sigmoidoscopy or colonoscopy	Every 3–5 years Once	
Counseling to encourage:		
Smoking cessation	Every visit	COPD, many cancers, CAD
Regular dental visits	Annually	Malnutrition, oral cancers, edentulism
Low-fat, well-balanced diet	Annually	Obesity, CAD
Adequate calcium intake	Annually	Osteoporosis

(continued)

19.1 | Evidence-Based Preventive Services Recommended for Older Adults *(continued)*

PREVENTIVE ACTIVITY	FREQUENCY	CONDITION TO DETECT OR PREVENT
Physical activity	Annually	Immobility, CAD, osteoporosis
Injury prevention	Annually	Injurious falls, motor vehicle crashes, burns, other injuries
Immunization		
Influenza vaccination	Annually	Influenza
Pneumococcal vaccination	—^{c}	Pneumococcal disease
Tetanus booster	Every 10 years	Tetanus
Chemoprophylaxis		
Aspirin therapy	Daily	Recurrent MI, TIA, or stroke

Note: CAD = coronary artery disease; COPD = chronic obstructive pulmonary disease; MI = myocardial infarction; TIA = transient ischemic attack.
[a]The optimal interval for screening is unknown.
[b]May stop screening at age 65 if patient has had regularly normal smears up to that age; if never tested prior to age 65, may stop after two normal annual smears.
[c]Vaccinate immunocompetent patients once at age 65; revaccination after 7–10 years may be appropriate.

as hyponatremia, hypokalemia, depression, confusion, or postural hypotension. This is especially true for the oldest-old and those who have multiple comorbidities and who are taking multiple medications.

Vision and Hearing Deficits

Routine screening with a Snellen chart is recommended by the U.S. Preventive Services Task Force (USPSTF). Undetected hearing loss can lead to social isolation and may indicate other underlying disorders. The USPSTF recommends periodically questioning older adults about their hearing and counseling them about the availability of hearing aid devices. Cerumen (ear wax) that blocks the eardrum is the most common cause of hearing impairment. Encouraging older adults to have their ears checked for wax buildup at least annually is an important nursing intervention to promote healthy and optimal hearing.

Alcoholism

All older adults should be screened for alcohol abuse. This can be done by asking the older adult how much they drink daily, socially, or by completing a screening questionnaire such as the CAGE (see Exhibit 19.1).

Osteoporosis

The USPSTF currently recommends that women age 65 and older be screened routinely for osteoporosis using bone density measurements. For those at high risk for osteoporotic fractures, screening should begin at age 60. Counseling regarding adequate calcium intake, smoking

19.1 | The CAGE Screening Test for Alcohol Problems

The CAGE screening test is used to screen for alcohol use problems in adults. However, it cannot be used to diagnose the disease. It only suggests that the disease may be present. Other tests are needed to diagnose alcohol dependence.

Screening test questions:

- Have you ever felt you ought to Cut down on your drinking or drug use?
- Do you get Annoyed at criticism of your drinking or drug use?
- Do you ever feel Guilty about your drinking or drug use?
- Do you ever take an Early-morning drink (eye-opener) or use drugs first thing in the morning ("a little hair of the dog that bit you") to get the day started or to eliminate the shakes?

A person who answers "yes," "sometimes," or "often" to two or more of the questions may have a problem with alcohol.

cessation, exercise, and avoidance of falls is also recommended (see Chapter 29, "Osteoporosis").

Cancer Screening

Mammography screening should cease at age 70, according to the USPSTF. With regard to colon cancer screening, however, the USPSTF recommends that individuals 50 years of age and older undergo annual screening. Screening for bowel cancer is particularly focused on identifying premalignant adenomatous polyps and may help identify premalignant lesions and prevent uncomfortable symptoms that might occur if left untreated (e.g., bowel obstruction). There is no single best test to screen for colon cancer; there are four options: Fecal occult blood test (FOBT), flexible sigmoidoscopy, colonoscopy, and double contrast barium enema. Stool DNA testing is a new approach for colorectal cancer screening. Initial testing of this approach indicated it was no better than FOBT. A new version of the screening, referred to as SDT-2, has a reported sensitivity of 40%. Ongoing research is needed to continue to explore the sensitivity and specificity of this measure.

The USPSTF and the American Cancer Society (ACS) recommend against screening women older than 65 for cervical cancer if they have had negative tests in the past and have no risk factors for cervical cancer (e.g., a history of cervical cancer, immunosuppression, diethyl stilbesterol exposure before birth, or documented human papilloma virus infection). Older women who have never had a prior Pap test should be screened annually until there are two negative tests. The USPSTF concluded that there was insufficient evidence to recommend for or against routine prostate-specific antigen screening for prostate cancer. In addition, the USPSTF currently recommends against the routine screening of adults for bladder, lung, oral, ovarian, pancreatic, skin, or testicular cancers.

Counseling
Smoking Cessation

Smoking cessation at any age reduces the rate of chronic obstructive pulmonary disease, many cancers, and coronary artery disease (CAD). All older adult smokers should be encouraged to and helped with smoking cessation at each office visit (see Chapter 37, "Substance Abuse," and Chapter 40, "Respiratory Diseases and Disorders").

Dental Care

Many common problems can be detected and effectively treated by regular dental visits, including periodontitis, xerostomia, and oral cancers (see Chapter 39, "Oral Diseases and Disorders").

Dietary Counseling

The importance of a well-balanced diet should be addressed routinely with older adults. An appropriate diet is high in fruits and vegetables, low in fat and salt, and has adequate calcium content. Also, it is important not to overly restrict the diet of those who are underweight or frail. Restrictions in these situations can be counterproductive and lead to increased morbidity (see Chapter 25, "Maintenance of Nutritional Status").

In addition to overall nutritional health, obesity should be addressed in older individuals as it can affect mobility and overall function, as well as be a risk factor for coronary heart disease and other chronic conditions. BMI is a reliable and valid measure of body fat. Overweight individuals are defined as those who have a BMI of 25 to 29.9 kg/m². Obesity is defined as a BMI of > 30. The BMI, however, is age-dependent and does not account for body fat distribution. Older adults at high risk of excess weight are likely to be underestimated because many have excess body fat that is counteracted by a loss of muscle mass with aging. Alternatively, waist circumference can be used: normal waist for men is 102 cm (40 inches) or less; for women, it is 88 cm (35 inches) or less. The most effective interventions for weight loss in older adults combine nutritional education, diet, and exercise counseling with behavioral interventions for weight loss as well as use of the Mediterranean diet, which is rich in healthy fats.

Physical Activity

Physical activity is one of the most effective ways in which older adults can maintain health, regardless of underlying physical condition or comorbidities. Currently, it is recommended that older adults engage in 30 minutes of moderate-level physical activity (i.e., 5 to 6 on a 10-point scale) a minimum of 5 days a week. This should be aerobic activity and can be done in 10 minute bouts. In addition, muscle strengthening activity should be done at least 2 days a week. Strengthening exercises should focus on all the major muscle groups (muscles in the chest, back, arms, and legs) with the individual performing 10–15 repetitions of each muscle group. Last, flexibility and balance exercise (for those at risk of falls) should be done at least 2 days a week (see Chapter 18, "Physical Activity").

Injury Prevention

Older adults experience the highest number of home-related injuries and deaths: 7,000 individuals annually. Falls are the leading cause of home injury; fires are second; poisoning is third. The USPSTF recommends counseling older persons on measures to reduce the risk of falling, on environmental hazard reduction, and on safety-related skills and behaviors. Exhibit 19.2 lists safety resources and interventions that are available through organizations such as the National Institute of Aging, AARP, and the Centers for Disease Control.

Fall prevention is a critical aspect of health maintenance among older adults and should include a focus on the individual as well as on his or her environment. Physical changes that affect gait and balance, whether related to normal age changes or disease (e.g., stroke or Parkinson's disease), cognitive changes, and environmental factors (e.g., tripping over something left on the floor) all can contribute to falls. Multifactorial approaches are effective interventions for fall prevention and should be encouraged (see Chapter 28, "Falls").

Environmental hazard reduction should be implemented to decrease the risk of fires, burns, and hypo or hyperthermia. Interventions include monitoring for ap-

propriate use of heating and cooling systems, appropriate water temperature to prevent serious burns, installing smoke detectors, and using alarms and automatic shut-off features on appliances. A home safety checklist or formal environmental assessment can facilitate injury prevention (see the home safety checklist listed in Exhibit 19.2).

Safety-Related Skills and Behaviors

Older adults should be encouraged to engage in safe behaviors regarding driving, sexual activity, and medication management (see Chapter 20, "Pharmacotherapy"). Unfortunately, older adults are nine times more likely to be involved in fatal accidents than are drivers aged 25 to 69; older individuals account for 13% of all traffic fatalities and 17% of all pedestrian fatalities. Health maintenance activities include the use of seat and lap belts in automobiles, safe driving evaluations, and the avoidance of alcohol or sedative-hypnotic medications when driving. Safe driving can be established through testing that involves physical as well as performance observations. These types of comprehensive driving evaluations are often performed by occupational therapists.

Sexual activity and intimacy can be an important aspect of health maintenance. Safe sexual activity needs to be addressed, particularly with regard to the prevention of sexually transmitted diseases (STDs) the most common being nongonococcal urethritis in men and genital herpes in women. The number of individuals over the age of 50 who are human immunodeficiency virus (HIV) positive has increased; older adults accounted for 15% of new cases reported in the United States in 2007. Unfortunately, older adults are less likely than younger adults to perceive themselves at risk for STDs and less likely to adopt safe sexual behaviors such as condom use or testing for infection prior to initiating sexual activity. Low-risk behaviors should be encouraged, such as practicing mutually monogamous relationships, partner reduction, and aggressive use of condoms (male and female versions).

Immunizations

Medicare covers the costs of influenza, pneumococcal, and tetanus immunizations.

Influenza Vaccine

The current influenza vaccine is a killed virus that is moderately immunogenic, with estimated efficacy rates in the general population of 70% for illness and 90%

19.2 | Safety Resources and Interventions

WEB PAGE	CONTENT AREA
http://app1.unmc.edu/intmed/geriatrics/index.cfm?L2_ID = 37&CONREF = 40&L1_ID = 11	Home safety checklist University of Nebraska
http://www.healthline.com/sw/hr-sr-home-safety-for-older-adults	Healthline Home safety information across all areas (driving, fires, diet)
http://www.cdc.gov/ncipc/factsheets/olderactivities.htm	Centers for Disease Control information on home safety
http://safety.fhwa.dot.gov/older_driver/index.htm	Federal highway administration on driving safety
http://www.nia.nih.gov/HealthInformation/Publications/drivers.htm	National Institute of Aging AgePage on driving safety
http://www1.aota.org/olderdriver/	American Occupational Therapy Association information on driving evaluations.
http://www.aarp.org/family/articles/older_drivers_and_auto_safety.html	AARP information on driving safety.
http://www.cdc.gov/ncipc/falls/default.htm	Centers for Disease Control Fall Prevention Programs
http://www.temple.edu/older_adult/fppmanual.html	Temple University Fall Prevention Program
http://www.healthyagingprograms.org/content.asp?sectionid = 69	Center for Healthy Aging Fall Prevention Program
http://www.masspro.org/HH/RACH/docs/education training/FastFactsJan07.pdf	MassPro Fall Prevention Information and Programs

for mortality. This means that 70% of the time it helps to decrease how sick individuals are with influenza and 90% of the time it helps to decrease death associated with influenza. Multiple evaluations of the vaccine's efficacy with older adults reveal that, although it does not completely protect these individuals against disease, it reduces rates of respiratory illness, hospitalization, and mortality. Annual vaccine administration must be provided because of the short-lived (4 to 5 months) protection provided by the vaccine. Current recommendations are that all residents age 65 or over or those under age 65 with underlying medical illnesses be immunized annually between October and mid-November, but any time from September to the end of influenza season is appropriate. Medical personnel and caregivers for high-risk residents should also be immunized. Potential adverse effects include fever, chills, myalgias, and malaise, but these are rare. Contraindications include anaphylactic egg hypersensitivity or allergic reactions following occupational exposure to egg protein. Live, attenuated influenza vaccines have been developed, appear to be more effective, and are likely to be approved for widespread use in the near future.

Pneumococcal Vaccination

Pneumococcal vaccination is indicated for all persons aged 65 years or older and for many persons under age 65 with comorbid conditions. If ≥ 5 years has elapsed since the first dose and the resident was vaccinated before the age of 65, a repeat vaccination is indicated.

Studies show that adverse events following revaccination are rare and mild. Thus, an unknown vaccination history should prompt administration of the pneumococcal vaccine. (When in doubt, vaccinate!) The vaccine does not prevent mucosal disease such as sinusitis and has unclear efficacy for preventing pneumonia. However, strong evidence suggests that the vaccine reduces the risk of invasive disease (i.e., bacteremia) and that it is cost-effective for older immune-competent adults.

Although the protective efficacy of the pneumococcal vaccine is estimated to be only 60% to 70% and studies have revealed mixed results regarding benefits in high-risk older adults, all residents aged 65 years and older should receive one dose at 0.5 mg intramuscular (IM). Studies suggest that people may benefit from revaccination every 7 to 10 years. Other than local soreness, adverse effects are usually minimal.

Tetanus Vaccination

More than 60% of tetanus infections occur in persons 60 years of age and older. There is evidence that the absorbed tetanus and diphtheria toxoids provide long-term protection 35 years after the primary series or booster. Older adults who have never been vaccinated should receive two doses, 0.5 mg IM 1 to 2 months apart, followed by an additional dose 6 to 12 months later. The optimal interval for booster doses is not established; the USPSTF and Canadian Task Force recommend booster vaccinations every 10 years. Local pain and swelling or, rarely, hypersensitivity may accompany vaccination. A neurologic or hypersensitivity reaction to a previous dose is an absolute contraindication for administration of tetanus vaccine.

PREVENTIVE SERVICES NOT INDICATED IN OLDER ADULTS

There is strong evidence that the general screening modality of the annual complete history and physical examination is not any more effective for improving outcomes than a more targeted approach of individual screening, counseling, immunoprophylaxis, and chemoprophylaxis. Current evidence does not support specific screening for lung, pancreatic, ovarian, bladder, or hematologic malignancies for the general population. However, promising new screening modalities, such as helical low-density computed tomography of the chest for lung cancer and homo-

cystinemia for heart disease, are being actively developed and investigated.

Older adults vary with regard to their willingness to engage in health maintenance activities. With aging, there seems to be less interest in engaging in health promotion activities for the purpose of lengthening life, and greater interest in engaging in these activities only if they improve current quality of life. Therefore, health maintenance activities with older adults should use an individualized approach. The goal is to provide older adults with the information needed for them to understand the risks and benefits associated with each health maintenance activity, and then to help them initiate and adhere to the activities in which they are interested and motivated (See Chapter 16, "Psychosocial Aspects of Aging," regarding self-efficacy theory; see also Exhibit 19.3).

19.3 | Preventive Services That Have Been Demonstrated Not to Be Beneficial

ANNUAL COMPLETE HISTORY AND PHYSICAL EXAMINATION

Screening for the following diseases:

Lung cancer

Pancreatic cancer

Ovarian cancer

Bladder cancer

Hematologic malignancies

Routine laboratory testing

Annual complete blood cell count

Annual blood chemistry panel

Annual electrocardiogram

Annual chest radiography

Chemoprophylaxis

Hormone replacement therapy

RESOURCES

Ahlquist, D.A., Sargent, D.J., Loprinzi, C.L., Levin, T.R., Rex, D.K., Ahnen, D.J., et al. (2008). Stool DNA and occult blood testing for screen detection of colorectal neoplasia. *Annals of Internal Medicine, 149*(7).

Assessment of nutritional health. (2008). Retrieved October 29, 2008, from http://www.co.dane.wi.us/aging//assessment.htm

Centers for Disease Control. (2008a). *Injury, violence and safety.* Retrieved October 29, 2008, from http://www.cdc.gov/Injury ViolenceSafety/

Centers for Disease Control. (2008b). *Prevention and control of influenza: Recommendations of the Advisory Committee on Immunization Practices (ACIP).* Retrieved December 1, 2008, from http://www.cdc.gov/mmwr/preview/mmwrhtml/rr5606a5601.htm

Ewing, J. (1984). Detecting alcoholism. The CAGE questionnaire. *Journal of the American Medical Association, 252,* 1905-1907.

Hara, M., Sakamoto, T., & Tanaka, K. (2008). Influenza vaccine effectiveness among elderly persons living in the community during the 2003-2004 season. *Vaccine, 26,* 6477-6480.

Medicare Stop Smoking Program. (2008). *Resources and information about the Medicare Stop Smoking Program.* Retrieved October 29, 2008, from http://www.medicare.gov/health/smoking.asp

Nelson, M.E., Rejeski, W.J., Blair, S.N., Duncan, P.W., Judge, J.O., King, A.C., et al. (2007). Physical activity and public health in older adults: recommendation from the American College of Sports Medicine and the American Heart Association. *Circulation, 116*(9), 1094-1105.

Resnick, B., & McClesky, S. (2008). Cancer screening across the aging continuum. *Journal of Managed Care Medicine, 14*(5), 267-276.

Resnick, B., Ory, M., Hora, K., Rogers, M., Page, P., Lyle, R., et al. (2008). A new screening paradigm and tool: The Exercise/Physical Activity Assessment and Screening for You (EASY). *Journal of the Aging and Physical Activity, 16*(2), 215-233.

The 2005 dietary guidelines for Americans. (2008). Retrieved July 6, 2008, from http://www.health.gov/DietaryGuidelines/

Thompson, P.D. (2005). Exercise prescription and proscription for patients with coronary artery disease. *Circulation, 112*(15), 2354-2363.

Thompson, P.D., Franklin B.A., Balady, G.J., Blair, S.N., Corrado, D., Estes, N.A. III, et al. (2007). Exercise and acute cardiovascular events placing the risks into perspective: A scientific statement from the American Heart Association Council on Nutrition, Physical Activity, and Metabolism and the Council on Clinical Cardiology. *Circulation, 115*(7), 2358-2388.

United States Preventive Services Task Force. (2008a). *Counseling to prevent tobacco use and tobacco-caused disease: Recommendation statement.* Retrieved October 292008, from http://www.ahrq.gov/clinic/3rduspstf/tobacccoun/tobcounrs.htm

United States Preventive Services Task Force. (2008b). Guide to clinical preventive services: Perceptions, barriers, and motivations. *Journal of Women and Aging, 17*(1-2), 37-53.

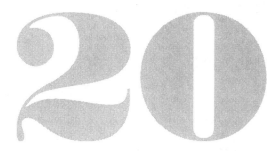

Pharmacotherapy

Todd P. Semla, Paula A. Rochon, and Barbara Resnick

As the most common treatment for acute and chronic diseases, drugs also are used to prevent many diseases and disorders experienced by the older adult. Successful pharmacotherapy requires ordering the correct drug for the correct disease or condition, at the correct dosage, at the correct time and route, and for the correct resident. Unfortunately, achieving optimal drug treatment of acute and chronic disease is not simple or easy. Many factors come into play: the individual's other disease states and medications; medical regimen adherence; personal beliefs about illness, health, and cure; functional status; physiologic changes due to aging and disease; and socioeconomic status (i.e., ability to afford the medication). Medication administration for older adults should be based on the basic principle of starting with a low dose and increasing this dose slowly (a start low and go slow approach).

UNDERSTANDING AGE-ASSOCIATED CHANGES IN PHARMACOKINETICS (HOW THE BODY USES MEDICATIONS)

Pharmacokinetic principles focus on the *absorption, distribution, metabolism,* and *elimination* of medication. The effects of aging on each parameter have been studied and formulated into principles of prescribing for the older adult.

Absorption

Aging does not affect drug absorption via the gastrointestinal tract to any clinically significant degree. The rate of absorption may be slowed with age, but the extent of absorption remains unchanged. Consequently, the peak blood concentration of a drug in the older adult may be lower, and the time to reach it may be delayed, but the overall amount absorbed (*bioavailability*) does not differ between younger and older adults. Exceptions include some drugs that go through multiple processes of elimination in the body (e.g., first via the liver and then via the kidney).

Factors that have a greater impact on drug absorption than do age-related effects include the way (i.e., route) a medication is taken, what it is taken with, and other medical illnesses. For example, the absorption of many fluoroquinolones (e.g., ciprofloxacin) is reduced when they are taken with calcium, magnesium, and iron, all of which are found in antacids, dairy products, or vitamins. Enteral feeding liquids interfere with the absorption of some drugs (e.g., phenytoin). An increase in gastric pH from proton-pump inhibitors, H_2 antagonists, or antacids may increase the absorption of some drugs, such as nifedipine and amoxicillin, and decrease the absorption of other drugs, such as the imidazole antifungals, ampicillin, cyanocobalamin, and indinavir. Agents that promote or delay gastrointestinal motility, such as stimulant laxatives and metoclopramide can, in theory, affect a drug's absorption by increasing or decreasing the time the drug sits in the area of the gastrointestinal tract where it could be absorbed.

Distribution

Distribution refers to the locations in the body that a drug penetrates and the time required for the drug to reach those locations. In older adults, drugs that are water soluble (*hydrophilic* [e.g., ethanol, lithium]) will not be efficiently distributed throughout the body because older adults have less body water and lean body mass. Digoxin binds to skeletal muscle; distribution is reduced in older adults who have reduced muscle mass. Distribution of drugs that are fat soluble (*lipophilic*) are higher in older adults because they have more fat stores, regardless of their weight, than do younger persons. Thus, it takes longer for a fat soluble medication to be effective and then it takes longer for that drug to be excreted. Examples of fat-soluble drugs include diazepam, flurazepam, thiopental, and trazodone.

The extent to which a drug is bound to *plasma proteins* also influences how it gets distributed. Albumin, the primary plasma protein to which drugs bind, is often decreased in older adults. This means that there will be a larger amount of the drug that is unbound; thus, it is pharmacologically active for a longer period of time. Drugs that bind to albumin in older adults include ceftriaxone, diazepam, lorazepam, phenytoin, valproic acid, and warfarin. Age-related decreases in the organ systems of elimination may result in the accumulation of unbound drugs in the body. Phenytoin is an example of the way an increase in an unbound drug can lead to an unnecessary and potentially harmful dosage increase. A resident with a low serum albumin (≤ 3 g/dL) whose phenytoin dose is increased because his or her total phenytoin concentration is subtherapeutic may develop symptoms and signs of phenytoin toxicity after a dose increase because the concentration of free phenytoin is elevated.

Metabolism

The liver is the most common site of drug metabolism, but metabolic conversion also can take place in the intestinal wall, lungs, skin, kidneys, and other organs. Aging affects the liver by decreasing liver blood flow as well as decreasing liver size and mass. Consequently, the metabolic clearance of drugs by the liver may be reduced. Drug clearance is also reduced for drugs that go through what are referred to as phase I pathways (mechanisms such as hydroxylation, oxidation, dealkylation, and reduction)—for example, diazepam. Drugs metabolized through the phase II pathways are converted to inactive compounds. Consequently, phase II drugs are generally preferred for older adults because their metabolites are not active and will not accumulate; this is why lorazepam is preferred over diazepam when treating anxiety in older adults.

Elimination

Elimination refers to a drug's final route(s) of exit from the body. For most drugs, this involves elimination by the kidney as either the parent compound or as a metabolite or metabolites. Terms used to express elimination are a drug's *half-life* and its *clearance*. A drug's half-life is the time it takes for its plasma or serum concentration to decline by 50%, for example, from 20 µg/mL to 10 µg/mL. Half-life is usually expressed in hours. Steady state is reached when the amount of drug entering systemic circulation is equal to the amount being eliminated. For a drug administered on a regular basis, 95% of steady state in the body is achieved after five half-lives of the drug.

Clearance is usually expressed as volume per unit of time (e.g., L/hour or mL/minute) and represents the volume of plasma or serum from which the drug is removed (i.e., cleared) per unit of time. Clearance can also be expressed as volume per weight per unit of time (L/kg/hour). Half-life and clearance can also refer to metabolic elimination.

The effects of aging on kidney function have been studied to a greater extent than have the effects of aging on liver function. Glomerular filtration declines as a consequence of a decrease in kidney size and renal blood flow and a decrease in functioning nephrons (cells of the kidney). On average, kidney function begins to decline when people reach their mid-30s. Serum creatinine is not an accurate reflection of creatinine clearance in older adults. Because of the age-related decline in lean muscle mass, production of creatinine is reduced. The decrease in the glomerular filtration rate counters the decreased production of creatinine, and serum creatinine stays within the normal range in older adults even when there is a decline in their kidney function. Measuring an older adult's 24-hour creatinine clearance would be the most accurate way to determine the appropriate dose, but it is generally not realistic for practical reasons to do a 24-hour urine test because so many older adults have some urinary incontinence, which would make the test not only difficult to do but useless if a full sample is not collected. Therefore, kidney function is estimated using the calculation in Exhibit 20.1.

20.1 | Cockroft and Gault Equation

$$CrCl = \frac{(140 \times age) \times weight}{72 \times serum\ creatinine}$$

Weight in kg; serum creatinine in mg/100 mL; 85% less in women.

20.2 | Factors Associated With Inappropriate Prescribing or Overprescribing

Resident factors

    Advanced age

    Female gender

    Lower educational level

    Rural residence

    Belief in using a pill for every ill

    Multiple health problems

    Use of multiple medications

    Use of multiple pharmacies

System factors

    Multiple prescribers for individual resident

    Poor record keeping

    Failure to review a resident's medication regimen at least annually

This calculated estimated of kidney function (the estimated glomerular filtration rate [GFR]) is provided by the laboratory following all lab drawings that include a blood urea nitrogen (BUN) and creatinine. In cases in which the resident's GFR is less than 60, the prescriber may decrease the dose from that normally recommended for adults or older adults with no kidney damage.

AGE-ASSOCIATED CHANGES IN PHARMACODYNAMICS

The pharmacodynamic action of a drug—that is, its time course and intensity of pharmacologic effect—may change with increasing age. An excellent example of such pharmacodynamic changes in older adults has been demonstrated with the benzodiazepines. On a psychomotor test, older adults are more sedated and have lower performance than younger adults following a single dose of triazolam. These differences are attributed to pharmacokinetic changes that result in a reduced clearance of this drug in older adults.

Pharmacodynamic and pharmacokinetic changes, alone or together, generally result in the older adult's increased sensitivity to medications. In older individuals, lower doses, longer intervals between doses, and longer periods between changes in dose are ways to successfully manage drug therapy and decrease the chances of medication intolerance or toxicity.

OPTIMIZING PRESCRIBING

Factors associated with inappropriate prescribing or overprescribing are listed in Exhibit 20.2. Simply limiting the number of medications for a given individual, however, is not always possible or desirable. For example, a resident with heart failure may be appropriately treated with three or four drugs: a diuretic, an angiotensin-converting enzyme (ACE) inhibitor, a β-blocker, and perhaps digoxin. If this resident has hyperlipidemia and diabetes mellitus, another two or three medications could be required. Hence, such a resident would be taking five to seven indicated medications for major medical conditions alone.

Underprescribing medications is also of concern and may result from an effort to avoid overprescribing, a complex medication regimen, or adverse effects. It may also result from the thinking that older adults will not benefit from medications intended as primary or secondary prevention, or from aggressive management of chronic conditions, such as hypertension and diabetes mellitus. Medications often cited as underprescribed in older adults include ACE inhibitors and β-blockers for heart failure, warfarin for atrial fibrillation, HMG–CoA reductase inhibitors for primary prevention of cardiovascular events, gastroprotective agents for residents at high risk for nonsteroidal anti-inflammatory drug–induced gastrointestinal bleeding, and narcotic analgesics for pain control.

ADVERSE DRUG EVENTS (ADEs)

An ADE is defined as an injury resulting from the use of a drug. Preventable ADEs are among the most serious consequences of inappropriate drug prescribing among older adults. An *adverse drug reaction* (ADR) is a type of ADE; it refers to harm that is directly caused by a drug at usual doses. Risk factors for ADEs in older adults are shown in Exhibit 20.3.

A *drug–drug interaction* (DDI) is defined as the pharmacologic or clinical response to the administration of a drug combination that differs from that anticipated from the known effects of either of the two agents when given alone. Drug–drug interactions are important because they may lead to ADEs. The likelihood of DDIs increases as the number of medications a person takes increases. Among prescription drugs, cardiovascular and psychotropic drugs are most commonly involved in DDIs. The most common adverse effects are neuropsychologic (primarily delirium), hypotension, and acute kidney failure. Drug combinations associated with increased risk for hospitalization for older adults are shown in Exhibit 20.4. Drugs commonly involved in DDIs in long-term care settings (e.g., nursing homes, assisted living) are listed in Exhibit 20.5. Risk factors associated with DDIs include the use of multiple medications, receiving care from several prescribing clinicians, and using more than one pharmacy.

20.3 | Risk Factors for Adverse Drug Events in Older Residents

- Age > 85 years

- Low body weight or body mass index

- ≥ 6 concurrent chronic diagnoses

- An estimated creatinine clearance < 50 mL per minute

- ≥ 9 medications

- ≥ 12 doses of medications per day

- A prior adverse drug reaction

20.4 | Most Common Drug–Drug Adverse Effects Identified Upon Hospitalization

COMBINATION	RISK
ACE inhibitor + diuretic	Hypotension, hyperkalemia
ACE inhibitor + potassium	Hyperkalemia
Antiarrhythmic + diuretic	Electrolyte imbalance; arrhythmias
Benzodiazepine + antidepressant	Confusion, sedation, falls
Benzodiazepine + antipsychotic	Confusion, sedation, falls
Benzodiazepine + benzodiazepine	Confusion, sedation, falls
Calcium channel blocker + diuretic	Hypotension
Calcium channel blocker + nitrate	Hypotension
Digitalis + antiarrhythmic	Bradycardia, arrhythmias
Diuretic + digitalis	Arrhythmias
Diuretic + diuretic	Dehydration, electrolyte imbalance
Diuretic + nitrate	Hypotension
Nitrate + vasodilator	Hypotension

Note: ACE = angiotensin-converting enzyme.
From "Drug-Drug Interactions Related to Hospital Admissions in Older Adults: A Prospective Study of 1000 Patients," by J. Doucet, P. Chassagne, C. Trivalle, I. Landrin, N. Kadri, J.F. Menard, et al. 1996, *Journal of the American Geriatrics Society, 44*(8), p. 944–948. Copyright ©1996 by *Journal of the American Geriatrics Society.* Reprinted with permission.

20.5 | Dangerous Drugs Involved in Drug–Drug Interactions in Long-Term Care

MEDICATION	INTERACTING MEDICATIONS
Angiotensin-converting enzyme inhibitors	Potassium supplements, potassium-sparing diuretics
Digoxin	Antiarrhythmics, verapamil
Quinolones	Theophylline, warfarin
Warfarin	Sulfa drugs, macrolides, quinolones, nonsteroidal anti-inflammatory drugs, phenytoin

Drug interactions can take many forms. For example, absorption can be enhanced or diminished (as described previously), drugs with similar or opposite pharmacologic effects can result in exaggerated or impaired effects, and drug metabolism (i.e., how that drug is eliminated from the body) may be sped up or slowed down.

DRUG–DISEASE INTERACTIONS

Drug–disease combinations common in older adults can affect drug response and lead to ADEs. Obesity and ascites alter the distribution of lipophilic and hydrophilic drugs, and thereby change the effectiveness of those drugs. Residents with dementia may have increased sensitivity or paradoxical reactions to drugs that act on the central nervous system (sedative-hypnotic drugs such as sleeping pills) or drugs with anticholinergic activity (Exhibit 20.6). Residents with renal insufficiency or impaired hepatic function due to cirrhosis or hepatic congestion have impaired excretion of drugs, and drugs will therefore continue to be effective for longer than would have been anticipated.

20.6 | The Impact of Medications with Anticholinergic Side Effects

AREA OF IMPACT	POSSIBLE SIGNS AND SYMPTOMS ANTICHOLINERGIC EFFECTS
General effects	Ataxia; loss of coordination
	Decreased mucus production in the nose and throat; consequent dry, sore throat
	Xerostomia or dry mouth with possible acceleration of caries
	Cessation of perspiration; consequent decreased thermal dissipation through the skin leading to hot, red skin
	Increased body temperature
	Pupil dilation (mydriasis); consequent sensitivity to bright light (photophobia)
	Loss of accommodation (loss of focusing ability, blurred vision—cycloplegia)
	Double vision (diplopia)
	Increased heart rate (tachycardia)
	Urinary retention
	Diminished bowel movement, sometimes ileus
	Increased intraocular pressure, dangerous for people with narrow-angle glaucoma
	Shaking
Central nervous system	Confusion
	Disorientation
	Agitation
	Euphoria or dysphoria
	Respiratory depression

(continued)

20.6 | The Impact of Medications with Anticholinergic Side Effects *(continued)*

AREA OF IMPACT	POSSIBLE SIGNS AND SYMPTOMS ANTICHOLINERGIC EFFECTS
	Memory problems
	Inability to concentrate
	Wandering thoughts; inability to sustain a train of thought
	Incoherent speech
	Wakeful myoclonic jerking
	Unusual sensitivity to sudden sounds
	Illogical thinking
	Photophobia
	Visual disturbances
	Periodic flashes of light
	Periodic changes in visual field
	Visual snow
	Restricted or tunnel vision
	Visual, auditory, or other sensory hallucinations
	Warping or waving of surfaces and edges
	Textured surfaces
	Dancing lines; spiders, insects
	Lifelike objects indistinguishable from reality
	Hallucinated presence of people not actually there
	Rarely: seizures, coma and death

PRINCIPLES OF PRESCRIBING

Principles of prescribing for older adults are shown in Exhibit 20.7. This basic approach applies primarily to medications that will be used to treat chronic conditions for which an immediate, complete therapeutic response is not necessary. A dose adjustment may still be needed for medications used to treat conditions requiring an immediate response (e.g., when prescribing antibiotics for a resident with impaired kidney function).

Overprescribing can be prevented by reviewing a resident's medications on a regular basis and each time a new medication is started or a dose is changed. The importance of maintaining accurate records of all medications taken by the resident cannot be overemphasized. Knowing what the resident has been prescribed as well as what he or she is taking over-the-counter (OTC, including herbals) and documenting all of this in the resident's records is crucial. Many residents do not consider vitamins, herbal preparations, or OTCs (even aspirin) to be medications; therefore, a specific question must be asked when inquiring about a resident's use of other medications/medicaments. In the assisted living (AL) setting, approximately 3.4 OTCs are used, on average per resident, among which are nutritional supplements, stomach/bowel medications, pain killers, herbals, cold remedies, and topical ointments. Fifty-one percent of these are misused (i.e., they resulted in duplication in treatment or caused DDIs).

NONADHERENCE

Nonadherence and underadherence to medications are a huge and often unrecognized problem in drug therapy. It is estimated that nonadherence (formerly known as noncompliance) among older adults may be as high as 50%. Residents may be reluctant to admit that they are not taking medications or not following directions. If nonadherence is suspected (by virtue of observing some symptoms), the nurse should consider the resident's financial, cognitive, and functional status, as well as his or her health literacy and beliefs about, and understanding of, medications and diseases.

Prescription drug costs have increased substantially. Medicare Part D and other supplemental prescription drug benefit plans may leave the older adult with an unaffordable co-payment. Cognitive impairment may also cause nonadherence, as residents forget to take medications or confuse them. Simplifying the regimen and simple oversight by setting up medications in a pill box (if permitted in the state) can optimize adherence

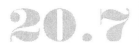 **20.7** Principles of Safe Use of Medications Among Older Adults

The basics:

- Start with a low dose.

- Titrate the dose upward slowly, as tolerated by the resident.

- Try not to start two drugs at the same time.

Determine the following before prescribing a new medication:

- Is the medication necessary? Are there nonpharmacologic ways to treat the condition?

- What are the therapeutic end points and how will they be assessed?

- Do the benefits outweigh the risks of the medication?

- Is one medication being used to treat the adverse effects of another?

- Is there one medication that could be prescribed to treat two conditions?

- Are there potential drug–drug or drug–disease interactions?

- Will the new medication's administration times be the same as those of existing medications?

- Do the resident and caregiver understand what the medication is for, how to take it, how long to take it, when it should start to work, possible adverse effects that it might cause, and what to do if they occur?

At least annually:

- Ask the resident to bring in all medications (prescription, over-the-counter, supplements, and herbal preparations) to the office; for new residents, conduct a detailed medication history.

- For prescription medications, determine whether the label directions and dose match those in the resident's chart; ask the resident how each medication is being taken.

- Ask about medication side effects.

- Note who else is prescribing medications for the resident and what the medications are and their indications.

- Look for medications with duplicate therapeutic, pharmacologic, or adverse effect profiles.

- Screen for drug–drug and drug–disease interactions.

- Eliminate unnecessary medications; confer with other prescribers if necessary.

- Simplify the medication regimen; use the fewest possible number of medications and doses per day.

- Always review any changes with the resident and caregiver; provide the changes in writing.

and ensure safe medication use. The resident's ability to read labels, open containers, or pour medications or even a glass of water may be impaired; therefore, functional assessment can be useful. Some residents may need additional education or reinforcement about the purpose of a medication, especially those used to treat conditions that are usually asymptomatic, such as diabetes mellitus and hypertension. They also may need reassurance regarding the safety and possible adverse effects of certain medications, particularly newly prescribed medications or those associated with serious adverse events, such as warfarin—and the dietary restrictions that apply. It would be important to estimate the effect of changed food intake on the resident's lifestyle preferences and the likelihood of nonadherence.

EVALUATING A RESIDENT FOR INDEPENDENT MEDICATION MANAGEMENT

There is no gold standard to evaluate a resident for safe, independent medication management. Moreover, the individuals permitted to conduct this evaluation vary by state. In some states, it can be done by any licensed health care provider; in other states it must be a physician. The evaluation should consider the functional ability of the resident (i.e., ability to open the pill bottle) as well as cognitive ability (i.e., ability to remember to take the medication). (See Chapter 10, "Medication Management," for a complete discussion of self-medication, and Chapter 1, "The Assisted Living Setting of Nursing Practice," for a discussion of health literacy.) Decisions about: (a) who can administer injectable medications, (b) who can administer suppositories, topical treatments, or other types of medications, and (c) who can administer *pro re nata* medications varies by state. In some states, unlicensed staff cannot assist with injectable medications (e.g., insulin), inhalers, suppositories or enemas, whereas in other states, assistance is acceptable if the resident is unable to do so independently. (See Chapter 10, "Medication Management," for description of reliable and valid tests/assessment of self-administration ability and discussion of medication administration by unlicensed personnel.)

DELEGATION OF MEDICATION ADMINISTRATION

The Nurse Practice Act stipulates what level of licensed nurse is authorized to delegate, what skilled nursing acts (such as medication administration) can be delegated, and to whom. There are five rights to safe and appropriate delegation: right task, right circumstances, right person, right direction/communication, and right supervision. (See also Chapter 9, "Staffing, Assignments, Delegation, and Time Management.") The nurse is *accountable* for the task that has been delegated; the person to whom the task was delegated (licensed or unlicensed) is *responsible*.

Understanding the normal age-related changes in older adults and how they influence drug absorption, distribution, and elimination is an important first step in safe oversight and administration of medication among AL residents. Knowing and implementing the regulations and guidelines around medication management in AL is the responsibility of the AL manager and delegating nurse. Technology will likely be increasingly used to optimize medication safety and facilitate the administration process, but it will not replace the nurse's knowledge and understanding of the medication being given and the impact of that drug in that specific older adult.

RESOURCES

Fick, D. M., Cooper, J. W., Wade, W. E., Waller, J. L., McClean, R., & Beers, M. H. (2003). Updating the Beers criteria for potentially inappropriate medication use in older adults: Results of a U.S. consensus panel of experts. *Archives of Internal Medicine, 163*(22), 2716–2724.

Goulding, M. R. (2004). Inappropriate medication prescribing for elderly ambulatory care patients. *Archives of Internal Medicine, 164*(3), 305–312.

Gurland, B. J., Cross, P., Chenn, J., Wilder, D. E., Pine, Z. M, Lantigua, R. A., et al. (2004). A new performance test of adaptive cognitive functioning: The Medication Management (MM) test. *International Journal of Geriatric Psychiatry, 9*(11), 875–885.

Gurwitz, J. H., Field, T. S., Harrold, L. R., Rothschild, J., Debellis, K., Seger, A. C., et al. (2003). Incidence and preventability of adverse drug events among older persons in the ambulatory setting. *Journal of the American Medical Association, 289*(9), 1107–1116.

Orwig, D., Brandt, N., & Gruber-Baldini, A. (2006). Medication Management assessment for older adults in the community. *The Gerontologist, 46,* 661–668.

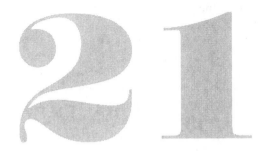

Chronic Pain and Persistent Pain

Jennifer Kapo, Debra K. Weiner, and Barbara Resnick

Pain, defined as an unpleasant sensory and emotional experience, is common in older adults. Chronic or persistent pain, in contrast to acute pain, is pain lasting 3 to 6 months or more after the original injury has healed, pain that is associated with a chronic medical condition, or pain that recurs at intervals of a month to years. Studies indicate that 25% to 50% of community-dwelling older adults and 45% to 80% of long-term care residents have chronic pain. The fact that pain is undertreated is due to several factors: some older adults tend to minimize or not report their symptoms and others are unable to report their pain because of language or cognitive impairments. Clinicians may inadequately assess pain, undertreat it with ineffective therapies, or encounter intolerable adverse effects with more effective therapies.

Chronic pain is complex, involving physical, social, and psychological factors. Untreated, it can result in difficulty performing activities of daily living, cognitive dysfunction, depression, anxiety, social isolation, appetite impairment, and sleep disorders.

ASSESSMENT OF CHRONIC PAIN

Assessment should include an examination of physical, emotional, and social function, recognizing the influence that each of these domains has on the experience of pain and suffering. Since there are no blood tests or im-

aging modalities to measure pain objectively, clinicians must rely on the resident, nursing staff, and family/friends' description of the pain as well as the demonstration of pain noted during a physical examination. It is necessary to identify the specific source of the pain (e.g., hip versus knee) so that it can be treated with the most effective, targeted, and specific treatment. Evaluation is complicated by several challenges, including underreporting of symptoms, existence of multiple medical comorbidities that exacerbate the pain and impair function, and the presence of cognitive impairment.

Initial and ongoing evaluation of pain should include consideration of the character of the pain (e.g., sharp, dull, burning), the course of its onset (e.g., sudden versus slowly worsening over time), duration, and location. The individual should be asked what relieves and what exacerbates his or her pain. Functional status needs to be carefully evaluated to determine ability to perform activities of daily living and instrumental activities of daily living. The resident's cognitive status, participation in social activities, mood, and quality of life are all components of a complete evaluation.

Pain intensity can be quantified using a pain intensity scale. Three commonly used validated scales are the Numeric Rating Scale (NRS), the Verbal Descriptor Scale (VDS), and the Faces Pain Scale (FPS). With the NRS, the individual is asked to rate his or her pain by assigning a numerical value wherein 0 indicates no pain and 10 represents the worst pain imaginable. The

VDS asks the person to describe his or her pain as "no pain" to "pain as bad as it could be." The FPS instructs the person to choose a face (from benign to grimacing) that best corresponds with or more reflects the pain that he or she is feeling. Choice of a scale depends, to some extent, on language comprehension and/or sensory impairment (e.g., vision impairment). For example, if the resident does not speak English well, the faces scale may be the best choice because it relies on pictures rather than words or numbers. The same scale should be used at follow-up examinations to evaluate how the pain has changed since the initial assessment. Physical examination of the older adult should focus on evaluation of the reported site of the pain (arm, shoulder, hip, knee, etc.).

Pain syndromes can be divided into at least three types: *nociceptive, neuropathic,* and *mixed* or unspecified. Nociceptive pain is pain due to trauma or some type of event that causes inflammation, swelling, or injury to the tissues; it can be defined further as either *somatic* or *visceral pain.* Somatic pain is well localized in skin, soft tissue, and bone and is commonly described as throbbing, aching, and stabbing. Visceral pain, due to cardiac, gastrointestinal, and lung injury, is not well localized and has been described as crampy, tearing, dull, and aching. Neuropathic pain, in contrast, is due to irritation in the nervous system (i.e., spinal column vertebrae causing nerve compression or peripheral neuropathy from diabetes) and is typically described as burning, numbness with pins and needles sensations, and shooting pains. Common causes of neuropathic pain include postherpetic neuralgia, poststroke pain, and phantom limb pain experienced following amputation.

Nociceptive pain is often adequately treated with common analgesics. Neuropathic pain responds unpredictably to opioid analgesia; it may respond well to nonopioid therapies such as anticonvulsants, tricyclic antidepressants (TCAs), and antiarrhythmic medications. Confusion between neuropathic pain and myofascial pain is possible, as older adults may describe both as burning. Careful physical examination will help to differentiate these disorders (i.e., taut bands and trigger points with myofascial pain and allodynia (pain from stimuli that are not normally painful) or hyperalgesia (an increased response to painful stimuli); both may exist in the same person.

Mixed or unspecified pain is common among older adults and has characteristics of both nociceptive and neuropathic pain (e.g., chronic headaches of unknown causes). Lower back pain, for example, is often a combination of pain due to musculoskeletal changes and misalignment of the spinal cord, and neurologic impingement due to compression of the vertebrae on nerves exiting the spinal column. Treatment may require trials of different medications or combinations of drugs.

ASSESSING AND TREATING PAIN IN COGNITIVELY IMPAIRED PERSONS

Older adults with mild to moderate dementia are often able to self-report pain and localize it. Those with severe cognitive impairment who are unable to verbally express themselves or express pain pose a challenge to the clinicians who care for them. The evaluation of pain among these individuals must depend on observation of the resident for possible pain. Exhibit 21.1 lists common pain behaviors in cognitively impaired older adults.

TREATMENT

Fundamental Approaches to Pain Treatment

For the older adult, education and involvement in treatment decisions are an important part of all treatment plans for chronic pain. They should be helped and encouraged to take medications for pain regularly. Nonpharmacologic treatments such as heat and cold application, massage therapy, acupuncture, and transcutaneous electrical nerve stimulation (TENS) might be effective. TENS is primarily used to treat nerve-related pain conditions by sending stimulating pulses across the surface of the skin and along the nerve strands. These pulses prevent pain signals from reaching the brain. TENS treatment also helps increase endorphin secretion of the body's own natural painkiller.

Cognitive behavioral therapy (see Chapter 34, "Depression and Other Mood Disorders") may be particularly useful in helping residents learn to cope with the stresses of chronic pain. When possible, family members and caregivers should be included in the therapy.

Regular physical activity can decrease pain, improve mood, improve functionality, and stabilize gait—all of which are associated with chronic pain. This is particularly true of pain due to arthritis as well as that from claudication. Exercise interventions will vary depending on the ability, level, and location of pain. *Non–weight bearing activities* such as swimming or water exercises, aerobics, and the use of a stationary bicycle may be necessary for older adults who are experiencing significant

21.1 | Common Pain Behaviors in Cognitively Impaired Older Adults

BEHAVIOR	EXAMPLES
Facial expressions	Slight frown—sad, frightened face; grimacing—wrinkled forehead, closed or tightened eyes; any distorted expression; and rapid blinking
Verbalizations, vocalizations	Sighing, moaning, groaning; grunting, chanting, calling out; noisy breathing; asking for help; and verbal abusiveness
Body movements	Rigid, tense body posture, guarding; fidgeting; increased pacing, rocking; restricted movement; and gait or mobility changes
Changes in interpersonal interactions	Aggressive, combative, resists care; decreased social interactions; socially inappropriate, disruptive; and withdrawn
Changes in activity patterns or routines	Refusing food, appetite change; increase in rest periods; sleep, rest pattern changes; sudden cessation of common routines; and increased wandering
Mental status changes	Crying or tears; increased confusion; and irritability or distress

Note. Some patients demonstrate little or no specific behavior associated with severe pain.
From "The Management of Persistent Pain in Older Persons," by American Geriatrics Society Panel on Persistent Pain in Older Persons, 2002, *Journal of American Geriatric Society, 50*(6 Suppl.), p. S211. Copyright ©2002 by American Geriatrics Society. Used with permission.

pain from lower extremity arthritis. *Resistance exercise* can strengthen the muscles around painful joints and support those joints. *Flexibility exercises* can improve motion and balance to optimally prevent falls as well as reduce pain (see Chapter 18, "Physical Activity").

Pharmacologic Therapy

Pharmacologic therapy for residents with chronic pain should be viewed not as an end but as a means to promote improved function and support adherence to additional interventions for pain management, such as exercise. When initiating pharmacologic therapy in older adults, it is important to consider the balance of risks and benefits of the treatment. If appropriate, local therapies should be tried first. For example, older adults who primarily have knee pain might respond to intra-articular corticosteroid injections: a direct injection of corticosteroid into the joint. This can decrease inflammation around the joint and relieve pain, without causing any drug side effects from the steroid. Individual

analgesics, their starting doses, and common adverse effects, are listed in Table 21.1.

Myofascial pain is musculoskeletal pain from specific trigger points that are locally tender when active. A trigger point or sensitive, painful area in the muscle or area around the muscle develops because of any number of causes, for example, trauma, repetitive use, excessive exercise, fatigue, or hormonal changes. Effective treatment (i.e., pain relief) is associated with local modalities such as massage, gentle stretching exercises, ultrasound, and trigger-point injections. Topical preparations such as capsaicin gel or lidocaine patches might be effective as primary or adjunctive therapy in treatment for neuropathic or myofascial pain syndromes.

If local treatments are ineffective, the next option is to begin systemic therapy that involves oral or parenteral administration of medications. Close monitoring is needed to ensure that the treatment is effective and adverse effects are minimized. Mild to moderate pain is commonly treated with acetaminophen or cautious use of nonsteroidal anti-inflammatory drugs (NSAIDs).

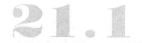

21.1 | Pharmacotherapy for Chronic Pain Management

DRUG	STARTING DOSE	COMMENTS
Acetaminophen (Tylenol)	325 mg q 4 h 500 mg q 6 h	Reduce maximum dose 50%–75% in patients with liver disease or a history of alcohol abuse
Carbamazepine[OL] (Tegretol)	100 mg qd	Monitor liver enzymes, CBC, BUN/Creat., electrolytes
Clonazepam[OL] (Klonopin)	0.25–0.5 mg hs	Monitor sedation, memory, and labs (CBC)
Gabapentin[OL] (Neurontin)	100 mg hs	Monitor sedation, ataxia, edema Approved for post-herpetic neuralgia; not approved for any other types of pain
Pregabalin (Lyrica)	25 mg tid	Monitor resident for dizziness and increased sleeping.
Baclofen[OL] (Lioresal)	5 mg	Monitor resident for muscle weakness, urinary function.
Choline magnesium trisalicylate (Tricosal, Trilisate)	500–750 mg q 8 h	Monitor for ringing in the ear and confusion.
Corticosteroids (prednisone) (e.g., Deltasone, Liquid Pred, Orasone)	5.0 mg qd	Monitor for fluid retention and elevated blood glucose.
Mexiletine[OL] (Mexitil)	150 mg	Avoid use in patients with a slow heart rate and monitor heart rate while on the medication
Tricyclic antidepressants: desipramine[OL] (Norpramin), nortriptyline[OL] (Aventyl, Pamelor)	10 mg hs	Significant risk of adverse effects in older patients; anticholinergic effects
Hydrocodone (e.g., Lorcet, Lortab, Vicodin, Vicoprofen)	5 mg q 4–6 h	Useful for acute recurrent, episodic, or breakthrough pain; monitor for side effects common with opioids
Hydromorphone (Dilaudid, Hydrostat)	2 mg q 3–4 h	For breakthrough pain; monitor for side effects common with opioids
Morphine, immediate release (e.g., MSIR, Roxanol)	2.5–10 mg q 4 h	Oral liquid concentrate recommended for breakthrough pain. Monitor for side effects common with opioids
Morphine, sustained release (e.g., MSContin, Kadian)	15 mg q 12 h	Monitor for side effects common with opioids
Oxycodone, immediate release (OxyIR)	5 mg q 4–6 h	Monitor for side effects common with opioids

(continued)

21.1   Pharmacotherapy for Chronic Pain Management *(continued)*

DRUG	STARTING DOSE	COMMENTS
Oxycodone, sustained release (OxyContin)	10 mg q 12 h	Monitor for side effects common with opioids
Tramadol (Ultram)	25 mg q 4–6 h	Monitor resident for serotonin syndrome when used with another serotonergic drug; monitor for seizures as Ultram lowers the seizure threshold.
Transdermal fentanyl (Duragesic)	25 μg/h patch q 72 h	Monitor for side effects common with opioids.

Note: ASA = acetylsalicylic acid; bid = twice daily; BUN = blood urea nitrogen; CBC = complete blood cell count; CNS = central nervous system; CrCl = creatinine clearance; Creat. = serum creatinine; CV = cardiovascular; DEA = U.S. Drug Enforcement Agency; ECG = electrocardiogram; FDA = U.S. Food and Drug Administration; GI = gastrointestinal; h = hour; hs = at bedtime; NA = not applicable; NSAIDs = nonsteroidal anti-inflammatory drugs; q = each, every; qd = daily; qid = four times daily; tid = three times daily.

Acetaminophen provides adequate analgesia for many mild to moderate pain syndromes, particularly musculoskeletal pain. No more than 4 grams (4,000 mg) of acetaminophen every 24 hours should be administered to older adults with normal hepatic and renal function, given the risk of liver toxicity. Caution should be taken when treating older adults with known liver disease and with those who have a history of heavy alcohol intake. In these older adults, the acetaminophen dose should be lowered by 50%.

NSAIDs are effective drugs for treatment of mild to moderate pain, particularly when the pain is due to inflammation such as occurs in muscles and bones after a fall. However, NSAID use can result in significant adverse effects, including renal dysfunction, gastrointestinal (GI) bleeding, impaired platelet function (i.e., decreased clotting ability), fluid retention, elevated blood pressure, and delirium. COX-2 inhibitors (i.e., nonsteroidal anti-inflammatory drugs such as celebrex) were developed to decrease the risk of GI bleeding, but they do not decrease the other potential risks associated with NSAIDs. Currently, older adults should receive a proton-pump inhibitor (i.e., drugs, such as prilosec or prevacid, that decrease acid production) to protect them from GI irritation and bleeding if they are taking NSAIDs, even for a short period of time.

Moderate to severe pain or pain that is not relieved by acetaminophen or an NSAID may need to be treated with opioid medications to provide sufficient relief. In general, continuous pain should be treated with a long-acting (24-hour) pain medication. A long-acting drug can be combined with a fast-onset medication with a short half-life to cover pain that breaks through the pain control of the longer-acting medication. All opioids provide similar analgesic efficacy. The cost of the medication and route of delivery can help guide the choice of medication.

Opioids are metabolized (broken down) by the liver and excreted (removed from the body) via the kidney. In kidney failure, the active components of morphine can accumulate, thus placing the older adult at increased risk for prolonged sedation. The dosing intervals should be increased or the dose lowered to reduce this risk in individuals with known kidney impairment.

Barriers to Using Opioids in Older Persons

Older adults (and their families) may have concerns about drug addiction that keep them from accepting adequate treatment for their pain. They may fear that opioid therapy for their current level of pain will result in the drugs' diminished effectiveness in the future when their pain becomes more severe. Physical dependence is an expected change in physiology when an older adult is receiving chronic, continuous opioid medication therapy. If opioids are discontinued suddenly, the physically dependent older adult will experience a withdrawal syndrome that can include restlessness, tachycardia, hypertension, fever, tremors, and lacrimation (excessive tearing of the eyes). These symptoms can be avoided, however, by tapering opioids carefully over days to weeks. *Tolerance* is a physiologic change resulting in the need to increase the dosage of opioid medicines over time to achieve adequate pain relief. There is limited cross-tolerance between different opioids, however, which means it is important to monitor the resident closely if his or her pain medication is switched from one opioid to another (e.g., morphine to oxycodone).

Psychological *dependence,* or true *addiction,* is a psychiatric state characterized by compulsive drug seeking and drug using with disregard for adverse social, physical, and economic consequences. It is very rare for older adults with chronic/persistent pain to become addicted to opioids. Addiction must be distinguished from *pseudo-addiction,* which occurs when a person with unrelieved pain adopts behaviors similar to those of truly addicted persons while seeking relief from pain.

Adverse Effects of Opioids

The most common adverse effect of opioid treatment is constipation, and this is due to multiple mechanisms, including dehydration, decreased GI tract secretions, and decreased motility of the GI tract. Although tolerance develops fairly rapidly to other adverse effects of opioids, such as respiratory depression and sedation, constipation usually complicates opioid use for the duration of treatment. Education regarding the probable need for a laxative is recommended for all individuals at the time opioid therapy is initiated. Simultaneously starting opioid treatment with a stimulant laxative (such as bisacodyl or senna) is the most effective way to avoid opioid-induced constipation. Several new laxatives specifically to treat opioid-induced constipation (e.g., methylnaltrexone and alvimopan) are purportedly effective, but they are expensive and methylnaltrexone has to be given subcutaneously.

Nausea and vomiting are common side effects of opioids. Opioids cause nausea because they have a direct effect on the part of the brain associated with the sensation of vomiting called the chemoreceptor trigger zone. Other common causes of nausea and vomiting include gastroparesis (i.e., slow movement of the GI tract), constipation, and renal and hepatic failure. Although the nausea and vomiting is usually self-limited to the first few doses, some individuals experience chronic, persistent nausea. After evaluation for reversible causes of nausea such as constipation, some individuals might benefit

from changing to an alternative opioid; others may need to be treated with chronic anti-emetics for the nausea.

Older adults might experience sedation, fatigue, and cognitive impairment with opioid treatment. The fatigue and sedation might be overcome over days to weeks as the person becomes tolerant to the medication. However, older adults need to be monitored closely for the risks of falls during the initial early treatment period. Some residents treated with opioids will experience persistent fatigue that limits their function significantly. In these cases, a different opioid could be tried as an alternative strategy.

Respiratory depression is a feared complication of opioid therapy. Older persons and those with a history of lung dysfunction are at particular risk when opioid doses are increased too rapidly. Naloxone, an opioid receptor antagonist, can reverse opioid-induced respiratory depression. Naloxone is generally not given unless the person's respiratory rate decreases to less than eight breaths per minute.

The principle of double effect, also known as the doctrine or rule of double effect (DBE) or the principle of secondary effect or unintentional effect is a set of ethical criteria. Nurses caring for people who are clearly dying and in extremis (e.g., pain, difficulty breathing) need to know that pain and symptom relief in exceptional circumstances is an ethical requirement of practice. First articulated by Thomas Aquinas, the principle holds that when a legitimate act, such as the relief of intractable pain, unintentionally causes what would ordinarily be impermissible, the person's death, that action is morally acceptable. When an action, such as administration of a high dosage opioid (e.g., morphine sulfate) has a known and foreseeable harmful effect that is almost inseparable from its beneficial effect, the action is justified if the nature of the act itself is good, that is, beneficial. The good effect is intended: to relieve pain (beneficence) and prevent further pain (i.e., nonmaleficence). The agent administering the medication—not uncommonly a nurse following a physician's orders—intended the good effect, not the bad—either as a means to the good end or as an end in and of itself.

Nonopioid Medication to Treat Chronic Pain

Nonopioid medications can also be tried either alone or in combination with opioids to manage chronic pain. These medications may be particularly useful in treating older adults with neuropathic pain or mixed pain syndromes. TCAs are the most commonly used medications for neuropathic pain, although this is changing to include the use of selective serotonin reuptake inhibitors (SSRIs) and neuroleptics (anti-epileptic medications). Studies report that TCAs are helpful in pain management particularly with regard to post-herpetic neuralgia (persistent pain following shingles). Unfortunately, TCAs are also associated with significant anticholinergic adverse effects in older adults, including constipation, urinary retention, dry mouth, cognitive impairment, tachycardia, and blurred vision. SSRIs are increasingly being used to manage chronic pain and the associated depression. Duloxetine, for example, which is an SSRI, is FDA approved as both an antidepressant *and* for the treatment of pain from diabetic neuropathy.

Antiepileptic drugs such as carbamazepine, gabapentin, and clonazepam are also commonly used to treat neuropathic pain. Gabapentin has demonstrated clinical efficacy in the treatment of post-herpetic neuralgia, and it has considerably fewer adverse effects than TCAs, although it costs substantially more. The main side effects of gabapentin are sedation and dizziness.

Corticosteroids are useful adjuvants to treat pain associated with swelling, inflammation, and tissue infiltration, as well as neuropathic pain. In addition to their analgesic properties, they can also increase appetite and improve energy. Adverse effects occurring with short-term use of steroids include confusion and psychosis, fluid retention, hair loss, loss of skin integrity, hyperglycemia, and immunosuppression.

Medications to Avoid in Older Persons

Several medications for pain relief should not be administered to older adults. Propoxyphene (Darvon) is an older opioid medication used to treat mild to moderate pain. Research and clinical experience has shown that the drug can accumulate and cause ataxia (i.e., impaired coordination) and dizziness as well as tremulousness and seizures. In addition, it has never been shown to be a more effective analgesic than a placebo medication. Meperidine (Demerol) is metabolized to normeperidine, a substance that has no analgesic properties but that can accumulate in residents with decreased kidney function and cause tremulousness and seizures. Neither of these medications is recommended for use in older persons.

Tramadol (Ultram) is being used increasingly in the management of acute and chronic pain in older adults. It can, however, lower the seizure threshold and is therefore not recommended for residents with a history of seizures or taking other medications that could lower the seizure threshold, such as SSRIs prescribed for depression. When taken together, these drugs can cause so-called serotonin syndrome (i.e., myoclonus, agitation, abdominal cramping, hyperpyrexia, hypertension, and potentially death). (See Chapter 34, "Depression and Other Mood Disorders".)

RESOURCES

American Geriatrics Society Panel on Persistent Pain in Older Persons. (2002). The management of persistent pain in older persons. *Journal of American Geriatric Society, 50*(6 Suppl.), S205–S224.
American medical directors clinical practice guideline: Pain management in the long term care setting. (n.d.). Retrieved November 3, 2008, from http://www.amda.com/tools/guidelines.cfm
National Guidelines Clearinghouse. (n.d.). *Pain management guideline.* Retrieved from http://www.guideline.gov/summary/summary.aspx?ss=15&doc_id=9744&nbr=5217

Syndromes

Geriatric syndromes are a group of related medical problems that the older adult experiences. Syndromes include such things as vision and hearing problems, urinary incontinence, dizziness, falls, delirium (i.e., acute confusion), sleep problems, and pressure ulcers. Geriatric syndromes usually have multiple causes and often involve several different body systems. A pres-sure ulcer, for example, may be due to poor circulation, changes in the musculoskeletal or neurological system, and changes in the skin. This section addresses some of the common geriatric syndromes and provides informa-tion about how to evaluate residents for these problems and how to prevent or manage them.

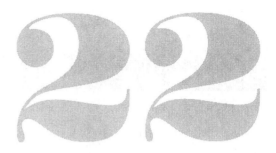

Visual Impairment

David Sarraf, Anne L. Coleman,
and Anne Scheve

Every aspect of life is linked to vision: relationships with others, navigating through the environment, the ability to perform activities of daily living, and staying safe and well. Most older adults experience changes in their vision that can negatively influence their ability to manage activities of daily living, to remain independent, and to engage in relationships—all aspects or values associated with quality of life. Falls, motor vehicle accidents, and other safety issues also are associated with impaired vision in older adults.

Visual impairment is defined as visual acuity less than 20/40. Typically, impairment increases with age, affecting 20% to 30% of those age 75 years or older. Blindness, defined as visual acuity of 20/200 or worse, affects 2% of those age 75 years and older. Among the blind population, 50% are age 65 or older. Presbyopia, cataracts, age-related macular degeneration, and glaucoma are the most common causes for vision loss commonly seen in the older adult population.

Normal age-related changes affect various structures of the eye (Table 22.1). The cornea, which allows light into the eye, becomes opaque and yellow with age; the lens increases in size and density resulting in increased stiffness and opacity; the iris (i.e., the eye muscle that regulates the amount of light that reaches the retina) becomes more rigid. Increased rigidity of the iris results in reduction of the size of the pupil thus interfering with the ability to respond to changes in light. The ciliary body that surrounds the lens of the eye is responsible for accommodation, the process that controls the abil-

ity to focus on near objects. With age, the ciliary body becomes stiffer and does not function as well resulting in loss of the ability to focus clearly on nearby objects. Taken together, age-related changes result in decreased visual acuity, decreased ability to respond to a dark environment, increased sensitivity to glare and a delayed ability to recover from glare, narrowing of the visual field, diminished depth perception, a decreased ability to focus on near objects, and altered color perception.

Presbyopia, decrease in near vision, is considered a normal age-related change: the eye cannot change the shape of the lens to focus on near objects, like print in a magazine; there is reduced ability to adapt to light (see Table 22.1).

DISEASES

Cataracts

Cataracts are a clouding of the crystalline lens and may cause blurred vision, lack of color contrast, and poor night vision (Figure 22.1). Untreated cataracts can cause a progressive yet painless loss of vision. More than 50% of older adults have cataracts. Cataracts can occur in one or both eyes. Risk factors include smoking, alcohol use, ultraviolet (UV) light exposure, diabetes, and hypertension. Surgical removal and lens implant (done on an outpatient basis) is effective and well tolerated in the majority of individuals; it is Medicare covered.

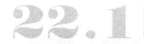 | Age-Related Changes to the Eye and the Effect on Vision

STRUCTURE	AGE-RELATED CHANGE	AFFECT ON VISION
Skin surrounding the eye	Increased thinning Decreased elasticity	Cosmetic Increased wrinkles (i.e., crow's feet)
Cornea	Increased opacity and yellowing	Decreased amount of light entering the eye Increased glare Altered color perception Decreased ability to focus on near objects
Lens	Increased size, density, stiffness, and opacity	Decreased light to the retina Diminished accommodation
Iris	Increased rigidity	Decreased ability to respond to changes in light and decreased acuity
Ciliary body	Increased stiffness	Narrowing of the visual field and increased sensitivity to glare

Age-Related Macular Degeneration (ARMD)

ARMD, the leading cause of central vision loss (and blindness) in older adults is the progressive accumulation of Drusen particles (i.e., submacular, extracellular, yellow deposits composed of by-products of metabolism). Risk factors include family history of ARMD, smoking and UV light exposure. ARMD is wet or dry. Dry ARMD is much more common and is characterized by deposits of Drusen under the macula. Drusen do not typically cause vision loss but are a marker for the wet form of ARMD characterized by angiogenesis or choroidal neovascularization (CNV) (i.e., new growth of blood vessels that cause a subsequent block in vision). The presence of larger, more numerous Drusen conveys the greatest risk for the development of CNV. Residents who develop sudden distortion or vision loss, signaling the development of CNV, require urgent evaluation. Severe vision loss or central visual blindness is usually caused by the wet form of ARMD identified by the presence of CNV.

The risk of development of CNV can be decreased by 25% when patients with high-risk Drusen are treated with high-dose oral multivitamin therapy containing beta-carotene 25,000 IU, vitamin E 400 IU, vitamin C 500 mg, and zinc 80 mg. This vitamin therapy, however, is contraindicated in smokers because of the risk of lung cancer in smokers who take beta-carotene sup-plements. The determination of Drusen risk as high or low is based on testing by the ophthalmologist. Slowing ARMD's progression from the intermediate stage to the advanced stage will save the vision of many people (*Facts About Age-Related Macular Degeneration*, 2008). Effective therapies also include laser treatments and phototherapy. Most recently, various types of inhibitors to vascular endothelial growth factor (VEGF) have been developed and approved for use by the Food and Drug Administration (FDA) for treatment of the wet form of ARMD. VEGF is administered via serial intravitreal injections, the need for which is based on the individual's response to treatment.

Glaucoma

Glaucoma, another progressive disease that leads to peripheral vision loss, is the second most common cause of blindness and the most common cause of blindness in African Americans. It is defined as optic nerve head damage and visual field loss. Elevated intraocular pressure (IOP) is no longer considered an absolute criterion, although it is a very important risk factor. Other risk factors include family history of glaucoma, African American heritage, diabetes, and hypertension. A variety of IOP-lowering medications in eye drop form and oral medications are available (see Figure 22.2).

Figure 22.1 Anatomy of the eye.

NURSING ASSESSMENT OF VISION CHANGES

It is important to assess vision and monitor for changes in vision over time. The goal of the nursing assessment is to identify risk factors for vision impairment, prevent further vision loss, and optimize function. In addition, as appropriate, nurses should encourage older adults to have an annual ophthalmologic exam every 1 to 2 years, and perhaps sooner if there are risk factors for eye disease, *and* at any time a change in vision is noted. The eye exam is a health promotion/disease prevention intervention that helps ensure that early problems can be identified and progression of eye disease prevented. Components of the nursing assessment include the following:

■ Observation of the resident's appearance and ability to negotiate the environment. Clues that vision may be diminished include wearing soiled clothing or relying on hands (instead of vision) to find objects.
■ Health history (several diseases can predispose older adults to vision impairments like diabetes and hypertension—both of which are leading causes of blindness due to retinopathy).
■ Vision history questions: date of last exam, vision difficulties, pain, dryness, use of glasses or contact lenses, and any recent change in vision.
■ Driving habits and any problems driving, especially at night. Many older adults fear losing their ability (and what they perceive as a right) to drive and may not answer truthfully. Ask a family member about the older adult's driving.

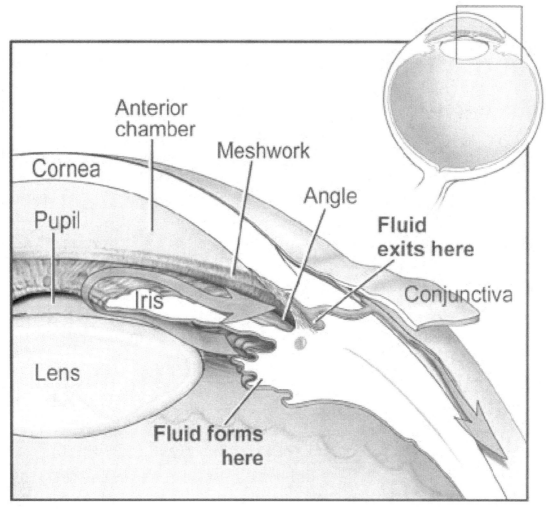

Figure 22.2   Glaucoma.

- Fall history in the past year.
- Eye examination including a general inspection of the eye: look for symmetry, proper eyelid alignment, and pupil focus.
- To assess vision:
  - ☐ Snellen Eye Chart: an accurate method to assess visual acuity. Instruct the older adult to stand 20 feet away from the mounted wall chart and cover one eye with an index card. Ask the person to read the line of print with the smallest letters that he or she can. If the older adult wears glasses, they can be on, except for reading glasses. Repeat with the other eye. Each line of print on the Snellen Eye Chart has a number assigned to it. The line of print that can be read correctly is the numerator of the vision score and the distance of 20 feet is the denominator. Therefore, if the resident can read line number 20 at the distance of 20 feet, visual acuity is 20/20.
  - ☐ The Near Vision Test measures the ability to read written material at normal distance. It is an important screening test since it can provide information as to whether or not the older adult can read medication bottle labels and written health care instructions. The Light House for the Blind (http://www. lighthouse.org) offers preprinted Near Vision Test screening cards with different size fonts, with instructions for the clinician. If these cards are not available, simply ask the resident to read from a magazine held about 14 inches away. Direct him

or her to cover one eye with an index card; test the other eye. Follow up is necessary if the older adult had difficulty reading at that distance. However, a literacy problem cannot be ruled out and needs to be checked. Presbyopia, the decreased ability to accommodate to near objects, is suspected if the older adult needs to move the card or magazine farther away.

NURSING INTERVENTIONS

Nursing interventions include identifying modifiable risk factors for vision loss, like sun exposure, cigarette smoking, hypertension, and diabetes, and establishing achievable goals with the resident to reduce these threats. Interventions focused on achievable goals include behaviors that the resident believes he/she can and wants to accomplish.

- Wearing protective UVA and UVB sunglasses while outside can limit damaging sun rays.
- Develop a smoking cessation program that the older adult believes he/she can follow.
- Control blood sugar and blood pressure.
- Educate the older adult on the importance of continuing the regimen for chronic eye disease management like eye drops for glaucoma.
- Encourage the older adult to schedule an annual dilated exam from an ophthalmologist and reiterate the importance of notifying his or her primary care provider of any acute change in vision.

Inform older adults and their families about the many resources and groups that can provide information about vision loss. Recommendations to modify the visual environment to maintain independence and maximize function are imperative. These include the following:

- Good lighting (increases in wattage to the recently available 170-watt incandescent lamps with ultra-high diffusion coatings to soften the light and minimize glare are an ideal lighting source)
- Encouragement and reminding to use eyeglasses and magnifiers
- Motion sensors to turn lights on when entering a room—or placing the light switch outside the room entrance
- Looking for areas where lighting is inconsistent and correcting the problem; shadows and dark areas can obscure objects and hazards

- Avoidance of glare (associated with highly polished floors or reflective surfaces); prevent glare with lamp shades and sheer curtains
- Using high contrast colors for signage and written instructions in large print that the resident can see
- Using extra lighting (as per previous recommendation) when working or reading
- Avoiding rugs with patterns to avoid visual clutter, which provides superfluous visual stimulation and is actually distracting
- Using bright/contrasting color tape or paint on step edges to signal that it is a step and change in orientation
- Low vision aids are available; investigate what works best for each person

SAFETY INTERVENTIONS

Safety issues are a major concern with vision loss. Motor vehicle accidents are the leading cause of accidental death in those 65 years and older. Therefore, it is very important to have vision screened and driving evaluated regularly. Most states require periodic vision screens for license renewal; few if any require a road test to renew a driver's license. Some states offer a driving safety course and evaluation for older drivers. AARP also offers a driving safety course. If concerned about the safety of the resident with visual impairment who is driving not willing to give it up, an option is to contact the Department of Motor Vehicles and have them pursue additional testing.

Falls are the leading cause of accidental death after age 75 and are associated with visual loss. Conduct a fall history and perform a falls risk assessment, physical performance maneuvers, and implement fall precautions (see Chapter 28, "Falls").

RESOURCES

Facts about age-related macular degeneration. (2008). Retrieved August 26, 2008, from http://www.nei.nih.gov/health/maculardegen/armd_facts.asp

Gorman, B. D. (2008). Glaucoma: Preventing the visual damage. *Cortlandt Forum, 21*(4), 21–24.

Gragoudas, E. S., Adamis, A. P., Cunningham, E. T., Jr., et al. (2004). Pegaptanib for neovascular age-related macular degeneration. *New England Journal of Medicine, 351*(27), 2805–2816.

Whiteside, M. M., Wallhagen, M. I., & Pettengill, E. (2006). A new look at the old. Sensory impairment in older adults: Part 2: Vision loss . . . 15th in a series. *American Journal of Nursing, 106*(11), 52–62.

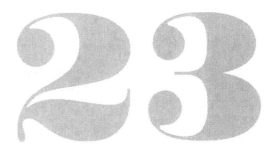

Hearing Impairment

Priscilla Faith Bade and Anne Scheve

Hearing, the process of decoding sounds, can change with aging. Hearing loss is reported to be the third most common chronic disease that affects older adults and can have a devastating influence on quality of life. Social isolation, loss of self-esteem, anger, and depression have been attributed to hearing loss. It has been suggested, as well, that there is an association between hearing loss and cognitive impairment, reduced mobility, and safety.

Factors in the environment and medication can predispose an older adult to hearing loss. Nursing assessments and interventions that promote improved hearing, communication, and maximizing function are discussed in this chapter.

HEARING AND AGE-RELATED CHANGES

The ear is divided into four parts, each of which plays a role in hearing. The outer ear collects and channels sound to the tympanic membrane. Cerumen, or earwax, lubricates the ear and facilitates the movement of sound. Age-related changes in the outer ear can interfere with hearing; specifically, there is an increase in cerumen production. The cerumen becomes drier because of decreased sweat gland activity, increased keratin, and longer and thicker hair in the outer ear; this makes it more difficult to expel the cerumen. As such, cerumen can become a mechanical barrier blocking the tympanic membrane and inhibiting sound vibrations to proceed to the middle ear.

The middle ear begins at the *tympanic membrane,* whose primary function is to transmit sound vibrations.

With age, the tympanic membrane becomes stiffer and thicker, decreasing the ability to transmit vibrations. Three small bones in the middle ear—the ossicles— are also responsible for passing vibrations through to the inner ear. The ossicles become calcified because of changes in the bone with aging, which results in a decrease in vibration transmission. In addition, muscles in the middle ear that are responsible for filtering out background noise become weak and stiff and thus make it more difficult to hear sounds.

The inner ear, the third part of the ear, contains the *cochlea* that contains the sensory organ for hearing: the organ of Corti. When the vibrations from the ossicles activate the tiny hair cells of the organ of Corti, it releases chemical messengers that excite the hearing nerves that carry sound to the brain. Reduced blood supply, reduced hair cells, and reduced neurons—all age-related changes—diminish the ability to hear.

The fourth part of the ear is the central auditory system. This is a complex network of neural pathways in the brain responsible for sound localization, speech discrimination in noisy listening situations, and other complex tasks. Normal age changes such as the loss of auditory receptors, the hair cells, results in profound changes in the structure and function of the central auditory system.

Risk Factors for Hearing Loss

In addition to age-related changes in the structure and physiology of the ear, many risk factors contribute to hearing loss in the older adult. These include heredity, the environment, lifestyle choices, and medications. Identifying the most significant preventable risks to hearing and establishing goals to reduce these threats should be part of the nursing plan of care.

Some older adults may be predisposed to hearing loss by virtue of genetics. Several genes have been linked to the ability to hear and are necessary for the production and function of sensory hair cells. Researchers have identified ways to stimulate regrowth of hair cells damaged by age-related processes. Many experts believe that this may be the key to reversing hearing loss. While genetic predisposition to hearing loss is not controllable, other risk factors can be modified to prevent further hearing loss.

The most prevalent environmental risk factor for impaired hearing is noise exposure. A lifetime of noise exposure can cause significant hearing loss. Both the decibel (i.e., loudness) and exposure time contribute to hearing loss. According to the Better Hearing Organization's Noise Thermometer, 2 hours of listening to loud music (defined as a noise level of 90dB[A]) on a head set can cause hearing loss.

Cigarette smoking or second-hand smoke is another modifiable risk factor that is associated with hearing loss. Certain chemicals in cigarette smoke are believed to break down the fine hair cells of the inner ear and result in hearing loss. The ability to hear high-pitched sounds, such as smoke detectors, is particularly important from a safety perspective.

Many medications can contribute to hearing loss; more than 130 drugs are reported to be potentially *ototoxic* and can cause either permanent or temporary structural damage in the inner ear. Among the drugs known to cause permanent damage are the aminoglycoside antibiotics and the cancer chemotherapeutic agents cisplatin and carboplatin. Those known to cause temporary damage are salicylate analgesics, quinine, and loop diuretics. In some instances, exposure to damaging noise while taking certain drugs will increase their ototoxicity.

Types of Hearing Loss

Three types of hearing loss are commonly seen in the older adult.

- Sensorineural hearing deficit is a common hearing loss due to damage to the inner ear, the cochlea, or the fibers of the eighth cranial nerve (the vestibulocochlear nerve). Causes of sensorineural hearing loss include: hereditary risk, viral or bacterial infections,

trauma, tumors, noise exposure, cardiovascular conditions, ototoxic drugs, and Ménière's disease.
- Presbycusis, a form of sensorineural hearing loss, is the most common age-related hearing deficit. It causes difficulty hearing high-pitched sounds like s, z, sh, and ch. Background noise further aggravates this hearing deficit and makes it more difficult to hear and interpret what is being said.
- Conductive hearing loss, commonly seen in older adults, involves the outer and/or middle ear. Sound is unable to travel to the inner ear. Conductive hearing loss can be caused by cerumen impactions (the most common and reversible cause of conductive hearing loss) or obstructions from foreign bodies, ruptured eardrum, otitis media, and otosclerosis.

Evaluation of Hearing

While working with older adults, nurses can often pick up behavioral cues that suggest hearing loss, such as inappropriate answers to questions, not following directions, or turning an ear toward the speaker. Many times, however, family members are the first ones to complain about hearing loss. They often report being frustrated trying to talk with their family member or complain that the television volume is too loud.

When hearing loss is reported or suspected, a nursing assessment is indicated. The Hearing Handicap Inventory for the Elderly takes about 5 minutes to administer, is valid and reliable, is easy to use, and assesses the effect of hearing impairment on common activities of daily living.

Since hearing loss can affect so many aspects of human interaction with people and the environment, it is important to explore with the older adult the impact of hearing loss on her quality of life. In what way(s) does her hearing loss prevent her for doing or enjoying the things she likes to do (e.g., listening to music; conversation; going to a movie)?

Several other assessment techniques can also be done to assess hearing loss. Before beginning these assessments it is important to create a quiet environment by bringing the person into a quiet room. The Whisper Test is a simple test to administer. Place a finger over the right ear and then use a staccato like motion to open and close the right ear while whispering three unrelated words (e.g., pen, watch, and ring) into the left ear. Normally, an older adult who does not have hearing loss should be able to hear these three words. The inability to discriminate the words may suggest hearing loss and the need for further evaluation.

INTERVENTION

Most older adults with hearing loss are treated with communication strategies and/or amplification.

- Eliminate background noise.
- Rephrase sentences; avoid complex statements and words that are polysyllabic.
- Face the person directly.
- Be sure that vision is also optimized (e.g., eye glasses).
- Use print communication to augment verbal communication.
- Use nonverbal body language to supplement verbal communication. For example, if you would like the person to sit in a chair, point to the specific chair you would like him to sit in or demonstrate sitting in the chair.
- Slow the rate of speech and speak in lower tones.

Technology and Hearing Loss

Assistive listening devices are small portable amplifiers that are not personalized and can be used by different people. They are usually battery operated and inexpensive. These devices are useful when trying to facilitate communicating with the older adult with hearing loss during interactions such as when obtaining a history and teaching nursing interventions.

For some persons with hearing impairment, a personal amplifier may be more useful than hearing aids. These pocket-sized devices are considerably less expensive than hearing aids. Headphones, although they may be more visible to others, stay on the head better and distribute sound between the two ears better than earbuds. The volume and microphone placement of the amplifier should be adjusted to find the best combination for a given user. Television listening devices can spare others from overly loud volume levels and enable the older adult with hearing loss to enjoy their TV programs without annoying others. Vibrating and flashing devices such as alarm clocks and timers, smoke alarms, doorbell alerts, and motion sensors can improve the hearing-impaired person's convenience and safety. These items can be purchased from catalog retailers of assistive listening devices.

State agencies for deaf and hard-of-hearing persons might provide amplified telephones, vibrating and flashing ringer alert devices, and text telephones (TTY) at no cost to hearing-impaired persons. Maryland, for example, offers a range of functional telephone equipment, from amplified phones to alerting emergency devices, through their Department of Information Technology, Assistive Telecommunication Equipment. This type of equipment is also available from electronics and telephone equipment stores.

An audiologist can more comprehensively evaluate hearing loss and determine what type of hearing aid might be best for the individual. Depending on the type of hearing loss, Medicare might pay for the hearing evaluation with an audiologist. *Hearing aids* are the most common form of amplification; they often improve ability to understand speech, particularly soft speech and conversational loud speech. Optimizing hearing may prevent the development of isolation and depression, and the labeling of an individual as confused or cognitively impaired because of misunderstandings associated with impaired hearing and communication. There are many different types of hearing aids available today. Many factors need to be considered in deciding whether or not to fit the person with a hearing aid. In addition to the nature and degree of hearing loss, motivation and ability to adapt to and physically manipulate the aid, degree of social support, and ability to afford the device must be considered.

Generally, two hearing aids are more beneficial than one. The first aid provides the most gain; the second one helps with speech discrimination and with localizing the source of sounds. In the presence of asymmetrical hearing loss or significant difficulty in understanding competing speech, it is possible that the older adult may receive greater benefit from a single hearing aid.

Unfortunately, not everyone benefits from a hearing aid. The type of sensorineural damage may mean that speech discrimination is poor even with amplification. Some older adults are unable to tolerate the placement of the hearing aid in the ear. Individuals with dementia may remove and lose the aid. It is important to be sure that the aid can be returned during an initial trial period, usually 30 days, without having to pay the full cost. Currently about 10 states and the District of Columbia have a 30-day trial period. It is equally important not to give up on the aid too soon, since the audiologist often can adjust it to improve comfort and sound quality. The audiologist should provide counseling for its optimum use.

Many different styles of hearing aids are available. Behind-the-ear and mini-behind-the-ear aids are connected directly to an ear mold that is customized to fit each person's ear. All-in-the-ear aids, in-the-canal, and completely-in-the-canal aids have the advantage of fitting closely to the ear drum and thus need less power to work and thereby produce less chance of feedback sound. The smaller hearing aids may have remote controls. Selection of aid style for each individual depends on the degree of hearing loss, available features, and the person's dexterity and motivation.

The choice of analog or digital hearing aids depends on the individual consumer. Analog hearing aids amplify speech and noise indiscriminately, although they may have features and adjustments that can modify the sounds differentially. Until recently, this was the basic technology of hearing aids. The analog aid is generally less expensive, but it cannot be reprogrammed if hearing changes over time. However, the digital technology hearing aid has improved sound quality, reduced size, and increased ability to customize the amplification of the aid to the needs of the user.

Older adults with profound hearing loss who gain little or no benefit from hearing aids may benefit from a *cochlear implant*: an electronic device that bypasses the function of damaged or absent cochlear hair cells by providing electrical stimulation to cochlear nerve fibers. A receiver-stimulator and an intracochlear electrode array are surgically implanted. A headset is worn behind the ear. The headset microphone transmits signals to the speech processor, which filters and digitizes the sound into coded signals. The coded signals are sent to the cochlear implant, which then stimulates auditory nerve fibers in the cochlea. Nerve signals are then sent through the auditory system to the brain. Going through a cochlear implant involves being able to safely tolerate general anesthesia and to participate in extensive preimplant testing and postimplant training. The procedure is covered by Medicare. In general, outcomes of cochlear implantation in persons age 65 and older have been comparable to those of younger adults, with patients obtaining excellent results by both audiologic and quality-of-life measures.

Despite the potential improvements that older adults can achieve in hearing when using hearing aids, many refuse to consider or utilize these devices for the following reasons:

■ Hearing aids are expensive, and even though Medicare pays for hearing evaluations they do not pay

for hearing aids. Some federal programs such as the Department of Veterans Affairs pay for hearing aids, depending on the recipient's eligibility for services.
■ Indiscriminate amplification of background noise is louder as well as conversations. Whistling sounds occur typically from feedback.
■ Friends who have hearing aids may recount negative experiences.
■ Ego and embarrassment can also be a factor.

RESOURCES

Beisel, K., Hansen, L., Soukup, G., & Fritzsch, B. (2008). Regenerating cochlear hair cells: Quo vadis stem cell. *Cell and Tissue Research, 333*(3), 373–379.

BHI: Noise thermometer poster. (2004). Retrieved August 26, 2008, from http://www.betterhearing.org/hearing_loss_prevention/noisethermometer.cfm

Hallberg, L. R., Hallberg, U., & Kramer, S. E. (2008). Self-reported hearing difficulties, communication strategies and psychological general well-being (quality of life) in patients with acquired hearing impairment. *Disability and Rehabilitation, 30*(3), 203–212.

Hearing aids. (2007). Retrieved August 26, 2008, from http://www.nidcd.nih.gov/health/hearing/hearingaid.asp

Horwitz, A. R., Ahlstrom, J. B., & Dubno, J. R. (2008). Factors affecting the benefits of high-frequency amplification. *Journal of Speech, Language and Hearing Research, 51*(3), 798–813.

Meister, H., Walger, M., Brehmer, D., Wedel, U. C., & von Wedel, H. (2008). The relationship between pre-fitting expectations and willingness to use hearing aids. *International Journal of Audiology, 47*(4), 153–159.

Noise-induced hearing loss. (2008). Retrieved August 26, 2008, from http://www.nidcd.nih.gov/health/hearing/noise.asp

Orabi, A. A., Mawman, D., Al-Zoubi, F., Saeed, S. R., & Ramsden, R. T. (2006). Cochlear implant outcomes and quality of life in the elderly: Manchester experience over 13 years. *Clinical Otolaryngology, 31*(2), 116–122.

Sumi, E., Takechi, H., Wada, T., Ishine, M., Wakatsuki, Y., Murayama, T., et al. (2006). Comprehensive geriatric assessment for outpatients is important for the detection of functional disabilities and depressive symptoms associated with sensory impairment as well as for the screening of cognitive impairment. *Geriatrics and Gerontology International, 6*(2), 94–100.

Wallhagen, M. I., Pettengill, E., & Whiteside, M. (2006). Sensory impairment in older adults: Part 1: Hearing loss. *American Journal of Nursing, 106*(10), 40–49.

24

Dizziness

Kurt Kroenke and Joan Gleba Carpenter

The prevalence of dizziness ranges from 13% to 38% among older adults. Several factors make dizziness a challenging symptom to evaluate and manage. First, precise classification of the cause is often difficult. Second, it is important to ascertain that there is not a serious cardiac or neurologic cause. Third, there is no easy cure for dizziness. Fourth, like other geriatric syndromes such as delirium and falls, dizziness may be related to multiple causes at least half of the time.

CLASSIFICATION

The following is a symptom-oriented approach to classifying dizziness:

(1) Vertigo (a sensation that room is spinning),
(2) Presyncope (impending faint),
(3) Disequilibrium (loss of balance), or
(4) Lightheadedness (none of the other symptoms).

Vertigo

The three most common problems associated with a sense of vertigo include: benign positional vertigo (BPV), labyrinthitis, and Ménière's disease. BPV is often aggravated or brought on by changes in position, such as turning, rolling over, getting in and out of bed, or bending over. BPV spells are often brief (5 to 15 seconds) and milder than the severe vertiginous attacks seen with disorders such as labyrinthitis and Ménière's disease. Labyrinthitis (sometimes called vestibular neu-

ronitis) occurs suddenly, lasts for several days, and resolves spontaneously. Ménière's disease is characterized by repeated episodes of tinnitus (i.e., ringing in the ears), fluctuating hearing loss, and severe vertigo accompanied eventually by progressive hearing loss. The frequency and severity of vertigo may actually improve as hearing impairment worsens. Brain tumors are found in less than 1% of persons complaining of dizziness, although this is slightly more prevalent (2% to 3%) among older adults.

Nonvertiginous Dizziness

Presyncope is the sensation of near fainting. Most presyncopal persons presenting with dizziness have symptoms that occur when they change position. Certain stimuli (e.g., micturition, defecation, coughing) can precipitate this sense of dizziness as well. This is due to autonomic changes that affect cardiac function. Thus, the elderly man who rises to urinate in the middle of the night, the older person straining to have a bowel movement, or the pulmonary patient having paroxysms of coughing can experience lightheadedness or even frank syncope.

Disequilibrium is a sensation of being unsteady when standing or, in particular, when walking. Balance depends not only on the vestibular system of the inner ear but also on the visual and sensory systems. Thus, multiple factors can contribute to imbalance, including chronic vestibular problems, visual problems (e.g., errors of refraction, cataract, loss of binocular vision, macular degeneration), musculoskeletal disorders (e.g., arthritis, muscle weaknesses), and sensory or gait deficits (e.g., neuropathies, previous strokes, cerebellar disease, Parkinson's disease, dementia).

Lightheadedness is a vaguer sensation best reserved for those who do not have vertigo (spinning), presyncope (fainting), or disequilibrium (falling). Although any cause of dizziness may occasionally produce a nondescript lightheaded type of sensation, the two most prominent considerations are psychiatric (primarily depressive, anxiety, or somatoform disorders) or idiopathic causes, which together account for up to a third of all cases of dizziness.

Among other causes, drug side effects may also contribute to dizziness in older adults. The use of at least three to five medications is a risk factor for dizziness, as are drugs that cause orthostatic hypotension (e.g., cardiovascular, antihypertensive, and psychotropic medications).

PROGNOSIS

Dizziness usually resolves within days to several months, but about one fourth of patients may experience chronic or recurrent symptoms. Chronic dizziness is associated with worse self-rated health, increased risk of falling, and depression.

EVALUATION

A brief, focused evaluation by the nurse initially, followed by the primary care practitioner, coupled with simple follow-up is warranted in most older adults rather than diagnostic testing or referral. Symptoms gradually improve in most people. More than 75% of the cases are diagnosed by history and physical examination alone, with the history contributing the most to the diagnosis.

History

Four questions are particularly helpful to elicit the appropriate information:

(1) Is the dizziness characterized by one of three key sensations: spinning, fainting, or falling? A potentially helpful question to ask a resident is "Does it feel like your head is spinning? Or are your feet spinning?" to elicit a starting point for more focused discussion.

(2) Is there a positional effect on the dizziness and related symptoms: "Does the dizziness occur when you change position?"
With BPV, the effect is almost always one of transient dizziness with change of head position (i.e., moving the head from side to side), lying down, or sitting up. The most common cause of presyncope is an orthostatic change in blood pressure, in which case the older adult reports that dizziness occurs on assuming a more upright position (supine to sitting or sitting to standing). Disequilibrium is manifested only when the person is walking or standing.

(3) What associated symptoms are experienced along with the dizziness?
Dizziness with an actual loss of consciousness may mean there is underlying cardiac disease that has caused the dizziness. Tinnitus or hearing changes, or both, are associated with certain vestibular disorders such as Ménière's disease or the rare tumors. Nausea and, in particular, vomiting suggests vertigo rather than a nonvertiginous cause of dizziness. A central cause (i.e., located in the brain) would generally be associated with other neurologic symptoms (e.g. numbness, balance problems, confusion). Psychological causes, such as depression or anxiety typically include fatigue, insomnia, pain, or other physical and emotional symptoms in addition to dizziness.

(4) What medications is the resident taking? Be particularly suspicious of new medications that were started around the time that symptoms of dizziness began.

Physical Examination

A focused physical examination would include the following steps:

- Blood pressure and pulse measurement while the person is lying down and taken again after standing for 2 to 3 minutes to detect orthostatic changes.
- Check heart rate and rhythm (is it regular or irregular?)
- Conduct a brief neurologic exam to check balance and memory.
- Observe walking and turning (for balance or gait difficulties).

Dizziness correlates best with postural hypotension: systolic blood pressure (BP) drop of 20 mm mercury or diastolic BP drop of 10 mm mercury. Postural hypotension is absent if BP normalizes within 2 minutes.

Screening for evidence of a vestibular problem can also be done; the exam takes about 1 minute and has three elements:

■ Primary position: Instruct the person to look straight ahead and check for *nystagmus* (i.e., shaking of the eyes; rapid side-to-side movement).
■ Gaze-evoked: Instruct the person to look to the right, left, up, and down, holding each position for 5 to 10 seconds. More than three to five beats of movement of the eyes back and forth is abnormal.
■ Head-shaking: Instruct the person to close his or her eyes, rapidly shake his or her head back and forth for 10 seconds, and then open his or her eyes. Look for nystagmus.

In the event that nystagmus is noted, the older adult should be sent to his or her primary health care provider for further evaluation.

MANAGEMENT

Although the evidence-base for dizziness therapies is limited, the natural history of dizziness is nonetheless often favorable. In half of all patients, dizziness spontaneously resolves or substantially improves within 2 weeks. In some cases, dizziness is an associated symptom of viral or other self-limited illnesses. Other times, dizziness is a result of dehydration or a medication's adverse effect. The two most common causes of vertigo—labyrinthitis and BPV—typically resolve within days or weeks, respectively. Types of dizziness for which specific management strategies may be helpful are briefly discussed in the following list.

■ *Acute vertigo attacks:* Attacks that occur with peripheral vestibular disorders such as labyrinthitis and Ménière's disease may benefit from medications such as meclizine and, if needed, a benzodiazepine. Unfortunately, older adults are at risk for adverse effects related to meclizine and benzodiazepines (e.g., Benadryl).
■ *BPV:* This usually can be treated with simple reassurance, since symptoms are typically mild and usually improve within weeks to several months. For individuals with persistent symptoms, it is helpful to encourage and instruct the individual in careful position change and possibly work with a physical and/or occupational therapist or specialist in this area to establish an exercise program.
■ *Ménière's disease:* Attacks of frequent or disabling dizziness may benefit from treatment with such things

as salt restriction or diuretic therapy to decrease fluid within the inner ear.
■ *Orthostatic hypotension:* Correct reversible causes (e.g., dehydration, anemia, medication adverse effects).
■ *Disequilibrium:* Advise the older adult with a chronic sense of disequilibrium to take measures to prevent falls such as using a cane, walker, or other assistive device.
■ *Psychological causes:* Psychological dizziness may be related to depression or anxiety. If suspected and confirmed, depression and anxiety should be treated with medications and behavioral interventions.
■ *Chronic vestibular disorders:* Vestibular rehabilitation—a type of physical therapy exercise program to decrease dizziness—may be beneficial in persons with persistent dizziness.

It is important to remember when managing a resident with dizziness that there may be multiple causes of dizziness including depressive or anxiety symptoms, impaired vision or hearing, the use of multiple medications, abnormal balance or gait, postural hypotension, diabetes mellitus, and past myocardial infarction (i.e., heart damage). A multifactorial intervention targeting such factors might reduce the frequency or severity of dizziness in older adults. For example, a resident may have complaints of dizziness described as feeling faint when standing, unsteadiness when walking, and a nagging lightheadedness unrelated to position. This resident might have orthostatic hypotension from medications, depression, and disequilibrium. It is important to identify the underlying cause and treat these problems (e.g., decrease and eliminate medications when possible).

PREVENTION

■ Evaluate the environment to decrease falls and to encourage increased physical activity in order to improve strength and conditioning (see Chapter 28, "Falls," and Chapter 18, "Physical Activity").
■ Identify hearing or vision deficits so that these sensory systems are optimized.
■ Maintain adequate nutrition and hydration. If not contraindicated, encourage fluids with medication administration and at meals.
■ Continually monitor for drug side effects and assess for nonessential medications. Some medications commonly used in older adults that can cause dizziness include: antihypertensives, diuretics, antihistamines,

psychotropics, seizure medications, and over-the-counter cold preparations.

■ Reduce caffeine and alcohol intake.

While dizziness is a common problem and can be persistent for some older adults, many interventions can decrease the symptoms and episodes of dizziness.

RESOURCES

Blakley, B. W., & Gulati, H. (2008). Identifying drugs that cause dizziness. *Journal of Otolaryngology Head and Neck Surgery, 37*(1), 11–15.

Johnson, M. A. (2006). When the report is dizziness. *Geriatric Nursing, 27*(1), 41–44.

Kovar, M., Jepson, T., & Jones, S. (2006). Diagnosing and treating benign paroxysmal positional vertigo. *Journal of Gerontological Nursing, 32*(12), 22–27.

Lawson, J., Bamiou, D. E., Cohen, H. S., & Newton, J. (2008). Positional vertigo in a falls service. *Age Ageing, 37*(5), 585–589.

Newman-Toker, D. E., Hsieh, Y. H., Camargo, C. A., Jr., Pelletier, A. J., Butchy, G. T., & Edlow, J. A. (2008). Spectrum of dizziness visits to US emergency departments: Cross-sectional analysis from a nationally representative sample. *Mayo Clinic Procedures, 83*(7), 765–775.

Parnes, L. S., Agrawal, S. K., & Atlas, J. (2003). Diagnosis and management of benign paroxysmal positional vertigo (BPPV). *Canadian Medical Association Journal, 169*(7), 681–693.

Polensek, S. H., Sterk, C. E., & Tusa, R. J. (2008). Screening for vestibular disorders: A study of clinicians' compliance with recommended practices. *Medical Science Monitor, 14*(5), CR238–CR242.

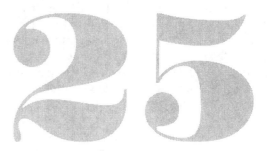

Maintenance of Nutritional Status

Colleen Christmas and Anna M. Mago-Sisic

Swallowing is an important and complex task that can be affected by normal aging processes, diseases, syndromes, and/or surgical/invasive interventions in older adults. *Dysphagia* is defined as an impairment of any part of the swallowing process. The estimation of the prevalence of dysphagia among community-dwelling older adults ranges from 7% to 22%; on average, it is 15%. However, among institutionalized older adults (i.e., in nursing homes, group homes, or assisted living facilities), prevalence of dysphagia dramatically increases to approximately 40%–50% of residents. Treatment of eating and feeding problems varies, depending on the identified etiology and other contributing factors.

SWALLOWING IN HEALTH AND DISEASE

Swallowing: Three Stages

Swallowing can be divided into three phases on the basis of anatomy. The preparatory or oral phase, which includes the oral propulsive phase, begins when the bolus (round mass of food) enters the oral cavity and mixes with saliva during mastication (i.e., chewing) to form a cohesive bolus. This stage is under voluntary control.

The second or pharyngeal phase is involuntary and begins as the cohesive bolus is propelled toward the oropharynx, thus initiating the swallow reflex. Soft palate elevation during this stage prevents food and liquids

from entering the nasopharynx. The epiglottis, a cartilage flap, closes and thereby prevents food from entering the airway (i.e., aspiration). The posterior tongue base propels the food through the pharynx with the assistance of the peristaltic contraction of the posterior pharyngeal wall. Execution of the oral and pharyngeal phases of swallowing requires the complex coordination of five cranial nerves and 50 pairs of muscles in the head and neck, with regulation from cortical input to the medullary swallow center, all in the appropriate sequence, usually within 1 second.

The third stage of swallowing, also involuntary, is the esophageal phase, during which food passes through the pharynx to the esophagus; the upper esophageal sphincter relaxes, thus allowing the bolus to pass through into the esophagus. The bolus is propelled down the esophagus by the action of skeletal muscle proximally and smooth muscle distally. The lower esophageal sphincter, located at the juncture of the esophagus and stomach, opens to allow the bolus entry into the stomach. This phase is regulated by its own intrinsic innervations. A delay or impairment in any stage of swallowing may result in dysphagia.

Aging and Swallowing

Normal aging is associated with several changes (e.g., dryness of the mucous membranes) that affect the older individual's ability to check, swallow, and enjoy eating. With age there is a decrease in the ability to taste but not of taste discrimination (i.e., an older person may be able to distinguish sweet from salty but may need to add more salt to food to taste it sufficiently). In addition, olfactory function decreases with age, further impairing taste sensations; there is a relationship between the smelling and tasting of food. *Xerostomia* (i.e., dry mouth) is a common complaint of older adults, usually owing to the adverse effects of medication. Loss of dentition greatly reduces chewing efficiency. The individual needs to chew for a longer period of time and with more chewing strokes to achieve the same level of food maceration; this is only partly improved with the use of dentures (see Chapter 39, "Oral Diseases and Disorders"). Sarcopenia, or age-related loss of lean muscle mass, may contribute to loss in chewing efficiency and to pharyngeal muscle weakness.

It is not clear exactly what changes commonly noted with swallowing in older adults are due to normal age-related changes and which are due to disease. Esophageal function is probably well-preserved, except, perhaps, in very advanced age (i.e., > 85 years). Other physiological changes that contribute to swallowing difficulty include: decreased tongue pressure and strength during bolus transfer; slower oral and pharyngeal bolus transit movement; delayed initiation of the pharyngeal reflex; reduced anteroposterior upper esophageal sphincter (UES) opening during swallowing; and a need for larger pharyngeal volumes to trigger a reflexive pharyngeal swallow. In total, these changes result in prolonged duration of each swallow. Furthermore, many diseases that produce dysphagia are more common in older adults (e.g., Parkinson's disease, stroke, Alzheimer's disease).

Dysphagia Stages and Symptoms

Dysphagia occurs when a disease affects any aspect of the three stages of swallowing function (oral, pharyngeal, or esophageal). Oral dysphagia occurs when there is difficulty with the voluntary transfer of food from the mouth to the pharynx. This might be diagnosed, for example, when the scrambled eggs served at breakfast are discovered in the cheeks of a resident shortly before lunch. Other symptoms of oral dysphagia may include frequent drooling, poor jaw movement, difficulty manipulating the bolus in the oral cavity, and loss of food from the mouth while eating.

In pharyngeal dysphagia, reflexive transfer of the food bolus from the pharynx to initiate the involuntary esophageal phase of swallowing—while simultaneously protecting the airway from misdirection of food—is difficult. The affected person may notice coughing, chok-

ing, or nasal regurgitation while eating and may also have to use repetitive swallows and throat clearing during the meal. A noticeable wet vocal quality may be heard when speaking after they have attempted to eat or drink something. There may also be complaints of food sticking in the throat or pain during swallowing. Overt symptoms of dysphagia that may not appear immediately include symptoms of aspiration, such as spiking a fever or a consistent low-grade fever and increased respirations with oral intake. History of frequent upper respiratory tract infections and pneumonia may also be symptoms of pharyngeal dysphagia. At least 50% of stroke patients experience pharyngeal dysphagia.

Esophageal dysmotility presents with three characteristic features: dysphagia (for solids and liquids), chest pain, and regurgitation. *Regurgitation* between meals or at night (described as mucus or bubbly saliva), with or without food particles, is suggestive of dysmotility. Unlike the regurgitation that is related to gastric reflux, the regurgitated fluid and/or food is not generally noxious to taste because it hasn't begun to be digested. The chest pain, described as heavy or crushing, is related to the spasm (i.e., achalasia) and may be difficult to distinguish from typical gastric reflux. The pain frequently occurs during meals but is generally unpredictable and is sometimes thought to be true chest pain from heart disease.

Whereas dysphagia for both solids and liquids suggests an esophageal motility disorder (e.g., spasm), dysphagia for solids only suggests a mechanical obstruction/structural disorder (e.g., tumor, esophageal ring, stenosis, stricture from mucosal irritation). Medication-induced esophagitis (which presents with odynophagia, or pain when swallowing) is commonly followed by dysphagia. Common causes of medication-induced esophagitis in older persons are potassium, nonsteroidal anti-inflammatory agents, biphosphonates, and tetracycline-related antibiotics.

Dysphagia and Aspiration

Recognizing aspiration—the misdirection of oral-pharyngeal contents into the airway—is essential in patients with dysphagia. Sources of aspiration include food, oropharyngeal flora/saliva, emesis/gastric contents, and tube feeding liquids. Aspiration may be observed as coughing and/or choking during meals, as well as drooling, gurgling or moist voice, or hoarseness. *Silent aspiration* is the absence of any symptoms at all. Aspiration pneumonia is believed to occur when bacteria arrive in the lungs from the pharynx in a large enough amount to overcome host defenses. Most often, local host defense mechanisms clear the lung of the offending aspirate without serious clinical impact. It is well established that many healthy individuals episodically aspirate without any significant consequences.

The typical symptoms of aspiration pneumonia (i.e., cough, fever/chills, sputum, and increased respiratory rate) may not be detected in the older adult. Rather, these individuals may present with delirium, falls, and changes in behavior. Right lower lobe pneumonias often are considered a primary clinical indicator of possible aspiration and suggest further evaluation. Older adults and individuals with neurological disorders (e.g., dementias, Parkinson's disease, strokes, multiple sclerosis, traumatic brain injury, etc.) are at high risk for dysphagia and possible aspiration. Individuals with a diminished gag reflex or any delay or weakness of swallowing mechanisms are also at risk for aspiration. These problems may occur following head and neck surgery or any surgery with general anesthesia, medications that decrease alertness, recent illness or debilitation, and medical conditions (e.g., heart failure, chronic obstructive pulmonary disease). Older adults without teeth, those with poorly fitting dentures, and those with poor oral hygiene are at risk for aspiration pneumonia.

Aspiration of oral contents or of gastric contents is *not* prevented by the placement of a feeding tube. Tube feeding is universally cited as a risk factor for major aspiration, and some patients who have never previously aspirated begin to do so after placement of a feeding tube. Further, there is no evidence to indicate that the placement of a jejunostomy tube as opposed to a gastrostomy tube results in lower rates of aspiration.

Assessment of Dysphagia

Several tools may be used to assess swallowing function when dysphagia is clinically suspected. Typically family, close friends, nurses, or nursing assistants are the first to recognize a resident's swallowing problem. In addition to notifying the resident's primary care provider, the nurse can also initiate the approaches summarized in *Try This: Preventing Aspiration in Older Adults With Dysphagia* (Metheny, 2007) to help decrease aspiration risk. Concerns about swallowing may lead to obtaining a more comprehensive swallowing evaluation from a speech-language therapist. However, clinical assessment alone underestimates the risk of aspiration by 50%. A more accurate estimation of aspiration risk is achieved by a videoradiographic swallow study, sometimes called the barium swallow, which can determine the presence, severity, and timing of aspiration. The patient is videotaped swallowing different food consistencies (e.g., apple sauce, pudding, eggs).

Depending on the results of the study, the therapist may recommend *swallow therapy* or diet modifications, or both. Swallow therapy may include techniques such as turning the head toward the weaker side while swallowing or doing exercises to improve the strength of the muscles involved in swallowing. Dietary recommendations generally consist of altering the amount of food the person tries to swallow at one time or changing the consistency of the food so that liquids are avoided. Residents with dysphagia who cannot safely swallow liquids should avoid mixing consistencies. Mixed consistencies typically have both a solid and a thin liquid consistency (e.g., canned fruit in water or juice, or cereal with milk). Ice cream and Jell-O are considered thin liquids.

The VitalStim dysphagia treatment (Chatanooga Group, Hixson, Tennessee) is an electrical stimulation treatment whereby the clinician stimulates the swallowing muscles directly to both strengthen and retrain these muscles. Also, adaptive feeding equipment may help facilitate safe swallowing. A dysphagia cup, shaped in such a way that it prevents tilting the head back while swallowing can help swallowing for some individuals. Last, good oral hygiene (brushing at least twice daily of permanent teeth or dentures) will decrease tooth decay and decrease the risk of aspiration pneumonia.

FEEDING

When an older adult experiences difficulty eating for reasons other than dysphagia, the treatment is either careful feeding by hand or by tube insertion. Consideration of the possible causes for difficulty eating include evaluating the resident for depression; infection; dehydration; dislike of the food and food choices; unpleasant or stressful eating environment; poor oral hygiene; missing, loose, or painful teeth; bad taste in the mouth due to disease or medications; xerostomia; movement disorders (i.e., hand or head tremor making eating difficult); or anorexia. The person with advanced dementia might forget how to eat and needs cueing to initiate eating and swallowing. These individuals may do well if they can model eating behavior. For example, eating with them or sitting them with others who are eating on their own might stimulate them to do likewise. Older individuals should have food that is easy to eat. Finger foods such as hunks of cheese, hard boiled eggs, sandwiches, muffins, energy bars, and other types of nutritious foods can be easily held and eaten. Retaining the ability to eat by mouth is essential to most people. This basic function not only satisfies nutritive needs but social and self-esteem needs as well. Through early identification and intervention, much can be done to help older adults with swallowing and eating difficulties to eat safely and enjoyably.

RESOURCES

Brady, A. (2008). Managing the patient with dysphagia. *Home Healthcare Nurse, 26*(1), 41–46.

Easterling, C.S., & Robbins, E. (2008). Dementia and dysphagia. *Geriatric Nursing, 29*(4), 265–282.

Marik, P.E., & Kaplan, D. (2003). Aspiration pneumonia and dysphagia in the elderly. *Chest, 124*(1), 328–336.

Metheny, P. (2007). *Try this: Preventing aspiration in older adults with dysphagia*. New York: Hartford Institute for Geriatric Nursing, New York University College of Nursing.

Mitchell, S.L., Kiely, D.K., & Lipsitz, L.A. (1998). Does artificial enteral nutrition prolong the survival of institutionalized elders with chewing and swallowing problems? *Journals of Gerontology Series A: Biological Sciences and Medical Sciences, 53*(3), M207–M213.

Palmer, J.L., & Metheny, N.A. (2008). Preventing aspiration in older adults with dysphagia. *American Journal of Nursing, 108*(2), 40–48.

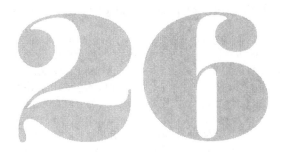

Urinary Incontinence

Catherine E. DuBeau and Barbara Resnick

Urinary incontinence (UI) is defined as the involuntary loss of urine, and is a significant problem both physically and psychologically for older adults in assisted living (AL) communities and nursing home settings. The overall costs and implications of UI are comprehensive and involve associated health risks including urinary tract infections, falls and fall-related injuries, skin breakdown, and the associated depression and withdrawal experienced by residents. While UI is a prevalent problem for older adults, it is not a normal consequence of aging. It has repeatedly been demonstrated that a comprehensive workup and management program can decrease the number of episodes of incontinence experienced by the older individual. Nurses in AL communities have the opportunity to work with residents and ensure that they have been adequately evaluated and matched with an appropriate treatment plan, and that the proposed plan of care is being implemented. In so doing, nurses can help to decrease the episodes of UI among residents and optimize quality of life.

PREVALENCE AND IMPACT

UI may cause morbidity, including cellulitis (i.e., skin infections), pressure ulcers, urinary tract infections, falls with fractures, sleep deprivation, social withdrawal, depression, and sexual dysfunction. It is not associated with increased risk of death, but it does impair quality of life, affecting the older adult's emotional well-being, social function, and general health. Incontinent persons often manage to maintain their activities, but with an increased burden of coping, embarrassment, and poor self-perception.

The prevalence of UI increases with age and affects women more than men (2:1 ratio) until age 80, after which men and women are equally affected. Of incontinent older adults age 65 years and over, 15% to 30% live in the community and at least 50% are in long-term care.

THE PATHOPHYSIOLOGY OF INCONTINENCE

Normal Micturition (Urination)

Continence requires effective functioning of the urinary tract, adequate cognitive and physical capability, motivation, and an appropriate environment such as accessible toilets that allow for safe transfers on and off the commode. The bladder is a loose sack that can accommodate a volume of urine up to a maximum of approximately 300–400 ml (i.e., cc) in normal adults. When the quantity of urine increases above the 300–400 ml range, tension in the bladder wall sends a message to the brain and the micturition reflex is triggered. When the individual has an appropriate place (e.g., bathroom, commode) in which to empty his or her bladder, the brain sends a signal to the external urethral sphincter muscle to allow the passage of urine from the body. Completion of bladder emptying is also facilitated by contraction of the abdominal wall and pelvic floor muscles.

Risk Factors for Urinary Incontinence

The many risk factors for UI in older adults include advanced age, (for women, number of birth children), depression, transient ischemic attack (TIA), stroke, Parkinson's disease, heart failure, fecal incontinence and constipation, obesity, chronic obstructive lung disease, chronic cough, diabetes mellitus, impaired mobility, and impaired activities of daily living. In addition, medications, as shown in Table 26.1, can contribute to UI.

Types of Urinary Incontinence

Urge Incontinence

Urge UI is the most common type of UI in older adults. It is characterized by abrupt urgency, frequency, and nocturia (i.e., frequent urination during the night). Urge UI is associated with uninhibited or uncontrolled bladder contractions, often referred to as *detrusor overactivity* (DO). The detrusor (i.e., the bladder muscle) contracts

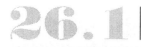 | Medications Commonly Associated With Incontinence

MEDICATION	EFFECT ON CONTINENCE
Alcohol	Frequency, urgency, sedation, delirium, immobility
α-Adrenergic agonists	Causes urinary retention with possible overflow
α-Adrenergic blockers	Relaxation of the urethra causes release of urine
Angiotensin-converting enzyme inhibitors	Associated cough with stress or stress-induced urge leakage

Anticholinergics:
    Antiarrhythmics (Norpace)
    Antidiarrheals (Lomotil)
    Antihistamines (Benadryl)
    Antiparkinsonians (Artane)
    Antispasmodics (Bentyl)
    Antidepressants (Elavil)
    Antipsychotics (Haldol)
    Sedative hypnotics (Ambien)
	Impaired emptying, retention, delirium, fecal impaction

Cholinesterase inhibitors (Aricept)	Urinary frequency and urgency
Diuretics	Polyuria, frequency, urgency
Narcotic analgesics	Urinary retention, fecal impaction, sedation, delirium
Drugs that cause edema: Nonsteroidal anti-inflammatory drugs, Diabetic medications, Thiazolidinediones, Antiseizure medications (neurontin), Hypertensive and other heart medications (calcium channel blockers)	Edema causing nocturnal frequency and incontinence
Caffeine	Urgency due to bladder irritation

unexpectedly while the bladder is filling, which then causes a large or small amount of leakage of urine. DO may be age related, secondary to changes in the brain that impair the individual's ability to stop this bladder activity (e.g., following a stroke), or it may be due to local bladder irritation (e.g., infection, bladder stones, inflammation, tumors).

Stress Incontinence

Stress UI, the second most common type of UI in older adults, is the result of failure of the *sphincter muscle* to maintain closure of the urinary outlet during bladder filling; hence, urine leakage occurs. Stress incontinence occurs when there is increased pressure in the abdomen that subsequently increases physical pressure on the pelvis, causing urine leakage. Coughing, sneezing, laughing, exercise, and even standing increase abdominal pressure as the abdominal muscles contract during these activities. A weak pelvic floor and a poorly supported urethral sphincter cause stress incontinence. Many women may have mixed UI, with both stress and urge symptoms.

Overflow Incontinence: Bladder Outlet Obstruction and Detrusor Underactivity

So-called overflow UI results from *detrusor underactivity* (i.e., impaired contractility) or bladder outlet obstruction, thus causing a back-up of urine and overflow, or both. Leakage is typically small in volume but continual. The postvoid residual (PVR) is the amount of urine that remains in the bladder after urinating. Symptoms may include dribbling, weak urinary stream, hesitancy, frequency, and nocturia.

Outlet obstruction is the second most common cause of UI in older men. Causes include benign prostatic hyperplasia (BPH, overgrowth of the prostate gland), prostate cancer, and urethral stricture (i.e., tightening of the urethra that stops the urine from passing through). In women, obstruction is uncommon but can occur after surgeries or may be associated with a large cystocele that kinks the urethra. When constipation occurs and the rectum is full of stool, this can put pressure on the urethra and cause a back-up of urine and overflow incontinence in both men and women.

Detrusor underactivity causing urinary retention and UI occurs in only 5% to 10% of older adults. Neurologic causes include peripheral neuropathy (associated with diabetes mellitus, vitamin B_{12} deficiency, alcoholism) or damage to the spinal cord, particularly when the damage affects the innervation of the bladder or detrusor muscle. This can occur when the resident has spinal disc herniation, spinal stenosis, tumor, or some type of degenerative neurologic disease.

ASSESSMENT AND MANAGEMENT

Like many geriatric syndromes, UI is multifactorial and requires a comprehensive diagnostic evaluation, with a careful search for all possible causes and precipitants beyond the genitourinary tract. The following sections describe ways in which nursing can assist with the diagnosis and management of this complex problem.

History

Always ask about UI symptoms: 50% of affected persons do not volunteer UI symptoms. Sudden, compelling urgency suggests detrusor overactivity; leakage that occurs while coughing is suggestive of stress UI. Frequency, nocturia, slow urine stream, hesitancy, interrupted voiding, straining, and terminal dribbling are common with DO, bladder outlet obstruction, and detrusor underactivity. Assess UI characteristics such as frequency, volume, timing, and precipitants (e.g., medications, caffeine, alcohol, physical activity, cough), and associated factors (such as bowel and sexual function, medical conditions and medications with temporal relation to UI, e.g., diuretics). Inquire how the person's quality of life is affected with respect to activities of daily living, social role, emotional and interpersonal relations (e.g., sexual), self-concept, and general health perception.

Physical Examination

The general examination must include cognition and functional status. Cardiovascular examination should include careful assessment of the amount of peripheral edema (i.e., swelling in the legs or arms). The abdomen should be evaluated for distension as this may indicate that the bladder is full and will not empty and/or that there is some constipation. If there is concern about fecal impaction, a rectal exam is indicated.

Testing

Urinalysis can be helpful. Dark urine is an indication that the individual may not be taking in sufficient fluid: the urine is irritating the bladder wall. Certainly, if there is an acute change in the individual's urinary problems then a test for infection should be considered.

A *bladder diary* provides data regarding baseline UI severity: timing and circumstances of incontinence and typical voided volume, voiding frequency, and the total day and nocturnal urine output (for a sample diary see http://www.healthinaging.org/public_education/blad der_diary.pdf). This can be difficult for a resident to independently obtain. Alternatively, staff can record the resident's continence status (dry, damp, soaked) every 2 hours over a 24-hour period to get a sense of his or her bladder activity. If there are increased episodes of incontinence at night and increased urinary volume, it may be due to edema that has accumulated during the course of the day, or to drinking alcohol, tea, or coffee in the evening. When UI occurs at a typical or predictable time of day, this suggests an association with medication, beverages, or activity.

PVR measurement is always very helpful, particularly when evaluating new onset UI. A PVR measurement can be obtained by having the resident empty his or her bladder and then either using a bladder scanner or via straight catheterization, immediately calculate the remaining amount of urine; it should be less than 300 ml.

A simple *stress test* can evaluate for stress UI. When the resident has a full bladder (i.e., he or she feels the need to urinate), have the resident stand up (preferably, while standing over the toilet/commode). Instruct the resident to do a single vigorous cough. If urinary leakage is instantaneous, it is specific for stress UI. If there is no clear cause of the UI and the resident would like to undergo a more extensive evaluation, this should be discussed further with the primary health care provider.

Management

Medical illnesses should be handled as optimally as possible; for example, to decrease edema, changing medications, if possible, and addressing problems such as constipation or insufficient fluid intake can often improve continence. Often, older adults will deliberately take in little fluid so that they do not need to urinate as often. However, the concentrated urine that occurs from this is a bladder irritant, will increase urgency, and even cause bladder spasm and thus release urine. Relieving the most bothersome aspects of UI for the person is key. A stepped strategy that moves from least to more invasive treatments should be used, with behavioral methods tried before medication, and both tried before surgery; this is an option for men and women. Treatment that simply decreases the number of UI episodes

may not be sufficient for persons most bothered by the timing of UI, nocturia, or leakage with exercise.

General management suggestions include avoiding excessively high fluid intake (> 2L/day), caffeinated beverages, alcohol, and minimizing evening intake if nocturnal UI is bothersome. The high fluid intake will not actually cause incontinence as much as make the symptoms (e.g., the number of incontinence episodes; increase in the amount of urine that the individual has to manage) of the underlying incontinence more bothersome. If pads and protective garments are used, they should be chosen on the basis of the patient's gender, the type and volume of UI, and cost. (These products are expensive; some users might not change them frequently enough.)

SPECIFIC TREATMENT STRATEGIES

Urge Incontinence

Behavioral treatment for urge UI employs two principles: (a) frequent voluntary voiding to keep bladder volume low and (b) retraining of the brain and the pelvic muscles to inhibit detrusor contractions and leakage. Cognitively intact persons can use *bladder retraining* with timed voiding while awake and suppression of urgency by relaxation techniques (see http://www. healthinaging.org/public_education/bladder_control. php for educational material for older adults). Initial toileting frequency can be every 2 hours or, based on a bladder diary, the shortest interval between voids. When the urgency occurs, the person is instructed to stand still or sit down, contract the pelvic muscles, and concentrate on making the urgency decrease and pass. The person should be instructed to take a deep breath and let it out slowly or to visualize the urgency as a wave that peaks and then falls. Once in control of the urgency, the person should walk slowly to a bathroom and void. After 2 days without leakage, the time between scheduled voids is increased by 30 to 60 minutes until the person voids every 3 to 4 hours without leakage. Successful bladder retraining usually takes several weeks; residents need support and encouragement to participate in this and reassurance to proceed despite any initial failure.

For cognitively impaired persons, behavioral methods include *habit training* (i.e., timed voiding, with the interval based on the person's usual voiding schedule), *scheduled voiding* (i.e., timed voiding usually every 2 to 3 hours), and *prompted voiding*. Prompted voiding has three components: regular monitoring with encouragement to report continence status, prompting to toilet on a scheduled basis, and praise and positive feedback when the person is continent and attempts to toilet. Persons most likely to respond to prompted voiding are those who void four or fewer times in 12 daytime hours and who toilet correctly over 75% of the time in an initial trial. These methods require training, motivation, and continued effort by residents and staff.

When behavioral methods alone are not sufficient, *bladder-suppressant medications* can be added. The combination of behavioral and drug therapy has higher efficacy than either route, alone. Antimuscarinic agents, of which there are many, are the primary source of drug treatment for urinary incontinence. These drugs work because their anticholinergic effects cause relaxation of the bladder muscle. All of them have proven efficacy in older adults, but they can have bothersome systemic anticholinergic side effects, especially dry mouth and constipation as well as indigestion. Patients with glaucoma should be warned about use of these medications and should be instructed to consult their ophthalmologist before initiating treatment. In addition, these medications can cause problems with memory and other central nervous system side effects. Maximum effect of antimuscarinic drugs may not be achieved for up to 1–2 months. Patients should therefore be educated to avoid unrealistic expectations about a quick cure and complete dryness. To maximize adherence, they should be told that many patients benefit from these drugs, some are cured, and that it may take several months to achieve the desired effect. Lack of response to one agent does not preclude response to another.

Other medications (propantheline, dicyclomine, imipramine, hyoscyamine, calcium channel blockers, and nonsteroidal anti-inflammatories) are sometimes used in more challenging UI situations. However, there is less support for the effectiveness of these drugs with older adults.

Stress Incontinence

Pelvic muscle exercise (PME) strengthens the muscles that support the bladder and the urethra and is one of the most important noninvasive treatments for stress UI. These exercises are isometric, that is, an exercise in which the muscle does not move through range of motion as is done when doing resistive exercise (e.g., weight lifting). To successfully do these exercises, the person must be cognitively intact and motivated. The PME known as the Kegel exercise is described in Exhibit 26.1.

Pessaries may benefit women with stress UI exacerbated by bladder or uterine prolapse (see Chapter 46,

26.1 | Kegel's Exercise: Instructions for the Resident

The resident should be encouraged to perform this exercise, hold the contraction for 6 to 8 seconds, and do it in sets of 8 to 12 contractions three or four times a week for at least 15 to 20 weeks.

Step 1. Isolate the appropriate muscle: stand up straight and place your hand on the front of your lower abdomen.

Step 2. While in this position, contract your pelvic floor muscles. The sensation will feel similar to when you need to urinate but are holding it in. Your pelvis should not move; this exercise is focusing on the internal muscle.

Step 3. Strengthen the muscle by tightening—hold for at least 3 seconds—then release. Repeat this 10 times. Once you can easily hold for a count of 3 seconds, try to increase this to hold for a count of up to 6 to 8 seconds.

Step 4. Recheck your technique—be sure that you are not holding your breath or clenching your abdominal muscle.

Step 5. Repeat this exercise 8 to 12 times a day, at least 3 or 4 days per week.

Step 6. Follow this regimen, and within 2 weeks you will see a noticeable difference in the length of time that you are able to hold the muscle—and an increase in bladder control!

Step 7. Keep at it for at least 15 to 20 weeks.

"Gynecologic Diseases and Sexual Disorders in Women and Men"). There is no strong evidence that the use of estrogen, either taking it orally or applying it directly to the vaginal wall, will help UI. There is some evidence, however, that maintaining the health of the vaginal area tissues with estrogen can help decrease episodes of stress UI and feelings of urgency.

Surgery provides the highest cure rates for stress UI in women. The standard surgical procedure is bladder neck suspension. Other treatments include injections of collagen, Teflon, or fat to the urethral area. For men who have had prostate surgery and have stress UI following that surgery, artificial sphincters have been used with some success. All surgical options should be discussed by the primary health care provider.

Bladder Outlet Obstruction

A range of medical and surgical alternatives are available for prostatic obstruction (see Chapter 47, "Prostate Diseases and Disorders"). Obstruction is also possible in women; after evaluation of constipation, there should be further evaluation for evidence of a prolapse (see Chapter 46, "Gynecologic Diseases and Sexual Disorders in Women and Men"). A pessary may help. Discussion of surgical options is also recommended.

Detrusor Underactivity

Treatment is supportive. Drugs that impair the bladder's ability to contract should be discontinued, if possible; constipation should be treated. Intermittent clean catheterization is effective for willing and able individuals. Sterile intermittent catheterization is recommended for frailer older adults and those in institutional settings. In some cases, bladder emptying may improve with *double voiding* or simply unhurried voiding. To double void, instruct the person to remain on the toilet until it feels as if the bladder is empty. Then, instruct him or her to stand up and sit down again, lean forward slightly at the knees, and try to urinate again.

Catheters and Catheter Care

Indwelling catheters (i.e., Foley's) cause significant medical problems, including bacteriuria (i.e., bacteria in the urine), recurrent febrile episodes, bladder and kidney stones, epididymitis (i.e., inflammation of the tip of the penis), chronic kidney inflammation and infection, and irritation of the meatal area (i.e., opening to the urethra). External collection devices (i.e., Texas catheters) also cause bacteriuria, infection, penile skin inflammation, and urinary retention if the condom twists or its external band is too tight.

Indwelling catheters should be reserved for the following situations:

■ Short-term use to rest the bladder after there has been an acute problem (e.g., sudden urinary retention for any number of reasons);

■ Chronic retention that cannot be managed surgically or medically;
■ Wounds that need protection from urine;
■ Care of a terminally ill or severely impaired patient who cannot tolerate garment changes; or
■ When there is persistent patient preference for catheter management despite risks.

Several general principles guide safe and effective catheter care. Bacteriuria and infection are reduced by closed drainage systems. It is important to note that bacteriuria will always be present in these individuals and should not be treated unless there are clear symptoms. In symptomatic patients (i.e., those with fever, pain, extremely foul smelling urine), cultures should be done after the old catheter is removed and a new catheter is inserted. When long-term catheter use is necessary, there is no need to change the catheter on a regular basis. The person should be monitored for symptoms of infection and adequate passage of urine. The problem of leakage around the catheter can be managed by changing the Foley and increasing the size of the lumen if tolerated by the resident. Alternatively, evaluate the resident for bacteriuria, constipation or impaction, or improper catheter positioning (e.g., kinking).

For *acute urinary retention*, standard treatment is to rest the bladder with an indwelling catheter for at least 7 days. Clamping the catheter should *not* be done. The Foley is then removed and the individual given a trial of voiding generally over 6 to 8 hours. Intermittent catheterizations every 6 to 8 hours should be ordered during the trial period or as needed (when the resident feels uncomfortable and there is at least 300 cc of urine in the bladder). A 7-day trial is sufficient to observe if the individual can empty his or her bladder.

RESOURCES

Fung, C.H., Spencer, B., Eslami, M., & Crandall, C. (2007). Quality indicators for the screening and care of urinary incontinence in vulnerable elders. *Journal of the American Geriatric Society, 55,* S443–S449.

Holroyd-Leduc, J.M., & Straus, S.E. (2004). Management of urinary incontinence in women. *Journal of the American Medical Association, 291,* 986–995.

Ouslander, J.G. (2004). Management of overactive bladder. *New England Journal of Medicine, 350,* 786–799.

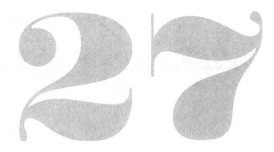

Gait Impairment

Neil B. Alexander and Kathleen Michael

Gait impairments are commonly associated with falls and disability in older adults. This chapter reviews the epidemiology of gait impairment, comorbidities that contribute to the disorder, and clinical assessments and interventions to reduce their functional impact.

EPIDEMIOLOGY

Limitations in walking increase with age. At least 20% of community-residing older adults admit to difficulty with walking or require the assistance of another person or special equipment to walk. Among older adults age 85 and over, the incidence of limitation in walking can be over 54%. Age-related gait changes such as decrease in speed are most apparent past age 75 or 80, but most gait disorders appear in connection with underlying diseases, particularly as disease severity increases. For example, with advanced age (i.e., the old-old; > 85 years), three or more chronic conditions at baseline, and the occurrence of stroke, hip fracture, or cancer, predict catastrophic loss of walking ability immediately after the catastrophic event and then persistent changes over time depending on recovery.

Determining that a gait is abnormal is difficult because there are no clearly accepted general standards of normal gait for older adults. Some clinicians believe that slowed gait speed suggests an underlying medical disorder (e.g., Parkinson's disease, dementia).

CONDITIONS THAT CONTRIBUTE TO GAIT IMPAIRMENT

Impaired gait may not be an inevitable consequence of aging but, rather, a reflection of the increased prevalence and severity of age-associated diseases. These diseases, both neurologic and nonneurologic, are major contributors to impaired gait. However, attributing a gait disorder to one disease rather than another in an older adult is particularly difficult because similar gait abnormalities are common to many diseases (see Exhibit 27.1).

Pain, stiffness, dizziness, numbness, weakness, and sensations of abnormal movement are the most common contributors to the older adult's walking difficulties, according to self-report. The most common conditions contributing to gait disorders are: degenerative joint disease, acquired musculoskeletal deformities, intermittent claudication, impairments following orthopedic surgery and stroke, and postural hypotension. Often, more than one contributing condition is found. Joint pain is one of the most common contributors to abnormal gait, followed by stroke, visual loss, dementia, and fear of falling. Neurologic-based disorders include frontal gait disorders (usually related to normal-pressure hydrocephalus and cerebrovascular processes), sensory disorders (also involving vestibular and visual function), myelopathy (spinal problems), previously undiagnosed Parkinson's disease or parkinsonian syndromes, and cerebellar disease. The most

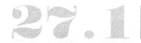 Description of Gait Abnormalities

TYPE OF GAIT	DESCRIPTION
Frontal lobe gait	Wide base of support Slightly flexed posture Small, shuffling, hesitant steps Poor initiation of gait; slipping clutch syndrome Turns by pivoting both feet in a small circle Cannot control changes in base of support
Sensory ataxic gait	Wide-based stance; foot-stamping walk High step/stamping walk Heel touches first, then foot stamps Visual input used to ambulate Positive Romberg's sign
Cerebellar ataxic gait	Wide-based stance Small, irregular, unsteady steps Drunken veering and lurching Impaired trunk control Difficulty with tandem gait En bloc turning
Spastic gait	Swings affected leg slowly in outward arc; circumduction of the leg Legs trace a semicircle when walking Feet scrape the ground Scissoring occurs Short steps Narrow base
Spastic gait	Legs move slowly and stiffly Short, labored steps with decreased hip and knee movement (bilateral circumduction—doesn't flex at the knee and hip but circles the leg around) Toes scrape the ground Scissoring occurs Short steps Narrow base
Steppage gait	Feet are lifted high off the ground to prevent scraping toes Toes hit first, then heels Head is down to observe foot placement
Peripheral vestibular imbalance	Unsteady gait
Antalgic and gonalgic gait	Reluctant to put weight on the joint Heel strike avoided on affected foot Push-off avoided Decreased stance and swing phases of gait Decreased walking velocity Knee and foot flexed Decreased hip and knee extension Limp due to leg length discrepancy

(continued)

27.1 Description of Gait Abnormalities *(continued)*

TYPE OF GAIT	DESCRIPTION
Podalgic gait	Pain with ambulation Toe contact occurs for three-quarters of the gait cycle
Dementia-related gait	Decreased walking speed Decreased step length Increased double-support time Increased step-to-step variability Increased postural sway Flexed posture Apraxic gait
Festinating gait	Symmetrical rapid shuffling of feet Trunk bent forward; hips and knees flexed Difficulty stepping
Parkinsonian gait	Festination Marche à petits pas; short, flat-footed shuffles Delayed gait initiation Body moves forward before feet Freezing Wide stance En bloc turning Loss of postural control Retropulsion; falls back in one piece like a log Propulsion
Waddling gait	Lateral trunk movement away from the foot, with exaggerated rotation of the pelvis and rolling of the hips Difficulty with stairs and chair rise
Vestibular ataxic gait	Broad based, with frequent sidestepping Drift toward the side of vestibular impairment Unsteady
Cautious gait	Flexed posture Decreased stride length Decreased walking speed Low center of gravity Wide base Short steps En bloc turning

severe gait impairments are generally due to hemiplegia and/or severe hip or knee disease.

Although older adults can maintain a relatively normal *gait pattern* well into their 80s, some slowing occurs. Decreased stride length thus becomes a common feature of an older adult's gait. Some clinicians suggest an age-related gait disorder, without accompanying clinical abnormalities: essential senile gait disorder. This gait pattern is described as broad-based with small steps, diminished arm swing, stooped posture, decreased flexion of the hips and knees, uncertainty and stiffness in turning, occasional difficulty initiating steps, and falls.

Tandem gait involves the ability to walk with one foot following the other and the toes of the back foot touching the heel of the front foot at each step. The inability to perform tandem gait is similar to gait patterns found in a number of other diseases, but the clinical abnormalities are insufficient to make a specific diagnosis. This so-called disorder may be a precursor to an as-yet-undiagnosed disease, such as Alzheimer's disease.

Factors that contribute to slowed gait speed are also considered contributors to gait disorders. These factors are commonly disease-associated (e.g., cardiopulmonary or musculoskeletal disease) and include reductions in leg strength, vision, aerobic function, standing balance, and decreased physical activity, as well as joint impairment, previous falls, and fear of falling. Combining these factors may result in an effect greater than the sum of the single impairments (such as combining balance and strength impairments). Furthermore, the effect of improved strength and aerobic capacity on gait speed may be nonlinear; that is, for very gait-impaired individuals, small improvements in strength or aerobic capacity yield relatively larger gains in gait speed, whereas these small improvements yield little gait speed change in healthy older adults. That is why it is so important for older adults to engage in regular physical activity, rehabilitation activities, and structured exercise classes.

ASSESSMENT

Gait disorders are divided into peripheral sensory impairment and peripheral motor dysfunction (i.e., lower extremity function disorders), including neurological and musculoskeletal disorders that cause weakness. With peripheral sensory impairment, unsteady and tentative gait is commonly caused by vestibular (inner ear) disorders, peripheral neuropathy (i.e., diminished sensation in the lower extremities), posterior column deficits (a proprioceptive issue: the ability to know where you are in space), or visual impairment. With peripheral motor impairment, a number of classical gait patterns emerge:

■ Trendelenburg gait: weight bearing shifts over to the weak hip, which then drops because of hip abductor weakness.
■ Antalgic gait: avoidance of weight-bearing leg and shortening of stance on one side because of pain.
■ Foot drop: due to ankle dorsiflexor weakness or the inability to point the toes to the floor and ceiling; frequently audible foot–floor contact with steppage gait

compensation, that is, excessive raising of the hip as if marching.

These gait impairments are the result of joint deformities, pain, and problems with muscle function or sensation. If the gait disorder is limited to this low sensorimotor level so that just the lower extremity is involved, the person will probably adapt fairly well to the gait disorder using adaptive equipment (e.g., canes and walkers) or by altering the environment (e.g., adding hand rails or avoiding the stairs). If the impairment is due to central involvement, as might occur after a stroke, the person may not be able to compensate as well because of problems such as impaired muscle innervations and balance. The person with central involvement therefore may not be able to maintain a functional gait to the point of being safe in his or her environment.

Gait impairments may also be due to spasticity (e.g., increased muscle tone due to diseases such as myelopathy, B_{12} deficiency, and stroke), parkinsonism (idiopathic as well as drug induced), and cerebellar disease (e.g., alcohol induced). A spastic gait occurs when there are fixed deformities in the range of motion of the lower extremities (i.e., generally contractures of the hip or the knee). The individual with a spastic gait will have leg circumduction, which means that he or she will make a circular motion with the leg rather than bending the leg at the knee or hip when walking. A flexed-forward, flat-footed, festinating gait (i.e., small shuffling steps) with reduced arm swing is classic for Parkinson's disease.

Frontal lobe lesions can cause even more significant gait disorders. The severity of the frontal lobe–related disorders runs a spectrum from difficulty with initiation of gait to the gait being so unsteady that it is neither practical nor safe for the individual to ambulate independently. Dementia and depression are also thought to cause abnormal gaits associated with frontal lobe impairment. With significant severity of the dementia, gait changes due to frontal lobe impairment progress such that the gait appears as described in Exhibit 27.1. A resident with significant dementia will be more likely to walk with a wide base and small shuffling steps. Table 27.1 describes aspects of gait associated with cerebellar, sensory, and frontal lobe impairment.

There is likely to be more than one disease or impairment present that contributes to a gait disorder: for example, a diabetic resident with peripheral neuropathy and a recent stroke who is now very fearful of falls. Medication (e.g., sedatives, tranquilizers, and anticonvulsants) and metabolic causes may result in changes to the central nervous system (i.e., affecting the brain in

27.1 | Aspects of Different Gait Patterns

ASPECT OF GAIT	CEREBELLAR ABNORMALITIES	SENSORY ABNORMALITIES	FRONTAL LOBE ABNORMALITIES
Trunk posture	Stooped—leans forward	Stooped—upright	Upright
Stance	Wide-based	Wide-based	Wide-based
Initiation of gait	Normal	Normal, wariness	Starts with hesitation
Postural reflexes	Generally intact	Intact	May be absent
Steps	Stagger-lurching	High-stepping-like marching	Small-shuffling
Stride length	Irregular	Regular	Short
Leg movement	Variable and uncoordinated	Variable—hesitant and slow	Stiff, rigid
Speed of movement	Normal to slow gait	Normal to slow gait	Very slow gait
Arm swing	Normal, exaggerated	Normal	Exaggerated
Turning corners	Veers away	Minimal effect—able to turn normally	Freezing-shuffling
Heel-toe test	Unable to perform	May be able to do this normally	Unable to perform
Romberg's test	Should be normal	Increased unsteadiness	Should be normal
Heel-shin test	Usually abnormal	Should be normal	Normal
Falls	Uncommon	Common	Very common

sending messages to the muscles and joints) and the peripheral nervous system (the body's ability to respond to nerve innervations in the hands and the feet).

History and Physical Examination

A careful medical history will help elucidate the multiple factors contributing to the older adult's gait impairment. Physical examination should include an attempt to identify what might be causing a sense of dizziness and thus altering gait. Blood pressure should be measured with the resident both lying and standing to exclude orthostatic hypotension (see Chapter 43, "Hypertension"). Conduct a vision screening (see Chapter 22, "Visual Impairment"). The neck, spine, extremities, and feet should be evaluated for pain, deformities, and limitations in range of motion. *Leg-length* discrepancies can occur following a hip replacement. Leg length is measured from the ankle bone to the top of the hip bone with the person lying down. Ideally, a formal neurologic assessment should be performed to evaluate muscle strength and tone, sensation, coordination, and gait. In taking the history, ask the resident if he/she notices that the room is spinning or if he/she seems to be spinning. A sensation that the room is spinning is indicative of vertigo. This may be worse with changes in position and disappear when the individual lies down and keeps his or her head still.

INTERVENTIONS TO REDUCE GAIT DISORDERS

Even if a diagnosable condition is found when conducting gait evaluation, many conditions causing a gait disorder might be only partially treatable. Functional improvement, therefore, becomes the treatment goal. Gait disorders due to B_{12} deficiency, folate deficiency, hypothyroidism, hyperthyroidism, knee osteoarthritis, Parkinson's disease, and inflammatory polyneuropathy improve as a result of medical treatment. Physical therapy for diseases such as knee osteoarthritis and stroke also result in modest improvements in function, but the resident will likely have some persistent disability. Audio and visual cues for people with Parkinson's gait disorders, such as telling them to pick up their feet when walking, can improve gait speed. Treadmill walking can improve gait for individuals with total hip replacements, Parkinson's disease, and particularly for those who have had a stroke with residual hemiparesis. There may be some modest improvements in gait following some types of back surgery, following joint replacements (knee and hip), and following the placement of a shunt to drain fluid from the brain in normal-pressure hydrocephalus.

Use of orthoses and other mobility aids will help reduce the gait disorder. Although there are few data supporting their use, shoe lifts (either inside the shoe or on the bottom of shoe) to correct for limb length inequality may be provided in a conservative, gradually progressive manner. Ankle braces, shoe inserts, and shoe body and sole modifications are part of standard care for foot and ankle weakness, deformities, and pain but are beyond the scope of this review. In general, well-fitting walking shoes with low heels, relatively thin, firm (i.e., not soft rubber) soles, and, if possible, high, fixed heel collar support, are recommended to maximize balance and improve gait. Mobility aids such as canes and walkers reduce load on a painful joint and increase stability. Light touch on any firm surface like walls or leaning lightly on furniture (i.e., so-called furniture surfing) provides feedback to the individual and enhances balance.

RESOURCES

Le Masurier, G.C., Bauman, A.E., Corbin, C.B., Konopack, J.F., Umstattd, R.M., & Van Emmerik, R.E. (2008). Assessing walking behaviors of selected subpopulations. *Medicine Science Sports and Exercise, 40*(7 Suppl.), S594–S602.

Nutt, J.G. (2001). Classification of gait and balance disorders. In E. Ruzicka, M. Hallet, & J. Jankovic (Eds.), *Gait disorders. Advances in neurology* (vol. 87). Philadelphia, PA: Lippincott, Williams and Wilkins.

Van Hook, F.W., Demonbreun, D., & Weiss, B.D. (2003). Ambulatory devices for chronic gait disorders in the elderly. *American Family Physician, 67*(8), 1717–1724.

Verghese, J., Robbins, M., Holtzer, R., Zimmerman, M., Wang, C., Xue, X., et al. (2008). Gait dysfunction in mild cognitive impairment syndromes. *Journal of the American Geriatric Society, 56*(7), 1244–1251.

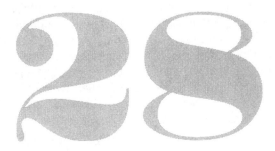

Falls

Douglas P. Kiel and Barbara Resnick

Falls are among the most common and serious health problems of older people. Falls in the elderly are multifactorial events and include intrinsic (resident-related) and extrinsic (environment-related) factors. In addition, falls result in multiple consequences, both physical and psychosocial, that can potentially have a long-term impact on older individuals. Fortunately there are many interventions that can be implemented to prevent a fall. These interventions are both intrinsic to the individual and extrinsic. Intrinsic interventions are focused on strengthening the individual physically and decreasing the likelihood he or she will experience a drop in blood pressure that could cause dizziness and a fall. Extrinsic interventions include such things as environmental changes to prevent a fall. Nursing can have an important impact on fall prevention by helping older adults adhere to important fall prevention interventions. This chapter provides an overview of falls, the potential consequences of falls, and reviews the many interventions to prevent a fall and thereby improve the quality of life of the assisted living residents.

PREVALENCE AND MORBIDITY

A fall is one of the most common events threatening the independence of older adults. By definition, a fall is considered to have occurred when a person comes to rest inadvertently on the ground or a lower level. Most falls are not associated with syncope. Incidence of falls increases with age and varies according to living status. Each year, between 30% and 40% of community-dwelling older adults age 65 years and older will fall. Among those with a history of a fall in the previous 12 months, the annual incidence of falls is close to 60%. In long-term-care settings, about half of all residents fall in 1 year.

Most falls result in an injury of some type, usually minor soft-tissue injuries, such as bruises and scrapes. However, 10% to 15% of falls result in fracture or other serious injury. Complications resulting from falls are the leading cause of death from injury in men and women age 65 and older. The death rate attributable to falls increases with age: White men age 85 years and older have the highest death rate (> 180 deaths per 100,000 population). In general, falls are associated with subsequent decline in functional status, greater likelihood of nursing-home placement, increased use of medical services, and development of a fear of falling. Of those older adults who fall, only half are able to get up without help, thus experiencing the so-called long lie that is associated with lasting decline in functional status.

The true cost of falls in health care dollars is difficult to ascertain. It is estimated that the lifetime costs of fall-related injuries for persons age 65 and older is $12.6 billion in the United States. Since many falls result in injury, there is a significant use of emergency department facilities among fallers.

CAUSES OF FALLS

Falls, incontinence, delirium, and other geriatric syndromes are the result of the accumulated effects of impairments in multiple domains (e.g., physical function, cognitive changes); they are rarely due to a single cause. Typically, there is often a complex interaction among factors intrinsic to the individual (e.g., chronic disease, acute illness, medications), challenges to postural control such as occurs when transferring from a chair to the bed or walking to the bathroom, and mediating factors (e.g., risk-taking behaviors such as using a step stool or maneuvering stairs while holding multiple packages).

Many risk factors are consistently associated with falls including age, cognitive impairment, female gender, past history of a fall, lower-extremity weakness, gait problems, foot disorders, balance problems, low levels of vitamin D, psychotropic drug use, arthritis, and Parkinson's disease. These multiple risk factors highlight the multifactorial nature of falls and suggest that there may also be unique circumstances surrounding falls. In general, the risk of falling increases with the number of risk factors, although some persons with no risk factors experience falls.

Successful prevention of falls begins with knowledge of age-related changes that increase the risk of falls. Thus, with aging, there are declines in the visual, proprioceptive, and vestibular systems. For example, the older individual may have reduced visual acuity, depth perception, contrast sensitivity, and dark adaptation. Changes in the proprioceptive system cause lessened sensitivity in the lower extremities and loss of ability to achieve and maintain balance. The vestibular system undergoes loss of labyrinthine hair cells, vestibular ganglion cells, and nerve fibers that can cause vertigo or dizziness. With age, older adults also tend to use the proximal muscles (i.e., those close to the center of the body), such as the quadriceps, before using the more distal muscles (i.e., those further from the central body) such as ankle muscles. This change reduces the older adult's ability to maintain or regain balance when pushed or put off balance.

An important physiologic contributor to the successful maintenance of upright posture is blood pressure. Failure to perfuse the brain, a sequelae of hypotension, increases the risk of a fall, usually in association with syncope. In addition, there are age-related declines in the function of baroreceptors that control the body's ability to respond to changes in position in terms of maintaining blood pressure. Reduction in total body water, another age-related change, increases the risk of dehydration, which, in the presence of acute illness, diuretic use, or hot weather, can cause orthostatic hypotension (see Chapter 42, "Cardiovascular Diseases and Disorders") and precipitate a fall.

A number of age-related chronic conditions warrant special mention because of their association with fall risk. Parkinson's disease, in particular, increases the risk of falls because of the associated rigidity of the lower extremity musculature, the gait changes that occur, hypotensive drug effects (e.g., side effect of Sinemet), and, in some cases, cognitive impairment. Osteoarthritis of the knee may affect mobility, the ability to step over and maneuver between objects, and increase the tendency to avoid complete weight bearing on a painful joint. Although not always a contributor to falls, specific classes of medications, such as the benzodiazepines, antidepressants (including selective serotonin-reuptake inhibitors and tricyclic antidepressants), sedative hypnotics, and antipsychotic drugs, have been associated with an increased risk of falls and hip fracture. An increased risk of falling is associated with changes in the dose of a medication and the total number of prescriptions.

The relative importance of environmental factors to the risk of falling appears to be much less than intrinsic factors in the individual. Nevertheless, attention to safety hazards in the home environment is certainly worthwhile, particularly if there is evidence of an environmental hazard, such as the different surface heights of an area rug and the bare floor. However, removal of seeming environmental hazards—if the individual is aware of them and knows how to ambulate on or near them appropriately—may decrease quality of life and not reduce falls.

DIAGNOSTIC APPROACH

History and Physical Examination

It is important to do a falls risk assessment (Exhibit 28.1) on admission or after significant change in condition (e.g., hip fracture, pneumonia, stroke). The most important point in risk assessment is the previous history of a fall: a strong risk factor for future falls. For residents who experience a fall, it is important to do a complete history or exploration of the fall as close to the time it occurred as is possible (Exhibit 28.2). Components of the fall history at the time of the fall include the activity of the faller at the time the incident occurred, evidence of prodromal symptoms (e.g., lightheadedness, imbalance, dizziness), location of the fall, and time of the fall. Loss of consciousness is associated with injurious falls and should raise important considerations, such as orthostatic hypotension or cardiac or neurologic disease (see Chapter 24, "Dizziness"). A complete

28.1 | Falls Risk Assessment

RESIDENT	DATE	
RISK	YES	NO
Previous fall		
Fear of falling		
Cardiac arrhythmia		
Transient ischemic attacks		
Stroke		
Parkinson's disease		
Delirium		
Dementia		
Depression		
Musculoskeletal problems (degenerative joint disease)		
Mobility/gait problems		
History of fractures		
Orthostatic hypotension		
Bowel/bladder incontinence		
Visual or auditory impairments		
Dizziness		
Dehydration		
Acute medical illness		
Use of restraint		
Hypoglycemia		
Polypharmacy		
Alcohol use		
Total		

Score: 0–5 in the "yes" column is low risk; 6–10 in the "yes" column is moderate risk; 11+ in the "yes" column is high risk.

28.2 | Evaluation of Fall Incident

NAME	DATE	DESCRIPTION OF FALL:
Variable		
Fall location		
Room		
Outside (e.g., parking lot, entrance, walking path)		
Bathroom		
Dining Room		
Hallway		
Activity room		
Other (Elevator, front lobby, store, stairs)		
Activity related to fall		
Walking		
Transferring		
Dressing		
Bathing		
Toileting		
Exercising (independently, in group)		
Cooking or cleaning		
Doing laundry		
Time of fall		
12:01 P.M.–6 P.M.		
6:01 P.M.–12 midnight		
12:01 A.M.–6 A.M.		
6:01 A.M.–12 noon		
Breakfast, lunch, and/or dinner		

(continued)

 | Evaluation of Fall Incident *(continued)*

NAME	DATE	DESCRIPTION OF FALL:

Loss of consciousness

  Yes

  No

Dizziness

  Yes

  No

Alcohol/sedative hypnotic use at time of fall

  Yes

  No

Outcome of fall

  None

  Hematoma

  Swelling

  Skin Tear

  Fracture

  Musculoskeletal pain

  Laceration

medication history should focus specifically on the use of vasodilators, diuretics, and sedative hypnotics because these agents have been associated with increased risk of falls. It is useful, also, to consider and explore the use of alcohol before the fall. In addition to inquiring about the circumstances surrounding the fall, attempt to identify possible contributory environmental factors, such as lighting, floor covering, surface conditions (e.g., wet floor), door thresholds, railings, footwear, and furniture.

Physical examination should focus on identification of any consequences associated with the fall and any physical factors that may have contributed to the fall (e.g., heart rate greater than 120 or low blood pressure) (Exhibit 28.3). Areas of pain, swelling and/or hematoma guide the possible need for tests/X-rays. A check of the range of motion of each major joint is

recommended, as is determination if the individual is able to come to a standing position and ambulate. If the individual has acute pain when bearing weight on the leg, he or she should be placed in a sitting or lying position and further evaluation for fracture should be considered. Definitive signs of hip fracture are that the entire leg seems shorter and is rotated outward. Attempts at weight bearing or standing should be avoided as this can cause further injury. Obtaining information specifically about where there is pain, with and without weight bearing, can guide the health care provider toward further testing (e.g., what part of the body to x-ray). Information obtained from these assessments should be used to develop appropriate interventions to manage the outcomes of the current fall and—equally importantly—to implement interventions to prevent future falls.

TREATMENT AND PREVENTION

Interventions to prevent falls and fall-related injuries include the following:

- Education about apartment and community/assisted living community hazards
- Exercise or physical therapy (see Chapter 18, "Physical Activity")
- Cognitive-behavioral interventions (to build confidence around physical activity see Chapter 16, "Psychosocial Aspects of Aging")
- Medication withdrawal or adjustment
- Nutritional or vitamin supplementation
- Referral for correction of visual impairment
- Cardiac pacemaker insertion for syncope-associated falls
- Use of hip protectors

Using the initial risk assessment and assessments of subsequent falls to guide interventions is the most effective way to decrease falls. For example, decreasing clutter in a resident's environment, having him or her participate in daily exercise activities, and avoiding excessive intake of alcohol can all be critical interventions to decrease fall risk. Once fall prevention strategies are developed for the resident and integrated into his or her service plan, ongoing monitoring and encouragement from staff is needed to be sure he or she is adhering to those interventions (see Exhibit 28.4; see also Chapter 16, "Psychosocial Aspects of Aging," for discussion about self-efficacy and mastery).

28.3 | Physical Assessment and Evaluation Following the Fall

Name_____ Date of fall_____

I.   Vital signs:

    a. Heart rate _____

    b. Heart rhythm: regular_____   irregular_____

    c. Blood pressure: lying_____   standing_____

II.   Physical exam

    a. Active, or independent range of motion

      1. Neck   _____yes   _____no

      2. Shoulders Rt: _____yes   _____no   Lt: _____yes   _____no

      3. Wrists Rt: _____yes   _____no   Lt: _____yes   _____no

      4. Hands Rt: _____yes   _____no   Lt: _____yes   _____no

      5. Hips Rt: _____yes   _____no   Lt: _____yes   _____no

      6. Knees Rt: _____yes   _____no   Lt: _____yes   _____no

      7. Ankles Rt: _____yes   _____no   Lt: _____yes   _____no

      8. Feet Rt: _____yes   _____no   Lt: _____yes   _____no

    b. Observations of resident:

      1. Shortening and external rotation of lower extremities: Rt_____ Lt_____

      2. Swelling: Location_____

      3. Redness/bruising: Location_____

      4. Abrasions: Location_____

      5. Pain on movement: Location_____

      6. Shortness of breath: yes _____   no _____

      7. Impaired balance: yes _____   no _____

      8. Loss of consciousness: yes _____   no _____

      9. Change in cognition: yes _____   no _____

    c. Assessment of the environment

      1. Dim lighting: yes _____   no _____

      2. Glare: yes _____   no _____

      3. Uneven flooring: yes _____   no _____

      4. Wet or slippery floor: yes _____   no _____

      5. Poor fit of seating device: yes _____   no _____

      6. Inappropriate footwear: yes _____   no _____

      7. Inappropriate eye wear: yes _____   no _____

      8. Loose carpet or throw rugs: yes _____   no _____

      9. Use of full length side rails in bed: yes _____   no _____

      10. Lack of hallway rails in area of fall: yes _____   no _____

      11. Inappropriate assistive devices (fit or condition):   yes _____   no _____

      12. Lack of grab bars in bathroom: yes _____   no _____

      13. Cluttered areas: yes _____   no _____

      14. Other environmental causes: _____

III.   Underlying medical problems:

      a. Orthostatic hypotension   yes _____   no _____: Management _____

      b. Balance problems: yes _____   no _____: Management _____

      c. Dizziness/vertigo: yes _____   no _____: Management _____

      d. Other: _____: yes _____   no _____: Management: _____

IV.   Medications:

      a. Drugs that may contribute to fall:

        Diuretics: yes _____   no _____: Management _____

        Cardiovascular medications: yes _____   no _____: Management _____

        Antipsychotics: yes _____   no _____: Management _____

        Antianxiety agents: yes _____   no _____: Management _____

        Sleeping agents: yes _____   no _____: Management _____

        Antidepressants: yes _____   no _____: Management _____

V.   Functional status:

      a. Impaired sitting balance: yes _____   no _____: Management _____

      b. Impaired standing balance: yes _____   no _____: Management _____

      c. Independent ambulation: yes _____   no _____: Management _____

      d. Independent toileting: yes _____   no _____: Management _____

VI.   Sensory problems:

      a. Evidence of impaired vision: yes _____   no _____: Management _____

      b. Evidence of impaired sensation: yes _____   no _____: Management _____

      c. Evidence of impaired hearing: yes _____   no _____: Management _____

VII.   Psychological status:

      a. Evidence of depression: yes _____   no _____: Management _____

      b. Evidence of change in cognition: yes _____   no _____: Management _____

      c. Evidence of impaired judgment: yes _____   no _____: Management _____

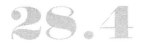 Description of the Interventions to Facilitate Adherence to Fall Prevention Interventions for Older Adults

Mastery experiences	Mastery: an effective way to increase adherence to a behavior that will make the individual feel confident about that behavior. This can be done by creating a strong sense of self-efficacy by helping the individual master the activity. Mastery involves the actual performance and successful completion of an activity.
	• Staff should provide opportunities for residents to do a functional task for themselves rather than simply doing it for residents (e.g., comb hair, wash face, put arm in shirt sleeve, drink with a no-spill cup, feed self with an adaptive utensil).
	• Personal care staff will be taught to encourage the residents to engage in exercise activities (e.g., this might be exercise classes if available, walking, balance activities) (see Chapter 18, "Physical Activity").
Vicarious experience	Role-modeling: can be used to show residents that other residents are using walkers, for example, or going to and enjoying a certain exercise class. In addition, the nurses and personal care staff can demonstrate how to do activities (functional tasks as well as exercises) and can share their own personal efforts and activities to prevent falls in their own lives.
	• Demonstration of performance of an activity (e.g., putting on a shirt in the case of an individual with cognitive impairment) or doing a certain balance exercise.
	• Demonstration of techniques to encourage participation: music as a motivator; encouraging resident activities that are consistent with past life experience, such as folding clothes or packing a briefcase.
	• Demonstration of an exercise routine (e.g., range of motion; small group activities with functional/physical activity focus).
Verbal encouragement	Can be done through education as well as direct verbal encouragement to participate in fall prevention activities (e.g., wearing appropriate footwear; going to exercise class).
	• Encouragement could include the use of humor.
	• Discuss with the resident how to incorporate fall prevention activities into his or her daily routine.
	• Establish relevant fall prevention goals and write these on a goal identification form.
Physiological feedback	Physiological feedback during an activity can have a positive or a negative influence. If going to exercise causes the resident pain, this might result in negative physiological feedback, and the resident might refuse to participate in the exercise activity. Conversely, if exercise causes the resident to feel healthier and stronger, then he or she will continue to engage in the activity.
	• Monitor/observe the resident for evidence of negative physiological feedback (e.g., pain associated with activity or dislike of/unwillingness to use a walker for psychological reasons); implement interventions to decrease those sensations.
	• Focus on and increase the pleasant or positive sensations and experiences associated with fall prevention behaviors (e.g., less dizziness since cutting back on a sleeping pill or decreasing alcohol intake). Gently remind the resident of the pleasant sensations that he or she is now experiencing.

RESOURCES

Bonner, A., MacCulloch, P., Gardner, T., & Chase, C. W. (2007). A student-led demonstration project on fall prevention in a long-term care facility. *Geriatric Nursing, 28*(5), 312–318.

Hendriks, M. R., Bleijlevens, M. H., van Haastregt, J. C., de Bruijn, F. H., Diederiks, J. P., Mulder, W. J., et al. (2008). A multidisciplinary fall prevention program for elderly persons: A feasibility study. *Geriatric Nursing, 29*(3), 186–196.

MacCulloch, P. A., Gardner, T., & Bonner, A. (2007). Comprehensive fall prevention programs across settings: A review of the literature. *Geriatric Nursing, 28*(5), 306–311.

Mitty, E., & Flores, S. (2007). Fall prevention in assisted living: Assessment and strategies. *Geriatric Nursing, 28*(6), 349.

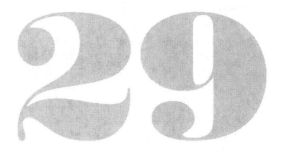

Osteoporosis

Karen M. Prestwood
and Andrea Brassard

Because osteoporosis is a result of unbalanced bone formation and resorption, and associated fractures usually involve a fall, optimal prevention and treatment also include strategies to minimize bone resorption and to reduce falls.

DEFINITION OF OSTEOPOROSIS

The World Health Organization (WHO) defines osteoporosis by bone mineral density (BMD) measurement. This means that an individual can be diagnosed and treated for osteoporosis prior to having a fracture. A BMD measurement at any site that is < 2.5 standard deviations below the young adult standard (i.e., T score of < -2.5) means that the individual has osteoporosis. A BMD measurement between -1 and -2.5 indicates osteopenia: the bone is thinning but has not deteriorated to the point of osteoporosis. Thus, the clinician can make the diagnosis of osteoporosis and begin the appropriate therapy before fracture in the older adult occurs. In addition, women with osteopenia can be placed on a preventive regimen and then followed carefully for further bone loss. Specific standards for definitions of osteoporosis have not been established for men or for racial and ethnic groups other than Whites, although it appears that similar standards apply to men and to Hispanic women.

EPIDEMIOLOGY AND IMPACT OF OSTEOPOROSIS

Osteoporosis is a major health threat in the United States. It is estimated that 55% of women and men over age 50 have low bone mass and that one of two women and one in five men will suffer an osteoporosis-related fracture. The incidence of osteoporotic fracture in women is greater than the incidence of heart attack, stroke, and breast cancer combined. The consequences of osteoporosis include diminished quality of life, decreased independence, and increased morbidity and mortality. Vertebral compression (crush) fractures are associated with pain, kyphosis, height loss, diminished quality of life, and reduced functional status (i.e., residents may be unable to bathe, dress, or walk independently). Approximately 50% of women with hip fracture do not fully recover prior function. Increased mortality is related primarily to hip fractures; 20% excess mortality occurs in older adults in the year following hip fracture.

BONE REMODELING AND BONE LOSS IN AGING

Bone tissue is able to repair itself by active remodeling (also called bone turnover) and bone resorption (i.e., breakdown of the bone) followed by bone formation. This process continues throughout the life span. Local signals, not yet fully understood, bring osteoclasts to specific areas of bone where resorption is initiated and resorption cavities are formed. Once osteoclasts have completed the resorption process, osteoblasts move into the area and begin to lay down osteoid and, later, to calcify the matrix. Under optimal conditions, once bone remodeling is completed in a specific area, the resorption spaces are completely filled with new bone. However, in postmenopausal women, and with the aging process in men and women, the remodeling cycle becomes unbalanced, and bone resorption increases more than bone formation, resulting in net bone loss. Most of the drug treatments for osteoporosis act to inhibit bone resorption rather than to increase bone formation.

Bone mass changes over the life span. In women, bone mass increases rapidly from puberty until the mid-20s to mid-30s, at which time peak bone mass is reached. At this time, a few years of stability are followed by a slow rate of bone loss, beginning well before the onset of menopause. After menopause, the rate of bone loss is quite rapid—as much as 7% per year—for up to 7 years—as a consequence of estrogen deficiency. In later life, bone loss continues, albeit at a slower rate, generally 1% to 2% per year; however, some older women may lose bone density at a higher rate. Data strongly suggest that reducing bone loss at any time will decrease fracture risk. It has been estimated that a 14% increase in bone density in a 70- to 80-year-old woman would halve the hip fracture risk. Although studies to date have focused primarily on women, men also lose bone with age at approximately the same rate. It is estimated that men aged 30 to 90 years lose approximately 1% per year in the radius and spine. Some men with risk factors for osteoporosis lose as much as 6% bone per year. Men have fewer vertebral fractures than women.

PATHOGENESIS OF OSTEOPOROSIS

Estrogen Deficiency in Women

The pathogenesis of osteoporosis in women is complex and involves factors that affect the level of peak bone mass, rate of bone resorption, and rate of bone formation. Peak bone mass appears to be 75% to 80% genetically determined, although the genes have not been identified. After menopause, in the presence of estrogen deficiency, a variety of factors that act locally on bone may lead to increased bone resorption.

Calcium Deficiency and Secondary Hyperparathyroidism

The mechanism by which older men and women continue to lose bone as they age is likely related to calcium deficiency (which causes secondary hyperparathyroidism). When parathyroid hormone (PTH) is elevated for long periods of time, it causes bone to breakdown. Aging skin and decreased exposure to sunlight reduce the body's ability to make vitamin D. Without vitamin D, it is impossible to absorb calcium, and thus the body cannot make new bone.

Androgens in Men

Androgens (i.e., male hormones such as testosterone) are important determinants for peak bone mass in men. Bone development is closely related to sexual maturity; men who had an abnormal or delayed puberty have reduced bone mass.

Changes in Bone Formation

In men and women, osteoblast activity appears to decrease with aging, compounding the bone loss that results from increased resorption associated with aging.

CAUSES OF OSTEOPOROSIS AND PREDICTION OF FRACTURE

Risk Factors

Risk factors for osteoporosis and osteoporotic fracture have been identified and have been used to determine who should be placed on preventive or therapeutic regimens. Exhibit 29.1 lists modifications of risk factors of osteoporosis—all of which should be addressed by the clinician as part of the routine care of an older adult. Risk factors should also be used to identify women younger than 65 years of age who should have BMD screening.

Secondary Causes

There are many secondary causes of osteoporosis. Laboratory tests are used to help clinicians determine what these causes are. These laboratory tests should be considered for persons who present with acute compression fracture or who present with a diagnosis of osteoporosis by BMD measurement. The most common

29.1 | Modifications to Reduce the Risk of Osteoporosis

Exercise: Encourage regular, weight-bearing exercise

Fall prevention: Use hip protectors in residents prone to falling

Nutrition: Encourage

- Adequate dietary intake of calcium and vitamin D

- Lower intake of animal protein

- Limit diet soda

- Limit caffeine

Calcium and vitamin D supplements

Smoking cessation

Minimize alcohol intake

Medications that may increase risk of osteoporosis—use with caution:

- Anticonvulsants

- Cyclosporine

- Glucocorticoids (> 5 mg/day of prednisone or equivalent for > 3 months)

- Long-term heparin

- Methotrexate

- Thiazolidinediones (glitazones)

- Thyroid hormone replacement (dose dependent)

---

causes of secondary osteoporosis in women are primary hyperparathyroidism and glucocorticoid use. Men are more likely than women to have a secondary cause of osteoporosis; as many as 50% of osteoporotic men may have a secondary cause. The most commonly reported secondary causes of osteoporosis in men are hypogonadism and malabsorption syndromes, including gastrectomy. Medications shown to adversely affect BMD in men and women include glucocorticoids, excess thyroid supplement, anticonvulsants, methotrexate, cyclosporine, thiazolidinediones (glitazones), and heparin; these meds should be given at the lowest doses possible or discontinued.

Glucocorticoids result in bone loss primarily through the direct suppression of bone formation, although they also further reduce sex hormone levels and cause secondary hyperparathyroidism through their effects on intestinal calcium absorption. The prevalence of vertebral fractures in persons taking glucocorticoids for 1 year is estimated to be 11%. The rate of trabecular bone (long bone) loss is dose dependent and generally occurs in the first 6 months of therapy. Although inhaled corticosteroids have not been as well studied, high doses of high-potency inhaled steroids may also result in bone loss. The best strategy for older persons who require long-term glucocorticoid therapy is to maximize bone health with a variety of interventions. It is important to use the lowest possible dose of glucocorticoids, to ensure adequate calcium and vitamin D intake (see "Prevention and Treatment of Osteoporosis" section, later in this chapter). Bisphosphonates such as alendronate[OL] and risedronate successfully prevent bone loss that is due to glucocorticoid therapy when they are initiated at the same time as the steroids (see "Prevention and Treatment of Osteoporosis" section).

Bone Density Measurement

Bone mass measurement or BMD, is the best predictor of fracture and can be measured by a variety of techniques. The preferred method of BMD measurement of the hip, anterior-posterior spine, lateral spine, and wrist is dual-energy radiographic absorptiometry (DEXA). Other methods of measuring BMD are quantitative computed tomography, ultrasonography of the calcaneus, single radiographic absorptiometry of the calcaneus, and radiographic absorptiometry. The National Osteoporosis Foundation, in conjunction with numerous specialty organizations including the U.S. Preventive Services Task Force, recommends BMD testing for all women aged 65 years and over, regardless of risk-factor status; there are no data to determine the frequency of screening or the age at which to stop screening. For women between 60 and 64 years of age, the presence of additional risk factors, particularly low body weight and no estrogen replacement therapy (ERT), makes their risk of osteoporosis and fracture comparable to that of women over 65 years. Interpretation of BMD involves evaluating the quality of the DEXA as well as the T scores. The BMD of the individual older woman is compared with that of young women (25 to 35 years of age) who are considered to be at or near peak bone mass. For every standard deviation below the young adult mean, which is a decrease in 1 unit *T* score, fracture risk at the spine and hip approximately doubles. For example, if a woman has a *T* score of − 2, her risk of fracture is four times that of a woman with normal bone density (controlled for height and weight).

When evaluating the spine BMD over time, several considerations are important. Vertebral or arterial or lymph node calcification or any scoliosis may falsely increase BMD of the postero-anterior spine DEXA. Thus, a woman with osteoporosis of the spine may have a DEXA *T* score that is higher than − 2.5. Medicare will cover the cost for an initial screening and repeat screening every 2 years. DEXA scanning to evaluate the effectiveness of osteoporosis treatment is covered by Medicare every 1 to 2 years.

BMD testing is also used to establish the diagnosis and severity of osteoporosis in men and should be considered for men with low-trauma fractures, radiographic criteria consistent with low bone mass, or diseases known to place a person at risk for osteoporosis. Data relating BMD to fracture risk are derived from studies of women, but data suggest that similar associations may be valid for men. Several studies found that men with hip fractures are often not evaluated and treated for osteoporosis.

FRAX Algorithm

The National Osteoporosis Foundation Clinical Recommendations 2008 are based on the newly developed World Health Organization 10-year fracture risk model. The FRAX algorithm estimates the likelihood of a person breaking a bone during the next 10 years, thus hoping to ensure that people at risk of fracture receive treatment. The FRAX algorithm takes into account nine clinical risk factors in addition to bone mineral density and is available online at http://www.shef.ac.uk/FRAX.

PREVENTION AND TREATMENT OF OSTEOPOROSIS

The Role of Exercise

Exercise is an important component of osteoporosis treatment and prevention, although exercise alone is not adequate to prevent the rapid bone loss associated with estrogen deficiency in early menopause. Weight-bearing exercises such as walking and high-intensity strength training help maintain femoral neck BMD as well as improve muscle mass and strength. Marked decreases in physical activity or immobilization result in a decline in bone mass; accordingly, it is important to encourage older adults to be as active as possible. Older persons should be encouraged to start slowly and gradually increase both the number of days as well as the time spent walking each day. The Exercise and Screening for You (EASY) tool (available at http://www.easyforyou.info/) provides some excellent examples of aerobic and resistive exercise that will help bones and muscles.

Calcium and Vitamin D

Calcium and vitamin D are required for bone health at all ages. To maintain a positive calcium balance, current recommendation for calcium intake for postmenopausal women and men aged 65 years and older is at least 1,200 mg per day of elemental calcium (see Table 29.1 for information on the calcium contained in selected foods). The amount of vitamin D required is 800 IU per day. In older adults, regardless of climate or exposure to sunlight, a daily supplement of ≥ 800 IU per day of vitamin D is recommended because skin changes that occur with aging result in less efficient use of ultraviolet light by the skin to synthesize vitamin D precursors.

Pharmacologic Options

Dosing and special considerations for the medications used to prevent and treat osteoporosis are provided in Exhibit 29.2.

Bisphosphonates

Alendronate has been approved for osteoporosis prevention (women) and treatment (men and women), including glucocorticoid-induced osteoporosis. Postmenopausal women with severe osteoporosis who were treated with alendronate, compared with women on placebo, had increased bone density of the spine and hip, as well as decreased vertebral fracture rate (Fracture Intervention Trial; see Black et al., 1998). Regardless of the presence of vertebral fractures at baseline, alendronate was found to decrease the vertebral and hip fracture rates. Alendronate has also been approved for the prevention of osteoporosis in early postmenopausal women. The daily dose for prevention is lower than that for the treatment of osteoporosis. If treatment with a bisphosphonate alone is not effective (bone loss of > 4% or fracture within 3 months of initiation), additional treatments such as raloxifene or ERT may be

29.1 | Calcium-Containing Foods

FOOD	SERVING SIZE	CALCIUM (MG) PER SERVING
Dairy products		
Milk	1 cup	290–300
Yogurt	6 ounces (¾ cup)	180–300
Swiss cheese	1 ounce (1 slice)	250–270
American cheese	1 ounce (1 slice)	165–200
Ice cream	½ cup	90–100
Cottage cheese	½ cup	80–100
Parmesan cheese	1 tablespoon	70
Powdered nonfat milk	1 tablespoon	50
Other		
Sardines in oil with bones	3 ounces	370
Calcium-fortified orange juice	1 cup	300
Canned salmon with bones	3 ounces	170–210
Broccoli	1 cup, cooked	90–100
Tofu (soybean curd)	4 ounces	80–200
Collard greens	½ cup, cooked	150–175
Turnip greens	½ cup, cooked	100–125
Kale	½ cup, cooked	90–100
Pizza	1 slice	90–100
Other fortified foods (bread, cereal, fruit juices)	1 serving	Varies: read food label

Note: Food labels list calcium as a percentage of the daily value (DV), based on 1000 mg of calcium per day. For example: 30% DV equals 300 mg; 20% DV equals 200 mg; 15% DV equals 150 mg.

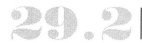

Instructions for Administration of Oral Bisphosphonates

- Take first thing in the morning before eating or drinking anything else

- Take with at least 8 ounces of plain tap water

- Take while upright in a chair or standing, and remain upright after ingestion for 30 minutes (alendronate and risedronate) to 1 hour (ibandronate)

- Do not eat or drink anything for 30 minutes (alendronate and risedronate) to 1 hour (ibandronate) after taking the medication

- Do not crush (alendronate is available in liquid form 75 ml followed with at least 2 ounces of plain tap water)

indicated. In women with lesser degrees of osteoporosis, alendronate has not been shown to prevent hip fracture. Alendronate is available in generic form. The optimal duration of treatment with bisphosphonates is unclear; one study indicated that the greatest increase in vertebral bone mass occurred during the first 5 years of treatment, and benefit was maintained for 10 years without undue risk.

The major adverse effects of bisphosphonates are gastrointestinal, including abdominal pain, dyspepsia, esophagitis, nausea, vomiting, and diarrhea. Musculoskeletal pain may also occur. Esophagitis, particularly erosive esophagitis, is seen most commonly in individuals who do not take the medication properly. The absorption of oral bisphosphonates is very poor; thus, it is extremely important to provide specific and detailed instructions for residents receiving any bisphosphonate therapy (Exhibit 29.2).

Risedronate, another bisphosphonate, has similar indication for osteoporosis prevention and treatment and has been approved for glucocorticoid-induced osteoporosis prevention and treatment. Alendronate and risedronate were the first two bisphosphonates available. Both have similar indication for osteoporosis prevention and treatment and both have been approved for glucocorticoid-induced osteoporosis prevention and treatment. Ibandronate, another bisphosphonate, is taken once a month and is approved for postmenopausal osteoporosis prevention and treatment. A 3-year study of postmenopausal women found that ibandronate re-

duced the incidence of vertebral fractures by 50%. However, ibandronate was not found to significantly reduce hip fracture incidence. A meta-analysis of 8,710 patients taking ibandronate found significant reduction in the relative risk of six nonvertebral fractures (clavicle, humerus, wrist, pelvis, hip, and leg) and delayed time to fracture compared to placebo. The newest available bisphosphonate, zoledronic acid, is administered as an intravenous infusion once a year. In a three year study of 7765 postmenopausal women, treatment with zoledronic acid reduced the risk of vertebral fracture by 70% and the risk of hip fracture by 40% compared to placebo.

Selective Estrogen Receptor Modulators

Selective estrogen receptor modulators are agents that act as estrogen agonists in bone and heart tissue but act as estrogen antagonists in breast and uterine tissue. These medications have the potential to prevent osteoporosis or cardiovascular disease without the increased risk of breast or uterine cancer. Tamoxifen, an agent used to treat breast cancer, has beneficial effects on bone, as reported in several studies, but it also has stimulatory effects on the uterus. Thus, tamoxifen is not indicated for osteoporosis treatment or prevention.

Raloxifene has been approved for the treatment and prevention of osteoporosis in postmenopausal women. Comparison of raloxifene with placebo in postmenopausal women with osteoporosis found that raloxifene decreases bone turnover and maintains hip and total body bone density. There were no differences between groups in breast abnormalities or endometrial thickness. Most importantly, data demonstrate that raloxifene (60 mg per day) reduces incident vertebral fractures by about 60%, despite only modest increases in bone density. In this study, raloxifene was not found to significantly reduce nonvertebral, hip, or wrist fractures. Reported adverse effects with raloxifene include flu-like symptoms, hot flashes, leg cramps, and peripheral edema.

Calcitonin

Calcitonin is a hormonal inhibitor of bone resorption that is approved for the treatment of osteoporosis in women. It is available as a subcutaneous injection and as a nasal spray. The nasal spray has fewer reported side effects and greater patient acceptance, but it may be less effective. Calcitonin increases bone density in the spine and reduces vertebral fractures. In epidemiologic studies, calcitonin reduces the incidence of hip fractures, although in clinical trials, hip bone density did not increase. Results of a 5-year study demonstrated that the incidence of vertebral fractures in women receiving 200 IU per day of nasal spray calcitonin was lower than that of women on placebo. The reduction in hip fracture incidence was not statistically significant in the group receiving calcitonin in comparison with the placebo group. Doses of 100 and 400 IU per day were studied as well, but they did not reduce incidence of vertebral fractures. In the same study, BMD changes at 3 years and changes in markers of bone turnover in the treatment and placebo groups were found not to be significantly different. Although there are no direct comparisons, calcitonin appears to be less effective than other antiresorptive drugs. There is some evidence that calcitonin produces an analgesic effect in some women with painful vertebral compression fractures.

Estrogen Replacement Therapy

ERT is an option for osteoporosis prevention; however, it is not recommended as a first-line choice for prevention. In case-control and cohort studies, ERT was associated with a 30% to 70% reduction in hip fracture incidence. Multiple studies have demonstrated that postmenopausal estrogen use prevents bone loss at the hip and spine when initiated within 10 years of menopause. However, in a cross-sectional study, BMD in women who initiated hormone replacement therapy (HRT) after age 60 was found not to be significantly different from in women who initiated HRT within 2 years of menopause. In the Postmenopausal Estrogen/ Progestin Intervention trial (Garg, 1995), older women, women with low initial BMD, and women who had not previously used HRT were found to gain more bone than did young women, women with higher baseline BMD, and those who had previously used HRT. Decreased incident vertebral fractures were seen in a small study of postmenopausal women using a transdermal estradiol preparation. Recent prospective data from the Women's Health Initiative (WHI) also demonstrated that postmenopausal women who took HRT for approximately 7 years had a decreased hip fracture risk; however, the dose and preparation of hormone therapy used also increased the risk of breast cancer, heart disease, stroke, and deep-vein thrombosis. Given the WHI findings, recent U.S. Preventive Services Task Force guidelines advise against the routine use of estrogen plus progesterone for the prevention of chronic conditions in postmenopausal women.

Parathyroid Hormone

PTH (teriparatide) is an anabolic (tissue-building) agent when administered by daily subcutaneous injection. It is approved for the treatment of osteoporosis in men and women who are at high risk for osteoporotic fracture and who are unable to tolerate other approved agents. PTH should not be used as a first-line therapy for osteoporosis. It has been shown to increase spinal BMD in osteoporotic men and women. In a 3-year randomized study of postmenopausal women with osteoporosis, the group receiving estrogen plus intermittent PTH had continuous increase in spinal bone mass over the study period, as well as decreased vertebral fracture rate. Bone mass of the hip and total body also increased significantly in the estrogen-plus-PTH group, in comparison with the group on estrogen alone. Recent studies have also demonstrated the effectiveness of PTH in reducing vertebral and nonvertebral fractures in postmenopausal women. In men with primary or hypogonadal osteoporosis, PTH also increased BMD at all sites. The safety and efficacy of PTH has not been demonstrated beyond two years of treatment.

WORKING WITH THE RESIDENT

Establishing and maintaining an optimal regimen usually requires considerable discussion with individual residents and is much easier when they and their families/proxies are well informed. The use of educational materials can be quite helpful, including medication administration reminders.

Adherence to the medication regimen is particularly important to help guide the interpretation of follow-up BMD measurements (every 1 to 2 years). If a resident is nonadherent to a medication, then additional treatment should not be added if the BMD does not improve at follow-up testing. Rather, focused interventions should be on improving behavioral and medication adherence.

MANAGEMENT OF VERTEBRAL FRACTURES

Most vertebral fractures are asymptomatic and are diagnosed by spinal radiographs. Over time, one may notice decreased height, increased kyphosis, or simply the fact that clothes no longer fit the person properly. Many older adults have chronic back pain due to the changes in the spine that occur with vertebral compression. In the case of symptomatic vertebral compression fractures, adequate pain control is essential. The pain usually lasts 2 to 4 weeks and can be quite debilitating. Nonsteroidal anti-inflammatory drugs and calcitonin can be tried; narcotics are commonly required to control the pain. Physical therapy is an important part of osteoporosis treatment programs for the management of acute and chronic pain, as well as for patient education. The physical therapist can provide postural exercises, alternative modalities for pain reduction, and information on changes in body mechanics that may help prevent future fractures. Newer treatments for vertebral fractures involve the injection of bone cement into the collapsed vertebra (vertebroplasty) or use of a balloon tamp into the fractured vertebrae (kyphoplasty). These methods can decrease pain and improve quality of life and function in some individuals.

RESOURCES

Black, D. M., Cummings, S. R., Karpf, D. B., Cauley, J. A., Thompson, D. E., Nevitt, M. C., et al. (1998). Effect of alendronate on risk of fracture in women with low bone density but without vertebral fractures. *The Journal of the American Medical Association, 280,* 2077–2082.

Black, D. M., Delmas, P. D., Eastell, R., Reid, I. R., Boonen, S., Cauley, J. A., et al. (2007). Once-yearly zoledronic acid for treatment of postmenopausal osteoporosis. *New England Journal of Medicine, 356*(18), 1809–1822.

Garg, A. (1995). The postmenopausal estrogen/progestin interventions trial. *Journal of American Medical Association, 274,* 1675–1676.

Meier, C., Kraenzlin, M., Bodmer, M., Jick, S. S., Jick, H., & Meier, C. R. (2007). Use of thiazolidinediones and fracture risk. *Archives of Internal Medicine, 168*(8), 820–825.

National Osteoporosis Foundation. (2008). *Clinician's guide to prevention and treatment of osteoporosis.* Retrieved December 1, 2008, from http://www.nof.org/prevention/index.htm

Parikh, S., Mogun, H., Avorn, J., & Solomon, D. H. (2008). Osteoporosis medication use in nursing home fractures in one US state. *Archives of Internal Medicine, 168*(10), 1111–1115.

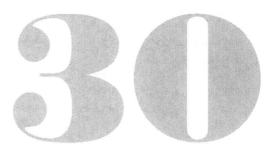

Behavior Problems in Dementia

Melinda S. Lantz, Constantine G. Lyketsos, and Elizabeth Galik

Most dementias are associated with a range of neuro-psychiatric and behavioral disturbances, with as many as 80% to 90% of sufferers developing at least one distressing symptom over the course of their illness. The development of behavioral disturbances or psychotic symptoms in dementia often precipitates placement in an assisted living community (ALC) or nursing home. These disturbances are potentially treatable, and it is vital that assisted living (AL) nurses anticipate, recognize, and use strategies to effectively manage them. If these symptoms become apparent, it is essential to perform a thorough assessment to identify contributing factors, target symptoms in need of treatment, and implement appropriate interventions for the resident and caregivers. Research that compares different treatment strategies for the behavioral and neuropsychiatric symptoms of dementia is growing in response to the great need for evidence-based treatment guidelines.

CLINICAL FEATURES

As the dementia progresses, a variety of psychiatric symptoms may develop, such as depression, delusions, hallucinations, and mania. Depressive symptoms are common in older adults with dementia; however, the clinical presentation is often different than it would be in a younger individual. Depression in the context of dementia often presents as apathy or anhedonia, that is, a lack of interest in previously enjoyable activities. Older adults with dementia and depression will often deny feeling sad but may be less hopeful about the future and make self-deprecating comments. This depressive syndrome may also include a loss of interest in self-care, eating, or interacting with peers. It is also common for these individuals to be quite irritable and impulsive. If these features become progressive, overt hostility or physical aggression may ensue. It is at this juncture that residents may be characterized as agitated, reflecting a loss of the ability to modulate their behavior in a socially acceptable way. Examples of such behavior are verbal outbursts, physical aggression, resistance to bathing or other care needs, and restless motor activity such as pacing or rocking. This type of overlap across symptoms, where some are associated with a depressive disorder but others such as hostility are considered atypical, often creates a significant challenge when assessing these residents. In this situation, the fairly nonspecific term *agitation* is commonly employed to describe the resident, but it may best be accompanied by additional description as to whether the problem is accompanied by simple irritability, vocal or physical aggression, or motor disturbances.

In some situations, agitation may occur when a resident demonstrates paranoia or delusional thinking, such as a fixed, false belief that caregivers are plotting to steal personal possessions or incur harm. When delusions occur, the resident is then characterized as suffering from psychotic symptoms. Hallucinations, sensory experiences without stimuli, are another type of psychotic symptom that may accompany episodes of agitated behavior. Visual and auditory hallucinations tend to be most common and often are threatening or frightening to the resident. For example, a resident may hear a baby crying at night when there are none present and try to leave her ALC apartment in order to find the baby. One way to conceptualize this complex condition is to consider the term *agitation* as a descriptor for the presence of abnormal behavior such as aggression, while the presence of psychosis (e.g., paranoid delusions) reflects the abnormal perceptions and beliefs that may lead to the agitated behavior. Depending on the degree of communication deficits in a given resident, the ability to discern the presence of psychosis is variable, and in many cases agitated behaviors may occur in the absence of clear evidence as to whether delusions or other psychoses are precipitating the disturbance.

Occasionally, a behavioral syndrome occurs that includes features of hyperactivity, euphoric mood, and grandiose beliefs that resemble a manic episode associated with bipolar affective disorder. The features are similar but less predictable than those seen in younger adults, and treatment strategies are more challenging. One key feature of the manic-like syndromes seen in dementia residents is the tendency to develop additional symptoms outside the typical course of a bipolar manic episode, such as agitated behaviors, defiance, and confusion.

Among the behavioral complications of dementia, the most severe disruptions in caregiving occur when residents develop physical behaviors such as hitting or wandering, or develop paranoid delusions that lead to hostility and altercations with caregivers or other residents. Caregivers, both professional and family, may use the word *agitation* to describe a variety of behaviors and psychological symptoms. The AL nurse must consider agitation to be a nonspecific complaint and pursue further history of the problem, including a description of specific behaviors and the time, course, frequency, and severity with which they occur. Environmental precipitants such as excessive stimuli or a change in the environment such as a new roommate may induce behavioral problems. The presenting complaint may relate to internal cues such as pain, hunger, thirst, or other needs that the resident is not able to express.

The complaints of family and professional caregivers in the ALC often arise from behavioral complications occurring during daily care that involve a resistance to bathing, dressing, or other routines. This type of overt resistance to care is most often seen in later stages of dementia, but it is important to note that behavioral problems may also be a first sign of cognitive decline in earlier stages as well. Neuropsychiatric symptoms such as apathy, poor self-care, or paranoia may be the first indication of dementia before cognitive decline is recognized. As such, evaluation for dementia in any resident who presents with new behavioral or emotional symptoms may reveal a previously undetected dementia syndrome.

ASSESSMENT

Comprehensive assessment of a resident with dementia and behavioral disturbance includes a history both from the resident and from an informant, such as a family member, and AL staff. The first step in assessment is to adequately describe the behavioral disturbance. This information should include a clear description of the behavior: when it began, the course and severity of the symptoms, associated circumstances, and its relationship to key environmental factors, such as caregiver status and recent stressors. The problem behaviors and symptoms should be then considered in the context of the resident's personal, social, and medical history.

Once the behavior is adequately described, the second step is to decide whether the disturbance is a symptom of a new or a preexisting medical condition or a medication adverse effect. Disturbances that are new, acute in onset, or evolving rapidly are most often due to a medical condition or medication toxicity. An isolated behavioral disturbance and change in mental status in a demented resident can be the *sole* presenting symptom for acute conditions such as pneumonia, urinary tract infection, arthritis, pain, angina, constipation, or poorly controlled diabetes mellitus. Additionally, the need to satisfy basic physical needs, such as hunger, sleepiness, thirst, boredom, or fatigue, which the resident cannot adequately communicate, may precipitate a behavioral disturbance. The need-driven dementia compromised behavior model provides a framework for understanding behavior problems that are precipitated by an unmet resident need. Medication toxicity due to new or existing medications might also present as behavioral symptoms alone. Treatment or stabilization of the medical or physical cause is often sufficient to resolve the disturbance. Older adults with dementia may require several weeks longer to recover from routine medical problems than those who are cognitively intact, as the associated exacerbation in cognitive function they experience will impair the recovery process (e.g., they may not be able to participate as well in rehabilitation activities).

The third step is to consider whether the behavioral disturbance is related to an environmental precipitant. These include disruptions in routine, time change (e.g., daylight savings time or travel across time zones), changes in the caregiving environment, new caregivers, a new roommate, or a life stressor (e.g., death of a spouse or family member). Other common environmental precipitants include overstimulation (e.g., too much noise, crowded rooms, close contact with too many people), understimulation (e.g., relative absence of people, spending too much time alone, use of television as a companion), and the disruptive behavior of other residents. For many disturbances, correcting an environmental precipitant or removing the stressor commonly improves the symptoms.

Another consideration is whether the disturbance results from stress in the resident–caregiver relationship. Caring for residents with dementia can be difficult and requires a degree of perseverance that most caregivers are capable of learning if proper guidance and support is provided. It is important for the AL nurse to assess the level of stress and burden on the staff and family caregiver as part of the evaluation of behavioral disturbances. Interventions to improve the resident–caregiver relationship and provide caregiver education and support are a vital part of treatment of behavioral disturbances in dementia. Staff and family caregivers may benefit from learning and practicing a *function focused philosophy of care* when working with older adults with dementia. Rather than simply having staff complete tasks, such as bathing or dressing a resident, a function focused care approach teaches caregivers to motivate and cue residents with dementia so that the residents actively participate in functional and physical activities. For example, rather than bathing a resident with cognitive impairment, standing in front of them and modeling washing behavior (i.e., having the caregiver demonstrate how to wash his or her own face) may stimulate the individual with cognitive impairment to wash as well. In end-stage dementia it is helpful to do hand-over-hand bathing so that the individual with dementia is washing his own face and body with assistance and thereby getting the range of motion associated with this activity. Because residents with dementia frequently misinterpret the touch of a caregiver as a threat, it is more effective to use strategies such as brief verbal cues to get them to bath themselves, role modeling, or at least hand-over-hand procedures when assisting residents with activities of daily living.

After medical, environmental, and caregiving causes are excluded, it might be concluded that the behavioral problem is a manifestation of the dementia and may not be amenable to a pharmacologic intervention. Such disturbances that are closely linked to the dementia syndrome take on the form of a *catastrophic reaction*: an acute behavioral, physical, or verbal reaction to environmental stressors that result from an inability to make routine adjustments in daily life. The reaction might include anger, emotional lability, or aggression when the resident is confronted with a deficit, such as the inability to find a word, or confusion about where she or he is or what she or he is supposed to do. Catastrophic reactions are best treated by identifying and avoiding their precipitants, by providing structured routines and activities, and by recognizing early signs of the impending catastrophic reaction so that the resident can be distracted and supported before reacting.

Behavioral disturbances may occur in all types of dementias, including Alzheimer's type, vascular, and mixed *frontotemporal dementia,* which is a less common type of dementia often associated with prominent disinhibition, compulsive behaviors, and social impairment due to more advanced frontal lobe degeneration. Another dementia associated with prominent psychiatric symptoms and behavioral disturbances is dementia with *Lewy bodies* (DLB). This form of dementia may be more common than previously thought. It is characterized by cognitive deterioration and parkinsonian features with prominent psychosis characterized by visual hallucinations. Individuals with DLB often suffer from distressing hallucinations and a fluctuating clinical course. These residents are extremely sensitive to the extrapyramidal side effects of antipsychotic medications (such as muscle rigidity and tremor) and often cannot tolerate even low doses of atypical agents.

TREATMENT: BASIC APPROACH

Treatment of the psychiatric and behavioral disturbances in dementia is complex and may require several interventions applied as part of a comprehensive plan of care. Specialists should be consulted in refractory cases. In general, treatment begins with appropriate environmental and caregiver interventions. Nonpharmacologic interventions should always be used as a first-line treatment in the management of disruptive, aggressive, or agitated behavior. Exhibit 30.1 provides a list of key behavioral interventions that might ameliorate behavioral symptoms in residents with dementia. The implementation of a daily routine and introduction of meaningful activities is vital. Residents with dementia may display a reduction in behavioral disturbances with the use of music, particularly during meals and bathing, and with light physical exercise, walking, and during active participation in activities of daily living. Massage, pet therapy, white noise, videotapes of family, and cognitive stimulation programs may also be helpful. If the disturbances persist despite best efforts, pharmacologic interventions for specific target symptoms are often necessary.

30.1 | Behavioral Interventions for Dementia Care

- Treat underlying medical problems

- Correct sensory deficits; make sure residents wear functioning hearing aids, eyeglasses, and dentures

- Remove offending medications, particularly anticholinergic agents

- Keep the environment comfortable, calm, and homelike with use of familiar possessions

- Provide regular daily activities, structure, and opportunities for exercise

- Monitor for acute medical problems

- Promote regular sleeping and eating patterns

- Install safety measures to prevent accidents

- Educate caregivers about practical aspects of dementia care and about behavioral disturbances

- Teach caregivers the skills of caregiving: communication skills, avoiding confrontational behavior management, techniques of ADL support, activities for dementia care

- Actively involve residents in their ADLs to promote maintenance of functional skills; use verbal cues and role modeling for bathing and dressing with the use of adaptive clothing and assistive devices if needed

Note: ADL = activity of daily living.

TREATMENTS FOR SPECIFIC DISTURBANCES

At the core of treatment is the identification of any possible underlying cause of the behavior change, with the recognition that multiple causes may be operating concurrently. First and foremost, managing pain, dehydration, hunger, thirst, and fatigue is paramount. Consider the possibilities of positional discomforts, oral pain from caries or severe gingivitis, or nausea secondary to medication effects, as these are common possible culprits. Environmental modifications can improve resident orientation. Good lighting, one-on-one attention, supportive care, and attention to personal needs and wants are also important aspects of treatment. If there is sleep–wake cycle disturbance, efforts should be made to stabilize the sleep cycle by maintaining a stable routine, using bright lights or sunlight, or prescribing short-term use of medications (see the section "Disturbances of Sleep" later in this chapter).

Mood Disturbances in Residents With Dementia

For residents experiencing mood symptoms, procedures similar to those used with other behavior disturbances should be employed, that is, optimize the environment by reducing adverse stimuli and assess physical health comprehensively. Recreation programs and activity therapies demonstrate positive results in improving mood in depressive symptoms in dementia. Criteria for the diagnosis of depression in Alzheimer's dementia have been proposed that note common features of irritability and social isolation or withdrawal. The waxing and waning course of mood symptoms in dementia is attributed to the cognitive loss and reduction in communication skills related to the dementia. Depression of 2 weeks duration resulting in significant distress should likely receive a trial of an antidepressant medication. Similarly, sustained depressive features lasting more than 2 months following the initiation of behavioral interventions warrant treatment with antidepressant medications. First-line agents are the selective serotonin-reuptake inhibitors, preferred for their favorable side effect profiles. Table 30.1 lists the antidepressants most commonly used to treat depressive symptoms in dementia.

The pharmacologic treatment of depression in dementia requires persistence. If a first agent has failed despite an adequate therapeutic dose for 8 to 12 weeks, an alternative agent should be tried. Venlafaxine, bupropion,

30.1 | Drugs to Treat Depressive Features of Behavioral Disturbances in Dementia

MEDICATION	DAILY DOSE	USES	PRECAUTIONS
Selective serotonin-reuptake inhibitors			
Citalopram	10–40 mg	Depression, anxiety[OL]	Gastrointestinal upset, nausea, insomnia, hyponatremia
Escitalopram	5–20 mg	Depression, anxiety	Gastrointestinal upset, nausea, insomnia, hyponatremia
Fluoxetine	10–40 mg	Depression, anxiety	Gastrointestinal upset, nausea, insomnia, hyponatremia
Paroxetine	10–40 mg	Depression, anxiety	Gastrointestinal upset, nausea, insomnia, hyponatremia, sedation
Sertraline	25–100 mg	Depression, anxiety	Gastrointestinal upset, nausea, insomnia, hyponatremia
Trazodone	25–150 mg	When sedation is desirable	Sedation, falls, hypotension, confusion
Serotonin norepinephrine-reuptake inhibitors			
Duloxetine	20–60 mg	Depression, diabetic neuropathy	Nausea, dry mouth, dizziness
Mirtazapine	7.5–30 mg	Useful for depression with insomnia	Sedation, hypotension
Venlafaxine	25–150 mg	Useful in severe depression	Hypertension may be a problem, sweating
Tricyclic antidepressants			
Desipramine	10–100 mg	Depression, anxiety	Anticholinergic effects, hypotension, sedation, cardiac arrhythmias
Nortriptyline	10–75 mg	High efficacy for depression if side effects are tolerable; therapeutic range 50–150 ng/dL	Anticholinergic effects, hypotension, sedation, cardiac arrhythmias

(continued)

30.1 | Drugs to Treat Depressive Features of Behavioral Disturbances in Dementia *(continued)*

MEDICATION	DAILY DOSE	USES	PRECAUTIONS
Other			
Bupropion	75–225 mg	More activating, lack of cardiac effects	Irritability, insomnia, contraindicated in residents with seizures

mirtazapine, and the tricyclic agents desipramine and nortriptyline might be considered. Tricyclics should be avoided if a bundle branch block or other significant cardiac conduction disturbance is present.

Manic-Like Behavioral Syndromes in Dementia Residents

Occasionally, mood syndromes may develop in dementia residents that are characterized by pressured speech, disinhibition, elevated mood, intrusiveness, hyperactivity, and reduced sleep. These syndromes resemble the manic episodes observed in the context of bipolar affective disorder in younger adults, although they are generally considered to be secondary to the dementing disorder. The important distinction in the dementia resident is the frequent co-occurrence with confusional states and a tendency to have more of a fluctuating mood; that is, the resident's mood may be irritable or hostile as opposed to euphoric. The appearance of hypersexual behaviors may be observed in this clinical scenario, although sexual disinhibition frequently occurs with dementia as a consequence of reduced frontal-executive functioning and may not necessarily be part of a manic syndrome. Treatment of manic-like states, emotional lability, disinhibition, or irritability typically begins with the use of mood-stabilizing agents such as divalproex sodium[OL] (see Table 30.2). Because of the potential adverse effects on the liver and thrombocytopenia, transaminase levels and a complete blood cell count (CBC) should be taken before therapy is initiated, rechecked with each dose increase, and repeated at least every 6 months while the resident remains on the drug. Alternatives to divalproex sodium are carbamazepine[OL], lamotrigine[OL], or lithium[OL]. Lithium is valu-

able as a mood stabilizer, but its use may be a problem in the older adult because of enhanced sensitivity to adverse effects. Elevated lithium levels may occur in the context of reduced renal function and dehydration, resulting in ataxia, tremor, gastrointestinal distress, and confusion.

Psychosis in Dementia: Delusions and Hallucinations

Delusions (i.e., fixed false beliefs) or hallucinations (i.e., false sensory perceptions), whether occurring independently or in association with mood syndromes, may require specific pharmacologic treatment if the resident is disturbed by these experiences, or if the experiences lead to disruptions in the resident's environment that cannot otherwise be controlled. Clinical criteria for the diagnosis of Alzheimer's dementia with psychosis specifies that the presence of delusions or hallucinations have to have occurred for at least 1 month, at least intermittently, and must cause distress for the person. Antipsychotic drugs and dosing information are listed in Table 30.3. The atypical agents risperidone[OL], olanzapine[OL], quetiapine[OL], and aripiprazole[OL] are being used more commonly than older agents such as haloperidol[OL]. The older agents are more likely to cause extrapyramidal side effects, such as parkinsonism and tardive dyskinesia.

Sedation, hypotension, and falls are common adverse effects with all antipsychotic agents. As these medications are more widely used, differences in side effect profile are emerging. An increased risk of cerebrovascular events in residents with dementia has been identified with use of atypical antipsychotics such as risperidone, olanzapine, and aripiprazole. The Food and

30.2 | Mood Stabilizers for Behavioral Disturbances in Dementia With Manic Features

DRUG	GERIATRIC DOSAGE	ADVERSE EFFECTS	COMMENTS
Carbamazepine[OL,a]	200–1000 mg/day (therapeutic level 4–12 µg/mL)	Nausea, fatigue, ataxia, blurred vision, hyponatremia	Poor tolerability in older adults; must monitor CBC, LFTs, electrolytes q 2 weeks for first 2 months, then q 3 months
Lithium[OL,a]	150–1000 mg/day (therapeutic level 0.5–0.8 mEq/L)	Nausea, vomiting, tremor, confusion, leukocytosis	Poor tolerability in older adults; toxicity at low serum levels; monitor thyroid and renal function
Divalproex sodium[OL,a]	250–2000 mg/day (therapeutic level 40–100 µg/mL)	Nausea, GI upset, ataxia, sedation	Requires monitoring of CBC, platelets, LFTs at baseline and q 6 months; better tolerated than other mood stabilizers in older adults

Note: CBC = complete blood cell count; GI = gastrointestinal; LFTs = liver function tests; q = every.
[a]Approved by the Food and Drug Administration for the treatment of bipolar disorder.

Drug Administration (FDA) has requested that the manufacturers of aripiprazole[OL], olanzapine[OL], quetiapine[OL], risperidone[OL], clozapine[OL], and ziprasidone[OL] add a boxed warning to their labeling describing an increased risk of mortality (reported in 17 placebo-controlled studies). In most cases the cause of death appeared to be heart-related or from infections (e.g., pneumonia). More information on this warning is available at http://www.fda.gov/cder/drug/infopage/antipsychotics/default.htm.

It also appears that traditional antipsychotics, such as haloperidol, possess similar risks.

Although antipsychotic agents have demonstrated efficacy in large controlled trials in the treatment of dementia with psychosis and aggression, it is important to note that the overall positive effects have been relatively modest. Although 45% to 55% of individuals improved on antipsychotic medications, placebo response ranged from 30% to 50% across studies. Antipsychotic agents clearly play an important role in the treatment of delusions, hallucinations, and aggression in dementia, but they must be part of a comprehensive treatment plan.

There is some evidence that cholinesterase inhibitors such as donepezil or galantamine may reduce the psychosis and behavioral disturbances of Alzheimer's disease. Studies comparing these agents with placebo in individuals with mild to moderate Alzheimer's disease suggest that they may reduce the rate of emergence of behavioral disturbances and psychosis.

Disturbances of Sleep

Treatment of insomnia and sleep-wake cycle disturbance should begin with improvement of sleep hygiene (see Exhibit 30.2 and Chapter 32, "Sleep Disorders"). This consists of efforts to get the resident to go to sleep

30.3 | Antipsychotic Agents for the Treatment of Psychosis (Hallucinations and Delusions) in Dementia

DRUG	DAILY DOSE	ADVERSE EFFECTS	COMMENTS	FORMULATIONS
Aripiprazole[OL]	5–15 mg	Mild sedation, mild hypotension	Warning about increased cerebrovascular events in dementia, possible hyperglycemia	Tablet, liquid concentrate
Clozapine[OL]	12.5–200 mg	Sedation, hypotension, anticholinergic effects, agranulocytosis	Weekly CBCs required, poorly tolerated by older adults, reserved for treatment of refractory cases, warning about hyperglycemia	Tablet, rapidly dissolving tablet
Olanzapine[OL]	2.5–10 mg	Sedation, falls, gait disturbance	Warning about hyperglycemia and cerebrovascular events in residents with dementia	Tablet, rapidly dissolving tablet, IM injection
Quetiapine[OL]	25–200 mg	Sedation, hypotension	Warning about hyperglycemia, ophthalmologic exam recommended every 6 months	Tablet
Risperidone[OL]	0.5–2 mg	Sedation, hypotension, EPS with doses > 1 mg/day	Warning about cerebrovascular events in residents with dementia, hyperglycemia warning	Tablet, rapidly dissolving tablet, liquid concentrate, depot IM injection
Ziprasidone[OL]	40–160 mg	Higher risk of QTc prolongation	Warning regarding increased QTc prolongation, possible hyperglycemia Little published information on use in older adults	Capsule, IM injection

Note: CBCs = complete blood cell counts; EPS = extrapyramidal symptoms; IM = intramuscular; QTc = corrected QT interval.

later every day, around 10:00 or 11:00 p.m., while keeping the environment calm, comfortable, and conducive to sleep, into the next morning. If the sleep disturbance is associated with depression, suspiciousness, or delusions, those conditions should be treated.

For primary sleep disturbances, when good sleep hygiene and increasing daytime activity level are not successful, trazodone[OL] (25 to 150 mg at bedtime) or mirtazapine[OL] (7.5 to 15 mg at bedtime) might be used. Benzodiazepines or antihistamines, such as diphenhydramine, should be avoided, since they carry a high risk for falls, hip fractures, disinhibition, and cognitive disturbance when prescribed for residents with dementia (see also Chapter 32, "Sleep Disorders").

30.2 | Behavioral Management of Insomnia

- Establish a stable routine for going to bed and awakening

- Optimize sleep environment (attention to noise, light, temperature)

- Increase daytime activity and exercise

- Reduce or eliminate caffeine, nicotine, alcohol

- Reduce evening fluid consumption to minimize nocturia

- Give activating medications early in the day

- Control nighttime pain

- Limit daytime napping to brief periods of 20 to 30 minutes

- Use relaxation, stress management, and breathing techniques to promote natural sleep

Zolpidem[OL] and zaleplon[OL] are short-acting non-benzodiazepine sedative hypnotics that may be helpful for sleep disturbances in the older adult, although there have been no controlled trials for their use in sleep disturbances secondary to dementia. Zolpidem has been studied in older adults without dementia and appears to be effective in improving sleep onset, although it does not improve sleep duration because of its short half-life. The recommended dose of zolpidem is 5 mg, as an increased risk of adverse effects appears to be dose related. Zaleplon has been less extensively studied in the older adult but appears to have similar properties.

Intermittent Aggression or Agitation

When disruptive behavior occurs, intermittently or episodically (i.e., once per week or less), behavioral interventions focusing on identifying the antecedents of the behavior and avoiding the triggers are often most useful. Behavior modification using positive reinforcement of desirable behavior is helpful—and it also helps encourage the caregiver to focus on times when behavior is not a problem. Reminiscence, validation therapy, aromatherapy, physical activity, and environmental modifications of light, sound, and space may all help promote positive behavior. Distraction techniques, activity therapies, and exercise also show promise in reducing troublesome behaviors. Physical restraint in any form should be avoided if at all possible.

RESOURCES

Alzheimer's Association. (2005). *Dementia care practice recommendations for assisted living residences and nursing homes.* Chicago: Alzheimer's Association Campaign for Quality Residential Care.

Galik, E. M., & Resnick, B. (2007). Restorative care with the cognitively impaired: Moving beyond behavior. *Topics in Geriatric Rehabilitation, 23*(2), 125–136.

McGonigal-Kenney, M. L., & Titler, M. G. (2006). Evidence-based guideline: Nonpharmacologic management of agitated behaviors in persons with Alzheimer disease and other chronic dementing conditions. *Journal of Gerontological Nursing, 32*(2), 9–14.

Penrod, J., Yu, F., Kolanowski, A., Fick, D. M., Loeb, S. J., & Hupcey, J. E. (2007). Reframing person-centered nursing care for persons with dementia. *Research and Theory for Nursing Practice, 21*(1), 57–72.

Rabins, P. V., Lyketsos, C. G., & Steele, C. D. (2006). *Practical dementia care* (2nd ed.). New York: Oxford University Press.

Zarowitz, B. J., & Tangalos, E. G. (2007). Application of evidence-based principles of care in older persons: Alzheimer's disease. *Journal of the American Medical Directors Association, 8*(3), 183–193.

31

Delirium

Elizabeth Galik

Delirium is a common and costly condition that affects older adults in a variety of settings. It has a rapid onset, fluctuating course, and results in a constellation of symptoms that may include disturbance in level of consciousness, attention, orientation, memory, thought process, perceptual disturbances, and sleep–wake pattern disruptions. Symptoms of delirium have been confused with symptoms of dementia; however, the onset of dementia is gradual and involves a slow, steady decline in cognitive function. This is quite different from the rapid onset and changes seen in delirium. Clinicians call delirium by many different names such as *acute confusional state*, *acute mental status change*, *altered mental status*, *organic brain syndrome*, and *reversible dementia*.

INCIDENCE AND OUTCOMES

Approximately one-third of patients aged 70 or older who are hospitalized on a general medical unit experience delirium; the prevalence of delirium in intensive care units can be as high as 80%. Approximately one-third of older adults presenting to the emergency department are delirious. In postacute skilled nursing facilities, 16%–23% of new admissions meet the full criteria for delirium, and an additional 49% may have some symptoms of delirium. Prevalence of delirium among older adults discharged from the hospital into community settings and assisted living remains unknown.

Although delirium is traditionally viewed as a transient phenomenon, there is growing evidence that it may persist for weeks to months in a substantial portion of affected persons. Risk factors for having a delirium that does not resolve in a short period of time include being older than 90 years of age and having preexisting cognitive impairment.

There is consistent evidence that delirium is strongly and independently associated with poor outcomes such as increased risk for death, infections, prolonged hospital length of stay, and greater need for skilled nursing care after the acute illness.

CLINICAL FEATURES AND CHARACTERISTICS OF DELIRIUM

- *Acute onset:* Symptoms of delirium develop quickly, often over a period of hours to days. Delirium can go undetected in older adults with dementia because related cognitive changes typically are assumed to be caused by progression of the dementing disorder.
- *Fluctuating course:* Prompt recognition of delirium is especially challenging and often missed in residential settings because of its varied presentation and fluctuating severity of symptoms in individuals over time. Fluctuations in level of consciousness, cognition, speech, and behavior can be unpredictable, but are often worse at night. Fluctuations caused by delirium may be observable during the course of a care interaction or over the course of a day or more. The resident can seem fine one minute and then confused and agitated the next.
- *Disturbance of consciousness:* Consciousness occurs on a continuum and is related to the level of alertness

of a resident. For example, a normal level of consciousness is often described as *alert,* while a resident who is restless, overly sensitive to stimuli and easily startled may be described as *hypervigilant.* A *lethargic* resident is drowsy but easily aroused, while someone who is *comatose* is unarousable.

■ *Inattention:* Residents with mild cases of delirium are particularly prone to problems with attention. The resident may be awake and alert but is easily distracted by stimuli occurring in her or his surrounding environment. The delirious resident may have difficulty keeping to a task in conversation and activity. Eye contact during an interview is typically poor.

■ *Changes in language:* Speech patterns may be poorly organized and difficult to follow. The resident may have difficulty finding the right words and may mispronounce words. Speech may also become slowed, slurred, and/or garbled. Knowing the resident's normal speech patterns is critical when assessing for changes in language due to delirium.

■ *Disorientation and memory impairment:* Memory loss and disorientation that suddenly worsens is often found in residents with delirium. Registration (i.e., encoding that involves receiving, processing, and combining received information) and recent memory are the most affected. Confabulation, or making up details, occurs in approximately 15% of older adults with delirium. There may also be a tendency to mistake someone or something that is unfamiliar for the familiar.

■ *Disordered thought:* Judgment and insight are acutely affected by delirium, as a result of which residents with delirium will often make poor decisions and exhibit unsafe behaviors. The ability to problem solve and think abstractly is impaired, and delusions (i.e., fixed false beliefs) of harm or persecution are common.

■ *Perceptual impairments:* A delirious resident will misperceive objects, people, and situations in the environment. A *distortion* is a perceptual impairment that results in the perception that objects have changed or are changing in shape, position, or motion. *Illusions* are misinterpretations of sensory stimuli, such as hearing a gun shot when a door slams. *Hallucinations* are sensory experiences without sensory stimulation and can be visual, auditory, tactile, gustatory, or olfactory. It is common for visual hallucinations to occur at night. Visual hallucinations can take the form of shapes, or light, or be more complex like people or animals.

■ *Behavioral disturbances:* Behavioral disturbances such as hyperactivity and verbal and physical aggression are common and may place the resident (as well as other residents and staff) at risk for injury.

■ *Alterations in sleep–wake patterns:* Delirium may first appear as a fragmentation or reduction of sleep at night. Residents then may begin to sleep more during the day. The resident with delirium may wake from a vivid dream or nightmare and believe that the dream was real.

Underrecognition of delirium is a major problem. Delirium may be mistaken for dementia or another psychiatric disorder, such as depression. To make this determination, the nurse must know the resident's baseline status. In the absence of baseline data, information from family members, caregivers, or others who know the resident is essential. An acute change in mental status from baseline is not consistent with dementia and suggests delirium. In addition, a rapidly fluctuating course (over minutes to hours) and an abnormal level of consciousness are also highly suggestive of delirium. Depression may also be confused with hypoactive or quiet delirium.

The Confusion Assessment Method (CAM) (Table 31.1) is a useful method to screen for the presence or absence of delirium in older adults. Another scale that may be useful in the assisted living community is the Delirium-O-Meter (DOM), a 12-item behavioral rating scale that determines delirium severity and is designed to be used primarily by nursing staff (Table 31.2). It is easy to use, takes about 3–5 minutes to administer, and measures the severity of both hypoactive and hyperactive symptoms of delirium.

THE SPECTRUM OF DELIRIUM

The classic presentation of delirium is presumed to be a wildly agitated resident. However, studies demonstrate that agitated or hyperactive delirium represents only 25% of all cases. More common, especially in older adults, is *hypoactive* or *quiet delirium,* or delirium with mixed features. Hypoactive delirium is less recognized and appropriately treated less frequently even than hyperactive delirium. The fluctuating nature of a delirium that changes from hypo- to hyperactive is also challenging to diagnose because nurses, and other health care providers, may fail to recognize that lucid intervals can still be characteristic of the disorder. Fluctuating symptoms of delirium make it difficult to detect for providers who spend only brief periods of time with residents. Nurses, who have more frequent

31.1 | The Confusion Assessment Method

CONFUSION ASSESSMENT METHOD

1. Acute change in mental status and fluctuating course
   —Is there evidence of an acute change in cognition from the resident's baseline?
   —Does the abnormal behavior fluctuate during the day, that is, tend to come and go, or increase and decrease in severity?

2. Inattention
   —Does the resident have difficulty focusing attention, for example, being easily distractible, or having difficulty keeping track of what is being said?

3. Disorganized thinking
   —Is the resident's thinking disorganized or incoherent, for example, rambling or irrelevant conversation, unclear or illogical flow of ideas, or unpredictable switching from subject to subject?

4. Altered level of consciousness
   —Is the resident's mental status anything besides alert, that is, vigilant (hyperalert), lethargic (drowsy, easily aroused), stuporous (difficult to arouse), or comatose (unarousable)?

The diagnosis of delirium requires the presence of features 1 and 2 and either 3 or 4

Source: http://www.hartfordign.org/uploads/File/trythis/issue13_cam.pdf.

and regular contact with residents, are often in the best position to document changes in alertness, cognition, and behavior.

RISK FACTORS

The cornerstone of management of delirium focuses on assessment and treatment of modifiable risk factors. Fortunately, research has identified several consistent risk factors for delirium in older adults. These risk factors classify into two groups: (a) baseline factors that predispose individuals to delirium and (b) acute factors that precipitate delirium. Among the predisposing factors, advanced age, preexisting dementia, preexisting functional impairment in activities of daily living, and high medical comorbidity are consistent risk factors. Male gender, sensory impairment (i.e., poor vision and hearing), and history of alcohol abuse have also been reported by some studies. Among acute precipitating factors, medications, especially those that are sedating or highly anticholinergic (e.g., drugs for Parkinson's disease or to treat urinary incontinence), uncontrolled pain, low hematocrit level, bed rest, and use of certain indwelling devices and restraints are associated with the development of delirium. A useful model suggests that delirium is precipitated when the sum of predisposing and precipitating factors crosses a certain threshold. In such a model, the greater the predisposing factors, the fewer precipitating factors are required to initiate delirium. This would explain why older, frail persons develop delirium in the face of stressors that are much less severe than those that can cause delirium in younger, healthy persons. A mnemonic for reversible risk factors for delirium is presented in Table 31.3.

POSTOPERATIVE DELIRIUM

Delirium may be the most common complication after surgery in older adults. Incidence is 15% after elective noncardiac surgery, and may exceed 50% after emergency procedures such as hip fracture repair. A prospectively validated clinical prediction rule for delirium after elective noncardiac surgery described *six risk factors* that can be identified preoperatively: advanced age, cognitive impairment, physical functional impairment, history of alcohol abuse, markedly abnormal serum chemistries, and specifically undergoing either intrathoracic surgery or surgery for an aortic aneurysm. Patients with none of these risk factors had a 2% risk of delirium; those with one or two risk factors had a 10% risk; those with three or more risk factors had a 50% risk.

In addition to baseline risk factors, postoperative management plays an important role in the development of delirium. Contrary to popular belief, the peak incidence of delirium is not immediately upon emergence from anesthesia, but on the second postoperative day. The stresses of surgery and anesthesia are not likely to be the sole precipitants of most cases of postoperative delirium.

Several studies demonstrate that the route of intraoperative anesthesia, whether general, spinal, epidural, or other, has little impact on the risk of delirium. Postoperative medication management plays a much more important role: benzodiazepines and certain opioids,

31.2 | Delirium-O-Meter

	0	1	2	3
1. Sustained attention	Is able to concentrate for longer periods of time during activities/conversation	Absent-minded, questions needs to be repeated sometimes	Easily distracted, questions need to be repeated most of the time	Not able to sustain attention at all, reacts to all kind of stimuli
2. Shifting attention	Switches between topics of conversation or activities without any problem	Occasionally continues talking about a previously discussed topic	Much difficulty shifting attention toward new activities/topics	Not at all able to raise attention or shift it toward new topics/activities
3. Orientation (test!)	Says correct date, knows where he is/his way around, recognizes persons	No problems other than saying the exact date and day of the week	Disoriented in time and place, doesn't find his own room, doesn't know where he is	Disoriented in time and place and person, recognizes family members insufficiently
4. Consciousness	Appears wide awake and alert during the day	Distracted look, as if he just woke up and is not quite well awake	Clearly appears to be sleepy, eyes are shut frequently, but does respond	Hard to awake, hardly responds when spoken to
5. Apathy	Starts conversation, shows interest, appears to be motivated to do something	Shows interest only when others invite him/her, but does not appear 'empty'	Almost no initiative and shows little interest in others (appears 'empty')	Does not do anything, appears to be emotionally 'empty'
6. Hypokinesia/psychomotor retardation	Normal spontaneous pattern of movements	Often sits inactively but just a little encouragement leads to activity	Little spontaneous movements, arms motionless or crossed before chest	No movement of arms or legs unless stimulated strongly
7. Incoherence	What the resident says is easy to understand even for someone who does not know him very well	What the resident says is not always easy to understand, sometimes jumps from one topic to another	Clearly hard to follow, associative, sentences appear unrelated, sometimes stops in the middle of a sentence	Not able to express a coherent thought, unfinished sentences, loose words, yells, moaning
8. Fluctuations in functioning	No diurnal variation in functioning, normal sleep–wake cycle	Minimal fluctuations (during the day or in sleep–wake cycle)	Moderate fluctuations (during daytime or in sleep–wake cycle)	Very marked diurnal variations or severely disrupted sleep–wake cycle
9. Restlessness	Is able to sit and relax, work on something or speak with someone without being restless	A little bit jumpy, fidgety, restless, rocks chair	Agitated, paces up and down the room, slightly irritated, restless arm movements	Extremely restless, irritated, plucking, oppositional behavior, pulls out catheter, restrictive measures used

(continued)

31.2 | Delirium-O-Meter *(continued)*

	0	**1**	**2**	**3**
10. Delusions (thinking)	Thoughts are 'in sync' with reality, no unfounded or unrealistic beliefs, no suspiciousness or, distrustful attitude	Somewhat distrustful, suspicious, sometimes thinks he is put behind, often asks "Why this . . ."	Clearly suspicious, has unrealistic, unfounded or bizarre ideas, for example, says he lives in the hospital	Is extremely suspicious or convinced of bizarre ideas and that makes it very hard to redirect the resident
11. Hallucinations (perceiving)	Perception; what he sees/hears/smells/senses/tastes matches reality	Occasional distorted perception of objects, for example, curtains/wallpaper motifs seen as little animals	Perceives persons, objects, smells, tastes, sounds or animals that are actually not there, can be redirected	Constantly perceives things that aren't there, can not be redirected, is hard to interact with
12. Anxiety/fear	Feels at ease, not anxious	Somewhat apprehensive about what is going on or what will happen	Clearly anxious, fearful, needs some reassurance	Extremely anxious, frightened, needs a lot of reassurance

Name_____ M/F   Date of birth_____ Total score_____
Observer_____ Unit_____   Date_____
Circle one: day-/ evening-/nightshift
From "Delirium-O-Meter: A Nurses' Rating Scale for Monitoring Delirium Severity in Geriatric Patients," by J. F. M. de Jonghe, K. J. Kalisvaart, J. F. M. Timmers, M. G. Kat, and J. C. Jackson, 2005, *International Journal of Geriatric Psychiatry, 20,* pp. 1158–1166. Copyright ©2005 by John Wiley & Sons, Ltd. Reprinted with permission.

31.3 | Mnemonic for Reversible Causes of Delirium

Drugs	Any new additions, increased doses, or interactions Consider over-the-counter drugs and alcohol Consider esp. high-risk drugs (see Table 31.6)
Electrolyte disturbances	Especially dehydration, sodium imbalance Thyroid abnormalities
Lack of drugs	Withdrawals from chronically used sedatives, including alcohol and sleeping pills Poorly controlled pain (lack of analgesia)
Infection	Especially urinary and respiratory tract infections
Reduced sensory input	Poor vision, poor hearing
Intracranial	Infection, hemorrhage, stroke, tumor Rare: consider only if new focal neurologic findings, suggestive history, or workup otherwise negative
Urinary, fecal	Urinary retention: cystocerebral syndrome Fecal impaction
Myocardial, pulmonary	Myocardial infarction, arrhythmia, exacerbation of heart failure, exacerbation of chronic obstructive pulmonary disease, hypoxia

especially meperidine, are strongly associated with development of delirium. Although pain medications can cause delirium, adequate pain management is also important, because high levels of postoperative pain have also been associated with delirium. Strategies to provide adequate analgesia with minimal doses of opioids should be employed. These include the use of scheduled rather than as-needed dosing, patient-controlled or regional analgesia, and opioid-sparing analgesics such as acetaminophen or nonpharmacologic approaches, such as ice packs. Low postoperative hematocrit level (< 30%) is associated with postoperative delirium. Appropriate transfusion of high-risk patients should be considered, especially after elective procedures for which autologous blood is available, though transfusions have not yet been shown to reduce delirium.

Several studies noted that there is a high incidence of cognitive dysfunction in patients who have had coronary artery bypass graft surgery (CABG). Although the exact nature and frequency of this dysfunction remains an area of active study, one large longitudinal study showed a 53% incidence of cognitive decline at hospital discharge, 36% at 6 weeks, and 24% at 6 months. None of the existing studies of cognitive outcomes after CABG explicitly assessed for delirium, thus the interplay between delirium and these more global measures of cognitive dysfunction remains unknown.

EVALUATION

All residents with newly diagnosed delirium require a careful history, physical examination, and targeted laboratory testing. Most of the treatable causes for delirium lie outside the central nervous system, and these should be investigated first. Because multiple contributing factors are often present, the workup should not be stopped because a single cause is identified. Key steps in the evaluation and management of delirium are summarized in Table 31.4.

The history should focus on the time course of the changes in mental status and their association with other symptoms or events (e.g., fever, shortness of breath, medication change). Inasmuch as medications are the most common and treatable cause of delirium, a careful medication history, using the nursing administration sheets in the hospital or a brown-bag review (i.e., when the individual brings all of his or her medications in a brown bag to his or her health care provider) in independent living settings, is important. In the assisted living setting the nurse has the opportunity to evaluate the resident's medications in the home setting. The resident's use of over-the-counter drugs and alcohol should not be overlooked. Physical examination should include vital signs and oxygen saturation, and a careful general physical assessment that includes a mental status examination (Table 31.5), gait, and functional assessment. The emphasis should be on identifying acute medical problems or exacerbations of chronic medical problems that might be contributing to delirium. Most residents with suspected delirium will require at least a complete blood cell count, electrolytes, and kidney function tests. Urinalysis, tests for liver function, serum drug levels, and arterial blood gases, as well as chest radiograms, electrocardiogram, and appropriate cultures are helpful in selected situations. Brain imaging is rarely helpful, except in cases of head trauma or new focal neurologic findings.

MANAGEMENT AND INTERVENTIONS

Older adults with delirium are particularly vulnerable to complications and poor outcomes and must be given special care. This requires a team effort that can, if possible, include the family. A multifactorial approach is the most successful since many factors contribute to delirium; thus, multiple interventions, even if individually small, may yield marked clinical improvement (see Table 31.4). Failure to identify and manage delirium properly may result in costly and life-threatening complications and long-term loss of function.

Modifying the risk factors that contribute to delirium is critically important. Some factors, such as age and prior cognitive impairment, cannot be modified. However, even some predisposing factors, such as sensory impairment, may be modifiable through proper use of eyeglasses and hearing aids. Drugs are the most common reversible causes of delirium. Anticholinergics, H_2-blockers, benzodiazepines, narcotics, and antipsychotic medications should be replaced with drugs that have no central nervous system effects. For example, an H_2-blocker, such as ranitidine (Zantac) may be replaced by antacids or proton-pump inhibitors, and regular dosing of 1 g of acetaminophen three times daily may reduce or eliminate the need for narcotic analgesics in many residents (see Table 31.6).

The delirious resident is susceptible to a wide range of secondary complications; careful surveillance is critical. Bowel and bladder function should be monitored closely, but urinary catheters, which can lead to urinary tract infection, are to be avoided unless treating urinary retention. Bowel stimulants and stool softeners can be used to prevent constipation, particularly in

31.4 | Management of Delirium

STEP	KEY ISSUES	PROPOSED TREATMENT
1. Identify and treat reversible contributors	Medications	Reduce or eliminate offending medications, or substitute less psychoactive medications
	Infections	Treat common infections: urinary, respiratory, soft-tissue
	Fluid balance disorders	Assess and treat dehydration, heart failure, electrolyte disorders
	Impaired CNS oxygenation	Treat severe anemia (transfusion), hypoxia, hypotension
	Severe pain	Assess and treat; use local measures and scheduled pain regimens that minimize narcotic analgesics
	Sensory deprivation	Use eyeglasses, hearing aid, portable amplifier
	Elimination problems	Assess and treat urinary retention and fecal impaction
2. Maintain behavioral control	Behavioral interventions	Teach staff appropriate interaction with delirious residents Encourage family visitation
	Pharmacologic interventions	Only if necessary, use low-dose antipsychotics
3. Anticipate and prevent or manage complications	Urinary incontinence	Implement scheduled toileting program
	Immobility and falls	Avoid physical restraints; mobilize with assistance; employ physical therapy
	Pressure ulcers	Mobilize Reposition immobilized resident frequently and monitor pressure points
	Sleep disturbance	Implement a nonpharmacologic sleep hygiene program, including a nighttime sleep protocol Avoid sedatives
	Feeding disorders	Assist with feeding; use aspiration precautions; provide nutritional supplementation as necessary
4. Restore function in delirious residents	Institutional environment	Reduce clutter and noise (esp. at night); provide adequate lighting; have familiar objects brought from home
	Ability to perform ADLs	As delirium clears, match performance to capacity
	Family education, support, and participation	Provide education about delirium, its causes, its reversibility, how to interact, and family's role in restoration of function

Note: ADLs = activities of daily living; CNS = central nervous system.

31.5 | Components of a Mental Status Exam

COMPONENT	METHOD OF ASSESSMENT
Level of consciousness	Is the resident alert, lethargic, hypervigilant, comatose? Is the resident able to remain engaged and focused during the interview without fluctuation in attention, concentration, and level of alertness?
Appearance and behavior	Is the resident clean and well groomed, or disheveled? Is the manner of dress appropriate for the temperature and season? Is the resident cooperative and engaged in the interview process, or agitated and restless? Describe the psychomotor behavior of the resident during the interview.
Speech and language	Describe the rate, rhythm, fluidity, spontaneity, and latency of speech.
Mood and affect	Describe the resident's mood in his own words (subjective mood) and the nurse's perception of mood (observed mood). Does the resident feel like his usual self (vital sense)? Describe the resident's perception of his self attitude. Are there any thoughts of a passive death wish or suicidal ideation?
Thought content and perceptions	Assess for the presence of hallucinations (sensory perceptions without a stimulus), illusions (misperceptions or distortions of sensory stimuli), and delusions (fixed false beliefs).
Insight and judgment	Is the resident aware and appreciative of his cognitive deficits? Does the resident display good judgment by being able to assess a situation, weigh the facts, and draw an appropriate conclusion?
Cognition	Use of a cognitive screening tool such as the Mini Mental State Examination (MMSE) is helpful when assessing: orientation, registration, calculation, recall, language, and visual spatial ability.

From "Mini-Mental State: A Practical Method for Grading the Cognitive State of Patients for the Clinician," by M. Folstein, S. Folstein, and P. McHugh, 1975, *Journal of Psychiatric Research, 2*, pp. 189–198. Copyright ©1975 by Pergamon Press. Reprinted with permission.

those who are taking narcotic analgesics. Complete bed rest should be avoided, as it may lead to increasing disability through muscle disuse, development of pressure ulcers, and atelectasis (i.e., lung collapse). Exercise and ambulation prevent the deconditioning often associated with decreased mobility. Malnutrition can be avoided with the use of nutritional supplements and careful attention to food and fluid intake. Some delirious residents may need cueing or hand-over-hand assistance with feeding. This involves guiding the resident's hand to self-feed rather than feeding the resident.

Managing behavioral problems while ensuring both the comfort and safety of the resident can be challenging. Nonpharmacologic behavioral measures can help provide orientation and a feeling of safety for the resi-dent. Ideally, try to normalize the resident's environment and routine. Orienting items such as a clock (with a real face), calendar, window view, familiar objects, and meaningful photographs should be made available. Limit background noise. For example, take the delirious resident out of the dining room when another resident starts yelling or when the clang of trays, dishes, and chairs gets to be overwhelming. Get the resident's attention before trying to communicate and give simple, one-step directions. Residents should also be encouraged and cued to wear their eyeglasses and hearing aids. Avoid the use of physical restraints with a resident who is delirious. Evidence from nursing home settings suggests that such restraints probably do not decrease the rate of falls by confused ambulatory residents, and

31.6 | Drugs to Reduce or Eliminate in the Management of Delirium

AGENT	ADVERSE EFFECTS	POSSIBLE SUBSTITUTES	COMMENTS
Alcohol	CNS sedation and withdrawal	If history of heavy intake, careful monitoring and benzodiazepines if withdrawal symptoms	Alcohol history is imperative
Anticholinergics (oxybutynin, benztropine)	Anticholinergic toxicity	A lower dose, behavioral measures	Rare at low doses
Anticonvulsants (esp. primidone, phenobarbital, phenytoin)	CNS sedation and withdrawal	Alternative agent or none	Toxic reactions can occur despite therapeutic drug levels
Antidepressants, esp. tricyclic agents (amitriptyline, imipramine, nortriptyline, desipramine)	Anticholinergic toxicity	SSRIs or other agents	Tricyclics may be used as treatment for chronic pain
Antihistamines (including diphenhydramine)	Anticholinergic toxicity	Nonpharmacologic protocol for sleep	Must take OTC medication history
Antiparkinsonian agents (levodopa-carbidopa, dopamine agonists, amantadine)	Dopaminergic toxicity	A lower dose; adjusted dosing schedule	Usually with end-stage disease and high doses
Antipsychotics, esp. low-potency anticholinergic agents and atypical agents (clozapine)	Anticholinergic toxicity; CNS sedation	No agents or, if necessary, low-dose high-potency agents	Increased risk of stroke and mortality associated with long-term use, primarily for agitation in dementia
Barbiturates	CNS sedation; severe withdrawal syndrome	Gradual discontinuation or benzodiazepine	In most cases, should no longer be prescribed; avoid inadvertent or abrupt discontinuation
Benzodiazepines, esp. long-acting (including diazepam, flurazepam, chlordiazepoxide)	CNS sedation	Nonpharmacologic sleep management; intermediate agents (lorazepam)	Associated with delirium in medical and surgical residents
Benzodiazepines: ultra short-acting (including triazolam, alprazolam)	CNS sedation and withdrawal	Nonpharmacologic sleep management; intermediate agents (lorazepam, temazepam)	Associated with delirium in case reports and series
Chloral hydrate	CNS sedation	Nonpharmacologic sleep protocol	No better for delirium than benzodiazepines

(continued)

31.6 | Drugs to Reduce or Eliminate in the Management of Delirium *(continued)*

AGENT	ADVERSE EFFECTS	POSSIBLE SUBSTITUTES	COMMENTS
H_2-blocking agents	Possible anticholinergic toxicity	A lower dosage; antacids or proton-pump inhibitors	Most common with high-dose intravenous infusions
Non-benzodiazepine hypnotics (e.g., zolpidem)	CNS sedation and withdrawal	Nonpharmacologic sleep protocol	Like other sedatives, can cause delirium
Opioid analgesics	Anticholinergic toxicity, CNS sedation, fecal impaction	Local measures and nonpsychoactive pain medications around the clock; opioids only for breakthrough and severe pain	Higher risk in residents with renal insufficiency; must titrate risks from drugs versus risks from pain
Almost any medication if time course is appropriate			**Consider risks and benefits of all medications in the older adult**

Note: CNS = central nervous system; OTC = over-the-counter; SSRI = selective serotonin-reuptake inhibitor.

may aggravate the underlying delirium and actually increase the risk of fall-related injury. Calm reassurance provided by a sitter or family member is much more effective than the use of physical restraints or drugs (such as antipsychotics).

Chemical intervention may be necessary for symptoms such as delusions or hallucinations that are frightening to the resident when verbal comfort and reassurance are not successful. Some delirious residents display behavior that is dangerous to themselves or others and cannot be calmed by providing a sitter or family companionship. However, the mere presence of delirium is not an indication for pharmacologic intervention. Indications for such interventions should be clearly identified, documented, and constantly reassessed.

When medications are used, antipsychotics are preferred. However, these medications must be used cautiously, as they may actually prolong delirium and may increase the risk of complications by converting a hyperactive, confused resident into a stuporous one whose risk of a fall or aspiration is increased. If antipsychotic medications are used, it is very important to assess for akathisia (i.e., motor restlessness) that

may be an adverse effect of high-potency antipsychotic medications—and can be confused with worsening delirium. The treatment for akathisia is less, not more, antipsychotic medication. Because of extrapyramidal effects, haloperidol should be avoided in older adults with parkinsonism, and a benzodiazepine such as lorazepam[OL] may be substituted. Low doses of atypical antipsychotic agents may be effective in delirium, as well. (The atypical antipsychotics are associated with increased risk of stroke and mortality, primarily in long-term use for agitation in dementia.) As with physical restraints, in all cases where pharmacologic restraints are used, the health care team must clearly identify the target symptoms necessitating their use, frequently review the efficacy of the sedative or antipsychotic in controlling the target symptoms, and assess the resident for adverse effects and complications.

It is important to stress to family members that delirium is usually not a permanent condition but, rather, improves over time. Unfortunately, the persistence of delirium is common. Thus, when counseling families, it is important to point out that many cognitive deficits associated with the delirium syndrome can continue, abating only weeks and even months following the illness. Advanced age (85 years or older), preexisting cognitive impairment, and severe illness are risk factors for slow recovery of cognitive function. Careful monitoring of mental status and provision of adequate functional supports during this period are necessary to give the resident the maximum chance of returning to his or her baseline level. Family members can play an important role in the assisted living community by providing appropriate orientation, support, and functional assistance.

PREVENTION

The most effective way to manage delirium is to prevent it from developing in the first place. A study demonstrated that a unit-based proactive multifactorial intervention reduced the incidence of delirium among older hospitalized patients age 70 or older by more than one-third. Six intervention components were used selectively on the basis of patient-specific risk factors determined at an admission assessment. These included interventions for cognitive impairment, sleep deprivation, immobility, visual impairment, hearing impairment, and dehydration. Among these, the most creative and successful intervention was a nonpharmacologic sleep protocol that involved trained volunteers offering patients warm milk, back rubs, and soothing music at bedtime; this intervention substantially reduced the use of sedative-hypnotic medication. Similar programs to prevent delirium should be developed and implemented in assisted living settings.

Multifactorial interventions are useful in preventing delirium. There are no standard guidelines or interventions that have been proven to best *treat* delirium in institutional settings. There is a critical need for more research on how to optimally manage the delirious individual and the development of novel approaches based on a better understanding of the pathophysiology of this common, debilitating, and costly syndrome.

RESOURCES

Bergmann, M. A., Murphy, K. M., Kiely, D. K., Jones, R. N., & Marcantonio, E. R. (2005). A model management of delirious post-acute care patients. *Journal of the American Geriatrics Society, 53,* 1817–1825.

Boockvar, K. S., Fridman, B., & Marturano, C. (2005). Ineffective communication of mental status information during care transfer of older adults. *Journal of General Internal Medicine, 20,* 1146–1150.

Cole, M. G., McCusker, J., Bellevance, F., Primeau, F. J., Bailey, R. F., Bonnycastle, M. J., et al. (2002). Systematic detection and multidisciplinary care of delirium in older medical inpatients: A randomized trial. *Canadian Medical Association Journal, 167*(7), 753–759.

de Jonghe, J. F. M., Kalisvaart, K. J., Timmers, J. F. M., Kat, M. G., & Jackson, J. C. (2005). Delirium-O-Meter: A nurses' rating scale for monitoring delirium severity in geriatric patients. *International Journal of Geriatric Psychiatry, 20,* 1158–1166.

Inouye, S. K., Foreman, M. D., Mion, L. C., Katz, K. H., & Cooney, L. M. (2001). Nurses' recognition of delirium and its symptoms. *Archives of Internal Medicine, 161*(20), 2467–2473.

Inouye, S. K., van Dyck, C. H., Alessi, C. A., Balkin, S., Siegal, A. P., Horwitz, R. I., et al. (1990). Clarifying confusion: the Confusion Assessment Method: a new method for detection of delirium. *Archives of Internal Medicine, 113*(12), 941–948.

Leslie, D. L., Zhang, Y., Bogardus, S. T., Holford, T. R., Leo-Summers, L. S., & Inouye, S. K. (2005). Consequences of preventing delirium in hospitalized older adults on nursing home costs. *Journal of the American Geriatrics Society, 53,* 405–409.

Naughton, B. J., Saltzman, S., Ramadan, F., Chadha, N., Priore, R., & Mylotte, J. M. (2005). A mutlifactoral intervention to reduce prevalence of delirium and shorten hospital length of stay. *Journal of the American Geriatrics Society, 53,* 18–23.

Voyer, P., McCusker, J., Cole, M. G., St-Jacques, S., & Khomenko, L. (2007). Factors associated with delirium severity among older patients. *Journal of Clinical Nursing, 16,* 819–831.

Voyer, P., Richard, S., Doucet, L., Danjou, C., & Carmichael, P. H. (2008). Detection of delirium by nurses among long-term care residents with dementia. *BioMed Central Nursing, 7,* 4.

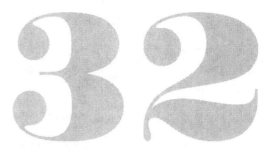

Sleep Disorders

Cathy A. Alessi and Ethel Mitty

Excessive sleepiness or excessive daytime somnolence (EDS) is a common syndrome affecting older adults. The three major causes are insomnia, restless leg syndrome (RLS), and obstructive sleep apnea (OSA). EDS is associated with circadian rhythm or sleep pattern disorder, insomnia, medications, lifestyle factors, psychological disorders, and medical illness. Many older adults as well as health care professionals regard daytime sleepiness as normal for older adults and believe that nothing can be done about it. This misperception prevents appropriate evaluation and treatments—many of which are quite effective (see Table 32.1).

EPIDEMIOLOGY

There is a high prevalence of sleeping problems among older adults. The most common sleeping complaints among community-dwelling older adults are difficulty falling asleep (37% of the sample), nighttime awakening (29%), and early morning awakening (19%). Daytime sleepiness is also common; 20% of community-dwelling older adults report that they are usually sleepy in the daytime. As a consequence of such complaints, at least one-half of community-dwelling older adults use either over-the-counter (OTC) or prescription sleeping medications.

Three large epidemiologic studies of older adults found an association between sleep complaints and risk factors for sleep disturbance (e.g., chronic illness, mood disturbance, less physical activity, and physical disability) but little association with older age, sug-

gesting that these risk factors, rather than aging per se, account for insomnia in the majority of those studied. However, some primary sleep disorders, such as sleep apnea and periodic limb movements in sleep, increase in prevalence with age. Although some studies have shown an increased risk of sleep complaints in women, others have not. Studies have shown that self-reported sleeping difficulties are more common in older Black Americans, particularly women and those with depression and chronic illness.

Unfortunately, late-life insomnia is commonly a chronic problem. A study of older people in Britain found that 36% of those with insomnia at baseline reported severely disrupted sleep 4 years later. Of those who reported the use of prescription hypnotics at baseline, 32% were still using these agents 4 years later. Another study of a volunteer sample of urban women aged 85 years and older found that all had health problems and sleeping difficulties, and the majority regularly used alcohol, OTC sleeping medication, or both, in an effort to improve their sleep. Previous research has suggested that insomnia is a predictor of death and nursing-home placement in older men, but not in older women.

Interestingly, the prevalence of insomnia among assisted living residents is similar to that reported among nursing home residents, that is, 70%. A study of assisted living residents found that 69% reported sleep disturbance: 42% described symptoms of insomnia, and almost 37% described EDS. Residents with insomnia performed better on the Mini-Mental Status Exam (MMSE) and on physical performance than did residents who did not report insomnia. One of the treatments for

Sleep Terminology

Bedtime	Actual time that a person starts to try to fall asleep; not the same as the time when the person got into bed.
Sleep latency	Amount of time between settling in for sleep and actually falling asleep (i.e., sleep onset).
Sleep efficiency	Entire period of time between when the lights were turned off and the person gets up for the final time in the morning; does not necessary mean up and out of bed. Mathematically: the amount of time asleep divided by the amount of time in bed expressed as a percentage. For example, slept 6 hours; in bed 8 hours = 75% sleep efficiency.
Number of awakenings	Number of times a person wakes up after falling asleep but is able to get back to sleep.
Wake after sleep onset	Sum of all wakefulness time after having fallen asleep the first time.
Total sleep time	Total amount of time asleep, including naps, in 24 hours.

depression is sleep deprivation; some data show that insomnia is associated with decreased mortality. However, other data indicate that daytime sleepiness (and daytime nap takers) have an increased mortality rate over 4 years and demonstrate less robust cognitive performance and functionality in comparison to those who do not exhibit daytime sleepiness. In this study, insomnia was treated with hypnotics and nonsedating antidepressants.

SLEEP ARCHITECTURE

Sleep architecture is a term used to describe the sleep cycle or stages—and wakefulness—during a single sleep period; it consists of rapid eye movement (REM) and non-REM sleep. Circadian rhythms (also known as biorhythms) regulate body temperature, metabolism, digestive processes, hormone secretion, and the quality and distribution of the stages of sleep. A circadian rhythm has a daily periodicity but is somewhat longer than 24 hours and varies between individuals. Circadian rhythms are present, as well, in plants and animals and are independent of time cues, per se. They are, however, dependent on light cues for the sleep–wake cycle. A consistent wake-up time helps the circadian rhythm remain aligned with the time of day. Although age-related changes in circadian rhythm do not result in

insomnia, older adults can become less responsive to changes in the light of day. As such, they might catnap in the early evening and then be unable to fall asleep or remain asleep when they go to bed (this is sometimes known as advanced sleep phase syndrome or ASPS). It is important to accurately describe and document the awake and sleep patterns of older adults who describe being unable to sleep or are wakeful at night. Overall, many older adults have decreased total sleep time and total sleep efficiency.

Sleep Stages

Sleep cycles last 90 to 110 minutes and typically consist of one non-REM and one REM stage. REM sleep occurs during the last third of total sleep. Non-REM sleep is associated with quality of the immune and digestive systems and consists of four stages:

- Stage 1: light sleep; duration: 5–10 minutes; occurs between being asleep and being awake; breathing: slow and regular; heart rate, slightly decreased; eyes roll slowly back and forth.
- Stage 2: true sleep; little muscle, eye, or body movement; fragmentary thoughts and images; approximately 50% of total sleep time.
- Stage 3: also known as delta sleep or slow wave sleep (SWS); very deep sleep stage; pulse and respiratory

rate further decreased; sleep-walking occurs during this delta stage.

- Stage 4: deepest sleep stage; usually occurs in the first third of total sleep time; also known as dream sleep or S-state sleep; only a few minutes long, at first, and then lengthens as sleeping continues.

Sufficient REM sleep is associated with emotional well-being, memory retention, and accounts for almost 20% of total sleep. Studies demonstrate that interrupting or denying REM sleep over a prolonged period can cause aberrant behavior, including psychosis. REM sleep is characterized by rapid eye movements (hence, its name); increased heart rate and irregular respirations; relaxed musculature of the upper airway; more oxygen consumption by the brain; and a disappearance of body temperature regulation. Vivid, active, complex dreams occur during REM sleep, as can penile erection. Two phases of REM are present in every stage:

- Tonic REM: body is virtually motionless, and there is increased cerebral blood flow.
- Phasic REM: respiratory and cardiac rate is irregular; rapid eye movement is present.

CHANGES IN SLEEP WITH AGING

Circadian rhythm changes with aging are subtle and do not result in insomnia. However, older adults can be less responsive to changes in the light of day and, as such, will feel sleepy in the early evening, go to sleep, wake up around 3 or 4 A.M., and then be unable to fall back asleep. Older adults have decreased sleep efficiency (time asleep divided by time in bed), stable or decreased total sleep time, and increased sleep latency (time to fall asleep). Older adults also report an earlier bedtime and earlier morning awakening, more arousals during the night, and more daytime napping. Significant age-related changes in sleep structure (architecture) as measured by polysomnography include a decrease in stage 3 and stage 4 sleep (the deeper stages of sleep). Stages 1 and 2 (the lighter stages of sleep) increase or remain the same. The decline in deep sleep seems to begin in early adulthood and progresses throughout life. In persons over age 90 years, stages 3 and 4 may disappear completely. Other common findings include an earlier onset of REM sleep and decreased total REM sleep. Older adults have more equal distribution of REM sleep throughout the night, whereas younger people have longer periods of REM sleep as the night progresses.

The significance of these changes in sleep is unclear. Most experts believe that the decreased sleep in older people is due to a decreased *ability* to sleep, rather than a decreased *need* for sleep. However, some research has shown that after a period of sleep deprivation older people show less daytime sleepiness, less evidence of decline in performance measures, and a quicker recovery of normal sleep structure than younger people. Older people have more sleep disturbance with jet lag and shift work, which may reflect physiologic changes in circadian rhythm with age. In addition, it is not clear to what extent changes in sleep are due to changes of normal aging or to pathologic changes from other processes. In studies comparing good sleepers with poor sleepers, poor sleepers take more medications, make more physician visits, and have poorer self-ratings of health.

ASSESSMENT OF SLEEP

The National Institutes of Health (NIH) consensus statement "Treatment of Sleep Disorders of Older People" (NIH, 1990) suggests that clinicians (e.g., nurses) ask some simple questions:

- Are you satisfied with your sleep?
- How difficult is it for you to fall asleep? To stay asleep? (Ask some probing questions, depending on the response: Do your legs jump around? Are you in pain? Do you have trouble breathing at night?)
- Does sleep or fatigue interfere with your daytime activities? (Probe: Do you think you are waking up too early/not getting enough sleep?)
- Does your bed partner or others (e.g., roommate) complain about your loud breathing during sleep, interrupted breathing, or leg movements?

Similar screening questions can be quite useful to identify sleep complaints in the older adult. Transient sleep problems (e.g., those lasting less than 2 to 3 weeks) are usually situational; persistent sleep problems are likely to require more detailed evaluation.

To obtain a careful description of the sleep complaint, ask the resident to keep a *sleep log* for 5–7 days, recording each morning the time spent in bed, the estimated amount of sleep, the number of awakenings, the time of morning awakening, and any symptoms he or she recalls having had during the night. This should be supplemented by information from the bed partner, or others who may have observed unusual symptoms during the night. Several validated sleep question-naires can be used. Reports (e.g., of painful joints) should be followed by a careful examination of the affected areas. Reports of nocturia that disrupts sleep should be followed by evaluation for cardiac, renal, or prostatic disease, or diabetes mellitus. Careful mental status testing is also indicated. The findings of the history and physical examination should guide laboratory testing.

Polysomnography is the gold standard and is indicated when the clinician suspects a primary sleep disorder, such as sleep apnea, periodic limb movement disorder, or violent or other unusual behaviors during sleep. Objective methods to measure sleep other than traditional polysomnography in a sleep laboratory have been developed and are being used more extensively in studies of sleep. *Portable monitoring systems* for use in the home have been developed and are used primarily to screen for sleep apnea. These systems generally measure pulse oximetry, heart rate, respiration, and nasal airflow. Although they are used extensively, research testing the validity of these systems is ongoing. Another methodology is a wrist-activity monitor, which estimates sleep versus wakefulness on the basis of the person's wrist activity. Some studies have demonstrated that the wrist monitor is sensitive enough to assess the efficacy of treatment for insomnia in older people.

The Epworth Sleepiness Scale (ESS) is a valid and reliable instrument to assess the severity of EDS and whether or not additional workup is needed. The ESS is easy to administer and score, and is available on the Internet. Respondents indicate—using a Likert-type scale—whether they would never doze (0), had a slight chance of dozing (1), a moderate chance of dozing (2), or a high chance of dozing (3) with regard to eight, very simply described situations, such as: sitting and reading, in a car while stopped in traffic, sitting inactively at a meeting or in the theatre, and so forth. The range of the numerical results indicate whether or not the individual is getting enough sleep or is at risk from sleeplessness. This is a subjective report of sleepiness; if the respondent is not sufficiently English-language literate, results could be inaccurate.

The Pittsburg Sleep Quality Index (PSQI) measures seven areas of sleep, including sleep quality, duration, and disturbances and obtains information about the person's use of sleep medications, his or her ability to function in the daytime over the preceding 30 days, his or her usual bedtime, length of time to fall asleep, usual arising time, and the hours spent actually sleeping (that

might be other than the hours spent in bed). Likert-type questions address the frequency in the past month that the older adult was unable to get to sleep in 30 minutes, woke in the middle of the night, felt too cold or too hot, had bad dreams, had been in pain, and so forth. As with the ESS, the PSQI has risks associated with language literacy; it is a subjective report. Nevertheless, both assessments/scales can be used for comparative measurements with older adults in a variety of settings including community-based living as well as to track the efficacy of specific interventions with a specific person in a specific setting. (This would appear to be the epitome of person-centered care.)

A *questionnaire for sleep apnea risk,* consisting of five questions, includes the ESS score, frequency of being told that one's snoring is disturbing others' sleep or that one has stopped breathing during sleep, being overweight, and medical history (including hypertension, heart disease, excessive fatigue, and difficulty concentrating or remaining awake during the day). Responding that all these events happen one to three times each week is indicative of sleep apnea risk and should lead to a recommendation to consult with the primary health care provider (physician, nurse practitioner).

CAUSES AND TREATMENT OF COMMON SLEEP DISORDERS

Insomnia is associated with a greater risk of falls than is the use of hypnotics to manage the condition itself. Defined as difficulty in initiating or maintaining sleep, insomnia is usually due to psychiatric, medical, or neurologic illness; EDS is usually due to a primary sleep disorder, such as sleep apnea. However, there is significant overlap among these symptoms. In one large study of patients of all ages referred to sleep disorders centers, insomnia was found to be most commonly due to psychiatric illness, psychophysiologic problems, drug or alcohol dependence, and restless legs syndrome; EDS was found to be most commonly due to sleep apnea, periodic limb movement disorder, or narcolepsy. However, patients referred to sleep centers are a select population, and the most common causes of excessive sleepiness in the community are probably chronic insufficient sleep (either voluntarily or because of work schedules), medical problems, or sleep-disruptive environmental conditions. Current treatment recommendations for older adults are use of a short-acting hypnotic in combination with treatment(s) for the likely causes of insomnia (e.g., pain, depression) *and* sleep hygiene measures.

Psychiatric Disorders and Psychosocial Problems

Many studies report that psychiatric disorders are the cause of sleep problems in more than half of all patients presenting with insomnia. Depression is a particularly common cause. Early morning awakening is a common pattern, although increased sleep latency and more nighttime wakefulness are also seen. However, these changes may not be present or may be less marked in depressed persons who do not seek medical care. Conversely, sleep disturbance in older people who are not currently depressed may be an important predictor of future depression. Treatment of depression may also improve the sleep abnormalities; several studies using electroencephalography have found that antidepressant medications alter sleep architecture (see Chapter 34, "Depression and Other Mood Disorders").

Bereavement can also affect sleep. Bereavement without major depression is not associated with significant changes in sleep measures, but people with bereavement and depression and those with major depression have identical sleep patterns. These sleep abnormalities improve with treatment of depression. Anxiety and stress can also be associated with sleeping difficulty, usually difficulty with initiating sleep or perhaps early awakening. Residents may have difficulty falling asleep because of excessive worrying at bedtime (see Chapter 35, "Anxiety Disorders"). Older adult caregivers report more sleep complaints than do similarly aged noncaregivers. In one study, nearly 40% of older women who were family caregivers of adults with dementia reported using a sleeping medication for themselves in the past month.

Drug and Alcohol Dependency

Drug and alcohol use account for 10% to 15% of cases of insomnia. Chronic use of sedatives may cause light, fragmented sleep. Many sleeping medications, when used chronically, lead to tolerance and the potential for increasing doses. When chronic hypnotic use is suddenly stopped, rebound insomnia may occur, and the person might start taking the medication again.

Alcohol abuse is often associated with lighter sleep of shorter duration. In addition, some persons try to treat their sleeping difficulties with alcohol. Older adults with poor sleep should be instructed to avoid nighttime alcohol because although alcohol causes an initial drowsiness, it can impair sleep later in the night. Finally, it is important to remember that sedatives and alcohol can worsen sleep apnea; the use of these respi-

ratory depressants should be avoided in older persons with documented or suspected untreated sleep apnea (see Chapter 37, "Substance Abuse").

Medical Problems

Treatable medical problems that may contribute to sleep difficulty in older adults include pain from arthritis and other conditions, paresthesias, cough, dyspnea from cardiac or pulmonary illness, gastroesophageal reflux, and nighttime urination (nocturia). In residents with sleeping difficulties who describe pain at night, assessment and management of the painful condition is the appropriate approach (see Chapter 21, "Chronic Pain and Persistent Pain"). Nocturia may be associated with sleep disorder, poorer quality of sleep, nighttime thirst, and increased fatigue in the daytime.

Sleep can be impaired by diuretics or stimulating agents (e.g., caffeine, sympathomimetics, and bronchodilators) taken near bedtime. Some antidepressants, antiparkinsonian agents, and antihypertensives (e.g., propranolol) can induce nightmares and impair sleep. Required medications that are sedating (e.g., sedating antidepressants) should be given at bedtime if possible.

Sleep Apnea

Sleep apnea is a disorder of periodic reductions in ventilation during sleep caused by pharyngeal obstruction that prevents air flow, lasting at least 10 seconds. Various terms have been used for this syndrome (e.g., *sleep-related breathing disorder, sleep-disordered breathing*), but *sleep apnea* remains the term used by most clinicians. Residents with OSA usually present with excessive daytime sleepiness and are typically unaware of their frequent arousals at night that are associated with reductions in ventilation. These individuals are often obese and may have morning headache, personality changes, poor memory, confusion, and irritability. A bed partner may report loud snoring, cessation of breathing, and choking sounds during sleep. Predisposing factors include normal age-related changes (e.g., diminished lung capacity and muscular endurance) and alteration in sleep architecture.

The reported prevalence of sleep apnea among older adults varies from 20% to 70%, depending on the population studied; prevalence increases with age. The most important predictor of OSA is large body mass. Other reported predictors identified in community-dwelling elderly adults include falling asleep at inappropriate times, male gender, and napping. The classic sleep apnea resident is the obese, sleepy snorer with hypertension. Large neck circumference has also been reported as a marker for OSA.

Alcoholism is an important risk factor for OSA; sleep-disordered breathing is a significant contributor to sleep disturbance in men over age 40 with a history of alcoholism. There appears to be an association between sleep apnea and dementia. One nursing home study found that the sleep disorder was positively correlated with severity of dementia in a nursing home study, but another study concluded that sleep-disordered breathing in Alzheimer's patients was mild and not associated with mental status or behavioral changes.

The importance of mild degrees of sleep-disordered breathing in elderly persons is unclear. One study found no association between mild or moderate sleep-disordered breathing and subjective sleep-wake disturbance. Residents suspected of having sleep apnea should be referred to a sleep laboratory for evaluation and, if the diagnosis is documented, a trial of treatment. Home-based diagnostic systems are also available, but the validity of such systems (in comparison with polysomnography in a sleep laboratory) is not clear. There is conflicting evidence as to whether or not older adults as well as middle-aged adults tolerate the gold standard treatment of OSA: nasal continuous positive airway pressure (CPAP). Careful efforts to use devices that improve comfort may improve adherence with CPAP. Unfortunately, there may be prejudice among clinicians against the use of nasal CPAP in older adults, perhaps because they assume that the treatment will not be tolerated or successful in this population. Oral appliances are an alternative treatment in some residents. Several upper airway surgical approaches have also been used.

Periodic Limb Movements During Sleep and Restless Legs Syndrome

Periodic limb movements during sleep (PLMS) is a condition of repetitive, involuntary flexion of the leg and foot that occurs in non-REM sleep. Leg movements occur every 20 to 40 seconds and can last hours or even much of the night, and each movement may be associated with an arousal. Occurrence of PLMS increases with age and can be present in as much as 30% of community-dwelling older adults. Correlates of PLMS included dissatisfaction with sleep, sleeping alone, and reported kicking at night. Some clinicians suggest that the high prevalence of PLMS with age is associated with delayed motor and sensory latencies noted on nerve conduction testing. PLMS may present as difficulty maintaining sleep or excessive daytime sleepiness. A bed partner may be aware of the leg movements, or

these movements may remain occult until identified in a sleep laboratory. When PLMS is associated with sleep complaints that are not explained by another sleep disorder, this is known as periodic limb movement disorder (PLMD). Polysomnography is required to establish a diagnosis of PLMD.

RLS is a condition of an uncontrollable urge to move one's legs at night in response to a disagreeable sensation. The symptoms occur while the person is awake, and symptoms can also involve the arms. It can be a side effect of some medications (e.g., tricyclic antidepressants, lithium, dopamine blockers) but is also caused by certain conditions: anemia, uremia, diabetes mellitus, Parkinson's disease, rheumatoid arthritis. Diagnosis is based on the individual's description of symptoms and the complaint of nighttime leg discomfort or difficulty in initiating sleep. Polysomnography is not required to make this diagnosis. There may be a family history of the condition and, in some cases, an underlying medical disorder (e.g., anemia, or renal or neurologic disease). Prevalence of RLS also increases with age; many older adults with the condition also have PLMS. In older adults with PLMD or RLS, dopaminergic agents are the initial agent of choice. An evening dose of a dopamine agonist (e.g., pramipexole[OL] or ropinirole) are commonly used for residents with frequent (e.g., nightly) symptoms. A nighttime dose of carbidopa-levodopa[OL] can be used for residents who need medication infrequently (i.e., for as-needed use). Some residents may describe a shift of their symptoms to daytime hours with successful treatment of symptoms at night. There is some evidence that individuals with RLS and a low serum ferritin level may improve with iron replacement therapy. Benzodiazepines, anticonvulsants, and narcotics have also been used for restless leg syndrome but likely have more adverse effects in older people than do the dopaminergic agents.

Disturbances in the Sleep–Wake Cycle

Disturbances in the sleep–wake cycle may be transient, as in jet lag, or associated with an obvious cause (e.g., shift work). Some older adults have persistent disturbance, with either a delayed sleep phase (fall asleep late and awaken late) or an advanced sleep phase (fall asleep early and awaken early). The advanced sleep phase is particularly common in older adults. Some older adults have persistent sleep-phase disturbance, in which circadian rhythms and sleeping period have become completely desynchronized (e.g., persons who are always asleep during the day and awake at night), or sleep–wake cycles are irregular and sleep habits are very disjointed. It is unclear to what degree, if any, changes in sleep pattern in older adults (such as increased daytime napping and disrupted nighttime sleep) are due to alterations in the circadian rhythm. Several studies have shown age-related decreases in hormonal levels and evidence of earlier circadian increases in certain hormones, suggesting the existence of age-related alteration in circadian rhythm. Problems related to an advanced sleep phase may respond to appropriately timed exposure to bright light (see the section "Nonpharmacologic Interventions," later in this chapter). Older adults with a significant sleep-phase cycle disturbance should be referred to a sleep laboratory for evaluation. Dementia and delirium may also cause sleep–wake disturbance, frequent nighttime awakenings, nighttime wandering, and nighttime agitation.

REM Sleep Behavior Disorder

REM sleep behavior disorder is characterized by excessive motor activities during sleep and a pathologic absence of the normal muscle atonia during REM sleep. Presenting symptoms are unusually vigorous sleep behaviors associated with vivid dreams. These behaviors may result in injury (to the individual or bed partner). The condition may be acute or chronic, and it is more common in older men. There may be a family predisposition. Transient REM sleep behavior disorder has been associated with toxic-metabolic abnormalities, primarily drug or alcohol withdrawal or intoxication. The chronic form of the disorder is usually idiopathic, or associated with a neurologic abnormality (e.g., drug intoxication, vascular disease, tumor, infection, neurodegeneration disorders such as Parkinson's disease, or trauma). Several psychiatric medications have been associated with this disorder, including tricyclic antidepressants, monoamine oxidase inhibitors, fluoxetine, venlafaxine, cholinesterase inhibitors, and other agents. Polysomnography is recommended to establish the diagnosis. Removal of the offending agent is indicated for drug-induced REM sleep behavior disorder. Clonazepam[OL] is reported to be effective for the treatment of REM sleep behavior disorder, with little evidence of tolerance or abuse over long periods of treatment, but some residents may have adverse effects from this agent. There is some evidence for the use of melatonin in the treatment of REM sleep behavior disorder in individuals with coexisting neurodegenerative disorders (e.g., Parkinson's disease, dementia with Lewy bodies). Environmental safety interventions are also indicated, such as removing dangerous objects from the bedroom, putting cushions on the floor around the bed, protecting windows, lowering bed height and, in some cases, putting the mattress on the floor.

CHANGES IN SLEEP WITH DEMENTIA

Most studies of sleep in dementia have focused on Alzheimer's disease. Unfortunately, the baseline slowing of electroencephalographic activity often seen with dementia can cloud the distinction between sleep and wakefulness and between the various stages of non-REM sleep in the sleep laboratory. Older adults with dementia have more sleep disruption and arousals, lower sleep efficiency, a higher percentage of stage 1 sleep, and decreases in stage 3 and 4 sleep than do nondemented older people. Interestingly, some studies suggest that older persons with dementia have less sleep disturbance than older depressed persons. Disturbances of the sleep–wake cycle are common with dementia, resulting in daytime sleep and nighttime wakefulness.

SLEEP DISTURBANCES IN THE HOSPITAL

Acute hospitalization is commonly cited as one of the stressors that can precipitate transient or short-term insomnia. This insomnia is likely multifactorial in origin and related to illness, medications, change from usual nighttime routines at home, and a sleep-disruptive hospital environment. Sleeping medications are commonly prescribed in hospitalized older adults, and at least 15% of patients who are newly prescribed a sleeping pill while in the hospital say that they plan to use the medication after discharge to home. There is little research comparing the use of different sleeping medications among hospitalized older adults. Benzodiazepine receptor agonists are very commonly used. Given the increased sensitivity in older adults, smaller doses may be effective as well as safer. Sedating antihistamines (e.g., diphenhydramine) should not be used as a sleep aid in hospitalized older adults because of possible complications related to anticholinergic adverse effects (e.g., delirium, urinary retention, and constipation).

Sleep-related breathing disorders may be common in hospitalized adults, particularly among those with cardiac illness and stroke. A variety of studies report shorter survival among patients with heart failure with central sleep apnea than among heart failure patients without evidence of this disorder; nearly one-fourth of hospitalized patients (mean age 74 years) with an acute stroke had normal oxygen levels during the daytime but 30 minutes or more of unexpected nocturnal hypoxia; significant sleep-disordered breathing in nearly half of patients (mean age 64 years) hospitalized with an acute stroke; one-third of severely obese (body mass index [kg/m^2] ≥ 35) hospitalized people had unexplained hypoventilation (mean PaCO$_2$ 52 mm Hg), which was associated with more reported sleepiness and excess morbidity and mortality than was found in severely obese persons without hypoventilation.

Nonpharmacologic interventions may also be important in the acute hospital. A large study testing the feasibility of a nonpharmacologic sleep protocol for hospitalized older patients (consisting of a back rub, warm drink, and relaxation tapes) administered by nurses was successful in reducing sedative hypnotic drug use; the sleep protocol was found to have a stronger association than sedative-hypnotic drugs with improved quality of sleep.

MANAGEMENT OF SLEEP PROBLEMS

The appropriate treatment of sleep problems must be guided by knowledge of likely causes and potential contributing factors. It is inappropriate to start an older adult complaining of persistent sleep problems on a sedative hypnotic agent without a careful clinical assessment to identify the cause. Sedative hypnotics have a documented association with falls, hip fracture, and daytime carryover symptoms in older people. If the initial history and physical examination do not suggest a serious underlying cause for the sleep problem, a trial of improved sleep habits (sleep hygiene) is usually the best first approach. If the older adult takes daytime naps, it is important to determine whether these are needed rest periods or are due to inactivity, boredom, or sedating medications. It is important to explain to the person that daytime naps will decrease nighttime sleep.

Short-term hypnotic therapy may be appropriate in conjunction with improved sleep habits in cases of transient, situational insomnia, particularly during bereavement, acute hospitalization, and other periods of temporary acute stress. People generally do not feel well if they do not sleep well. Sedative hypnotic medication should be prescribed in situations where it is clearly indicated; however, such medications should be used cautiously because of the complications associated with their long-term use (see the section "Chronic Hypnotic Use," later in this chapter). Continuing use of benzodiazepines can lead to dependence or cognitive impairment. Given the increasing debate among sleep experts on the risks and benefits of long-term use of sleeping medications in adults of all ages, there is good evidence

of increased risk of confusion, falls, and fracture with chronic sedative use by older adults. Regardless, in chronic insomnia, it is imperative that the clinician exclude primary sleep disorders and review medications and other medical conditions that may be contributory.

Sleep hygiene measures can restore healthy sleep patterns. Several cognitive-behavioral theories, such as self-efficacy theory, can frame the approach to sleep hygiene (see Chapter 16, "Psychosocial Aspects of Aging"). Sleep hygiene measures include the following:

- Consistent bedtime and awakening time.
- Using the bed only for sleeping and for (sexual) intimacy. Meals or snacks, watching TV, or listening to the radio should not be permitted in bed. (If the resident insists on having and making these choices, he or she needs to understand the likely impact on his or her sleep and wakefulness patterns.)
- Naps should be short and, if possible, taken in the early rather than late afternoon. A planned nap should be no longer than 1 hour.
- Encourage exposure to brightness and light (the sun!) during the day, especially in the early part of the day. Bright light therapy is used for circadian rhythm disturbances, especially for what is known as delayed phase sleep disorder or DPSD. Treatment consists of timed exposure to bright light; the amount of time and number of lumens is based on sleep results. Exposure for 30–60 minutes does not appear to be harmful.
- If unable to fall asleep after 15–20 minutes, get up and go to another room or space. Try to avoid watching TV because the screen is bright and stimulating.
- Avoid caffeine or nicotine after midday; no more than three alcoholic drinks in one day.
- Avoid strenuous exercise or a large meal just before bedtime.

It bears noting that excessive daytime napping could be a sign of boredom, social withdrawal, and depression and needs to be evaluated.

Nonpharmacologic Interventions

Trials have shown that nonpharmacologic interventions can be quite effective in improving sleep in older adults (see Table 32.2 for a summary of such interventions). Behavioral interventions for community-dwelling older adults with insomnia concluded that these interventions produce reliable and durable therapeutic benefits, including improved sleep efficiency, sleep continuity, and satisfaction with sleep; treatment is also helpful in reducing chronic hypnotic use. Stimulus control and sleep restriction, which focus on poor sleep habits, seem to be especially helpful for older adults with insomnia.

Cognitive and educational interventions are also important in changing inaccurate beliefs and attitudes about sleep. However, relaxation-based interventions seem less effective for older adults. One large randomized trial of insomniacs with a mean age of 65 years compared cognitive behavior therapy (stimulus control,

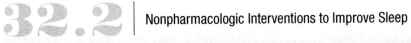 **32.2** | Nonpharmacologic Interventions to Improve Sleep

INTERVENTION	GOAL	DESCRIPTION
Stimulus control	To recondition maladaptive sleep-related behaviors	Resident is instructed to go to bed only when sleepy, not use the bed for eating or watching television, get out of bed if unable to fall asleep, return to bed only when sleepy, get up at the same time each morning, not take naps during the day.
Sleep restriction	To improve sleep efficiency by causing sleep deprivation	Resident first collects a 2-week sleep diary to determine average total daily sleep time, then stays in bed only that duration plus 15 minutes; gets up at same time each morning; takes no naps in the daytime; gradually increases time allowed in bed as sleep efficiency improves.
Cognitive interventions	To change misunderstandings and false beliefs regarding sleep	Resident's dysfunctional beliefs and attitudes about sleep are identified; resident is educated to change these false beliefs and attitudes, and learn about normal age-related changes in sleep and changes that are pathologic.
Relaxation techniques	To recognize and relieve tension and anxiety	In progressive muscle relaxation, resident is taught to tense and relax each muscle group. In electromyographic biofeedback, the resident is given feedback regarding muscle tension and learns techniques to relieve it. Meditation or imagery techniques are taught to relieve racing thoughts or anxiety.
Bright light	To correct circadian rhythm causes of sleeping difficulty (i.e., sleep-phase problems)	The resident is exposed to sunlight or a light box. Best evidence of effectives is from treatment of seasonal affective disorder. Light intensity (lux) and duration must be established by a clinician. Routine eye examination is recommended before treatment; light boxes with ultraviolet exposure are to be avoided.

sleep restriction, sleep hygiene, and cognitive therapy), pharmacotherapy (with temazepam), both cognitive behavioral therapy and pharmacotherapy, and placebo. All three active treatments were found to be effective in short-term follow-up in improving sleep, as indicated by sleep diaries and polysomnography. However, people reported more satisfaction with the cognitive behavioral therapy, and sleep improvements were found to be better sustained over time (up to 2 years) with behavioral treatment.

Several small studies tested the effectiveness of exposure to bright light (either natural sunlight or with commercially available light boxes) on the sleep of older adults with insomnia. Positive effects on sleep with light exposure of various intensities for various durations and at various times during the day were demonstrated. Evening exposure seems to be particularly useful in the older adult with an advanced sleep phase. However, even short durations of bright light in the morning reduce sleep complaints in healthy older adults. For demented residents with sleep and behavior problems, exposure to bright morning light was associated with better nighttime sleep and less daytime agitation.

Bathing before sleep enhances the quality of sleep of older adults, perhaps related to changes in body temperature with bathing. Moderate-intensity exercise also improved sleep among healthy, sedentary people age 50 and older who reported moderate sleep complaints at baseline. However, strenuous exercise should not be performed immediately before bedtime.

Another study of nursing home residents with dementia and behavioral problems found that a program of social interaction with nurses was effective in reducing behavioral problems and sleep–wake rhythm disorders in 30% of the residents. A small trial among incontinent nursing home residents demonstrated increased nighttime sleep and less agitation among those randomized to receive a combined daytime physical activity program plus nighttime intervention to decrease noise and light disruption. An enforced schedule of structured social and physical activity for 2 weeks in a small sample of assisted living residents found that those residents had enhanced SWS and improved performance in memory-oriented tasks.

Pharmacotherapy

Short-acting agents are recommended for residents with problems initiating sleep; intermediate-acting agents are recommended for problems with sleep maintenance. Short-acting agents have lower associations with falls and hip fractures. However, agents with rapid elimina-

tion, in general, also produce the most pronounced rebound and withdrawal syndromes after discontinuation. *Rebound insomnia* after cessation of short-acting agents is dose dependent and can be reduced by tapering the dosage prior to discontinuing the drug. Triazolam is a short-acting benzodiazepine that has been associated with nocturnal amnesia and confusion and is generally not recommended for older adults.

Zolpidem, zaleplon, and eszopiclone are nonbenzodiazepine hypnotics. These agents are structurally unrelated to the benzodiazepines, but they share some of the pharmacologic properties of benzodiazepines and have been shown to interact with the central nervous system γ-aminobutyric acid (GABA) receptor complex at benzodiazepine (GABA-BZ) receptors. The selectivity of these newer agents to the GABA-BZ receptor may account for their decreased muscle-relaxant, anxiolytic, and anticonvulsant effects in comparison with benzodiazepines in some studies. Zolpidem, a nonbenzodiazepine imidazopyridine that has been studied in older adults with insomnia does not produce rebound insomnia, agitation, or anxiety with cessation; does not seem to produce impaired daytime performance on cognitive and psychomotor performance tests; and may have a therapeutic effect that outlasts the period of drug treatment. Zaleplon, a nonbenzodiazepine hypnotic from the pyrazolopyrimidine class, has also been studied for short-term use by older adults with insomnia. Because of their rapid onset of action, zolpidem and zaleplon should be taken only immediately before bedtime or after the resident has gone to bed and has been unable to fall asleep. Eszopiclone is apparently effective in long-term management of insomnia and was recently approved by the Food and Drug Administration. Guidelines for zolpidem or zaleplon, like benzodiazepines, recommend that they be used only for a short term (2 or 3 weeks); if used longer, these agents should be used no more than 2 or 3 nights per week. Concerns remain regarding the risks of confusion, falls, and fracture with chronic use of these medications in older people, and caution is warranted even with these newer agents.

Low doses of sedating antidepressants such as trazodone[OL] or mirtazapine[OL] at bedtime may be used as a sleeping aid, particularly for residents with depression. These agents have been suggested for use as a nighttime adjuvant for sleep in depressed individuals receiving another antidepressant at therapeutic doses during the daytime. Other indications may be residents with a history of psychoactive substance use problems, failure with other sleeping medications, suspected untreated sleep apnea (where further respiratory depression is a concern), and fibromyalgia (where there is some evidence for antidepressant medication treatment effect). However, the adverse effects of sedating antidepressants may limit their usefulness.

Chronic Hypnotic Use

There is strong epidemiologic evidence for increased morbidity and mortality associated with chronic use of prescription sleeping pills; however, much of this evidence predates the availability of newer, nonbenzodiazepine hypnotics. Nightly use of prescription sleeping pills was associated with an increased mortality that is similar to the mortality hazard of smoking one to two packs of cigarettes per day. Tolerance to hypnotics after long-term use may actually make sleep worse. Additional research is needed to help clarify the consequences of long-term use of the newer, nonbenzodiazepine hypnotics in older people.

Several studies indicate that most prescription sleeping medication use is occurring among chronic users, and not those with transient sleeping difficulties. Chronic benzodiazepine use is greater among older adults than younger adults and among women more than men. The association between long-acting benzodiazepines and falls in older people has been known for some time.

Effective methods to help older chronic hypnotic users reduce or eliminate their use of these agents have been reported: slow reduction of dose over 2 to 6 weeks followed by full withdrawal was effective (over short-term follow-up) in eliminating hypnotic use without adverse effects on nighttime sleep, depressive symptoms, or daytime sleepiness.

Nonprescription Sleeping Agents

Nearly half of older adults report using nonprescription sleeping products. The most common treatments are antihistamines, acetaminophen, alcohol, and melatonin. Sedating antihistamines (e.g., diphenhydramine) are common ingredients in OTC agents as well as in combination with analgesic sleeping agents that are marketed for nighttime use. Diphenhydramine has potent anticholinergic effects, and tolerance to its sedating effects develops after several weeks; it is generally not recommended for older adults. Side effects commonly include such things as dry mouth, confusion, constipation, elevated blood pressure, or urinary retention. Those with mild pain that is stopping them from falling asleep may have adequate improvement in sleep with a simple pain reliever (e.g., acetaminophen) at bedtime and thus avoid risking the potential side effects of OTC sleeping agents, or agents that have both acetaminophen and diphen-

hydramine. Many older adults utilize alcohol intake at night believing it helps them with sleep. Unfortunately, although alcohol causes some initial drowsiness, it interferes with normal sleep cycles and can decrease the length of time that the individual actually stays asleep.

Evidence is mixed regarding the effectiveness of melatonin as a treatment for insomnia among older adults. There is some evidence that melatonin administration decreases sleep latency and wake time after sleep onset, and increases sleep efficiency. Because of mixed results regarding melatonin effectiveness and the lack of regulatory control in the currently available melatonin products, these products are generally not recommended. The exception may be for chronic hypnotic users, among whom there is some evidence for success in withdrawal of the hypnotic with concomitant use of melatonin. Valerian is an herbal product with mild sedative action that has been marketed for insomnia. The mechanism of action of valerian is uncertain; because it contains several potentially active compounds its use is not recommended.

RESOURCES

Alessi, C. A., Martin, J. L., Webber, A. P., Kim, E. C., Harker, J. O., & Josephson, K. R. (2005). Randomized control trial of a nonpharmacological intervention to improve abnormal sleep/ wakefulness pattern in nursing home residents. *Journal of the American Geriatrics Society, 53*(5), 803–810.

Ancoli-Israel, S., Martin, J. L., Kripke, D. F., Marler, M., & Klauber, M. R. (2002). Effect of light treatment on sleep and circadian rhythms in demented nursing home patients. *Journal of the American Geriatrics Society, 50*(2), 282–289.

Chasens, E. R., Williams, L. L., & Umlauf, M. G. (2008). Excessive sleepiness. In E. Capezuti, D. Zwicker, M. Mezey, & T. Fulmer (Eds.), *Evidence-based geriatric nursing protocols for best practice* (3rd ed., pp. 459–476). New York: Springer Publishing Company.

National Institutes of Health. (1990). The treatment of sleep disorders of older people. *NIH Consensus Statement Online, 8*(3): 1–22.

Rao, V., Spiro, J. R., Samus, Q. M., Rosenblatt, A., Steele, C., Baker, A., et al. (2007). Sleep disturbances in the elderly residing in assisted living: Findings from the Maryland Assisted Living Study. *International Journal of Geriatric Psychiatry, 20,* 956–966.

Sleep Disorders Center, University of Maryland Medical Center. (n.d.). *Questionnaire for sleep apnea risk.* Retrieved December 1, 2008, from http://www.umm.edu/sleep/apnea_risk.htm

Smyth, C. (1997). *Pittsburg Sleep Quality Index (PSQI). Try this 6.1.* Retrieved December 1, 2008, from http://www.consultgerirn.org/uploads/File/trythis/issue06_1.pdf

Smyth, C. (2007). *Epworth Sleepiness Scale (ESS). Try this 6.2.* Retrieved December 1, 2008, from http://www.consultgerirn.org/uploads/File/trythis/issue06.pdf

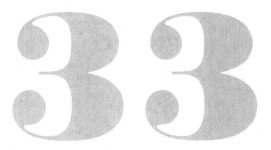

Pressure Ulcers

Anna M. Mago-Sisic and Courtney H. Lyder

Pressure ulcers are a serious and common problem for almost 1 million older adults. As the population ages, pressure ulcers will continue to be a major health care problem. The Surgeon General's "Healthy People 2010" document identified pressure ulcers as a national health issue for long-term care. The Centers for Medicare and Medicaid Services (CMS) has designated pressure ulcers as one of the three primary markers of quality of care in the long-term-care setting. Prevention and treatment of pressure ulcers requires the collaboration and skills of the entire interdisciplinary health care team.

EPIDEMIOLOGY

A pressure ulcer is defined as damage caused to skin and underlying soft tissue by unrelieved pressure when the tissue is compressed between a bony prominence and an external surface over a prolonged period of time. Because pressure is the major physiologic factor that leads to soft-tissue destruction, the term *pressure ulcer* is most widely used and preferred over *decubitus ulcer* or *bedsore*.

The causes of pressure ulcers are still not fully understood; most research has been conducted in animal models. Three main factors are believed to play a role in pressure-ulcer formation: *pressure, friction* (i.e., rubbing against a sheet) and *shear forces* (i.e., pulling a resident up in the bed). The amount of pressure, friction, or shear forces needed to create a pressure ulcer depends on quality of the tissue, blood flow, amount of pressure applied, and moisture. Hence, for residents with poor-quality tissue (i.e., tissue with inadequate blood perfusion), it may take less sustained pressure over a shorter period of time to develop a pressure ulcer. All of this is made worse when the skin is moist. Conversely, residents with good-quality tissue may be able to sustain higher loads of pressure over a longer period of time before an ulcer develops. Ulcers caused by shearing forces tend to develop deep in the tissue, whereas ulcers caused by friction tend to be quite superficial, starting in the most superficial to deeper layers of the skin.

Skin anatomy consists of the epidermis (outer layer) and dermis (inner layer). The *epidermis* is divided into five layers, is thin and avascular, and regenerates every 4–6 weeks. The epidermis's main function is protection. The *dermis* is the thickest layer of skin and is divided into two layers. It is composed of sparsely populated cells when compared with the epidermis. The dermis's main function is to provide strength, support, blood, and oxygen to the skin. Major proteins found in the dermal layer include collagen (providing strength) and elastin (giving skin its recoil). They are synthesized and secreted by fibroblasts. The dermal-epidermal junction, known as the *basement membrane zone*, separates the epidermis and dermis. Under the dermis is a layer of loose connective tissue, or *hypodermis*, which attaches the dermis to underlying structures. The hypodermis consists of adipose and connective tissue, blood and lymphatic vessels, and nerves. Its function is to provide blood supply to the dermis for regeneration.

With aging, the epidermis and basement membrane becomes thin. The skin becomes a less effective barrier against water loss and infection. Blood vessels become thinner and more fragile, leading to the appearance of hemorrhagic spots known as *senile purpura*; skin tears often occur at these sites. The dermis thins by approximately 20% and is probably the biggest contributing factor to *paperlike skin* (i.e., tissue paper skin) in an older adult. Decreases in skin cells, blood vessels, nerve endings, and collagen lead to altered sensation, thermoregulation, rigidity in the blood vessels, and moisture retention. Loss of subcutaneous tissue, primarily adipose or fat tissue, results in a loss of protection and insulation of the underlying tissue. These changes in aging skin with altered sensation and the resultant lowered tolerance to hypoxia may predispose the older person to pressure ulcer development.

The incidence and prevalence of pressure ulcers varies greatly, depending on the setting. In acute care, incidence rates range from 0.4% to 38%. Higher rates are noted in intensive care units, where residents are less mobile and have severe systemic illnesses. The Fourth National Pressure Ulcer Prevalence Survey reported an annual hospital prevalence rate of 10.1%. In the long-term care setting, incidence and prevalence rates range from 3% to 30%. Less is known about pressure ulcers in home care, but studies report incidence rates of 4% to 17% and prevalence rates of 5% to 15%.

The incidence of pressure ulcers not only differs by health care setting but also by stage of ulceration.

- *Stage I pressure ulcer (nonblanchable erythema)* is the most common, accounting for 47% of all pressure ulcers. Nonblanchable erythema can be evaluated at the bedside. Transient pressure against the skin causes paleness or pallor where blood flow to a specific area has stopped. After little more than 1 minute, the area will blanch (become white). When the pressure is relieved, the area becomes reddened or hyperemic as blood flows back and revitalizes the area. This rush of blood back into the area is called reactive hyperemia, the earliest sign of tissue compromise and pressure-related ischemia. If the pressure is prolonged, reactive hyperemia is not sufficient to revitalize ischemic tissue (i.e., tissue that has not gotten oxygen via blood supply). In healthy tissue, if pressure is applied to a hyperemic area, the skin will blanch as blood is pushed away from the area. It becomes erythemic again as blood rushes back to the area. In compromised tissue, the hyperemic area will not blanch. Nonblanching erythema is a serious sign that tissue is not receiving adequate oxygen and nutrients. This is a stage I pressure ulcer and should no longer be referred to as reactive hyperemia. In dark-skinned residents, reactive hyperemia can be evaluated by increased darkening of the skin over bony prominences and palpating these areas for warmth, edema, induration, or hardness.

- *Stage II pressure ulcer* is partial thickness loss involving only the epidermal and dermal layers and accounts for 33% of all pressure ulcers.

- *Stage III* (full-thickness skin loss involving subcutaneous tissue) and *Stage IV* (full thickness involving muscle, bone, tendon, or supporting structures) pressure ulcers comprise the remaining 20%. Several studies note that the incidence rates of pressure ulcers among African Americans and Whites may differ; African Americans tend to have a greater incidence of stage III and stage IV pressure ulcers than do Whites. This may be because it is more difficult to detect nonblanchable skin in dark-skinned individuals. Whether this can be attributed to structural skin changes, socioeconomic factors, or clinicians not identifying, for example, a stage I pressure ulcer in dark toned skin, is unknown because of the paucity of pressure ulcer research among minority groups in the United States.

RISK FACTORS AND RISK-ASSESSMENT SCALES

The literature abounds with lists of risk factors associated with pressure ulcer development. However, any disease process that renders an older adult immobile for an extended period of time will increase the risk for pressure ulcer development. *Intrinsic* and *extrinsic factors* determine the tolerance of soft tissue to the adverse effects of pressure. Intrinsic risk factors are physiologic factors or disease states such as age, poor nutritional status, and decreased arteriolar blood pressure. Some physiologic risk factors (e.g., diabetes mellitus, cerebral vascular accident [CVA], arterial disease) have been associated with microcirculatory impairment, thus leading to neural and endothelial compromise and increasing the risk of ulceration. Extrinsic factors are external factors that damage the skin, for example, friction and shear, moisture, and urinary or fecal incontinence or both. Variables that appear to be predictors of pressure ulcer development include age 70 or older, impaired mobility, smoking history, low body mass index, altered mental status (e.g., confusion), urinary and fecal incontinence, malnutrition, restraints, dehydration, depression, malignancy, diabetes mellitus, CVA, pneumonia, heart failure, fever, sepsis, hypotension, hypothyroid, kidney failure, dry and scaly skin, history of pressure ulcers, anemia, lymphopenia, and hypoalbuminemia.

Because of the myriad risk factors associated with pressure ulcer development, various scales have been developed to quantify a person's risk by identifying the presence of factors in several categories. The Braden Scale (Braden & Bergstrom, 2001) and the Norton Scale (Norton, McLaren, & Exton-Smith, 1962) are probably the most widely used and validated instruments for identifying older adults at risk for developing pressure ulcers. Both tools are recommended by the Agency for Healthcare Research and Quality (AHRQ). The Braden Scale has a sensitivity of 83% to 100% and a specificity of 64% to 77%; the Norton Scale has a sensitivity of 73% to 92% and a specificity of 61% to 94%.

The AHRQ guidelines for preventing pressure ulcers recommend that bed- and chair-bound residents or those with impaired ability to reposition themselves should be assessed upon admission to a hospital or long-term care facility for additional factors that increase the risk for developing pressure ulcers. Pressure ulcer risk should also be reassessed at periodic intervals and when there is a change in level of activity or mobility, such as with acute illness. Studies demonstrate that the incorporation of systematic risk-assessment tools significantly reduces the incidence of pressure ulcers. To date, the Braden Scale is the only tool to be validated in non-White populations. Use of risk-assessment tools does not guarantee that all older adults at risk for pressure ulcers will be identified.

PREVENTION

The AHRQ-sponsored clinical practice guidelines (CPC) for the prevention of pressure ulcers in adults is an excellent approach to evidenced-based pressure-ulcer prevention. *Pressure Ulcers in Adults: Prediction and Prevention* CPC is available from Agency for Health Care Policy and Research (1992).

Skin Care

There is limited evidence on the effectiveness of skin care in pressure ulcer prevention; most recommendations are based on expert opinion. After identification of the older adult at risk for pressure ulcers, the goal of skin care is to maintain and improve tissue tolerance to pressure in order to prevent tissue injury.

All older adults at risk should have a systematic skin inspection at least once a day, with emphasis on the bony prominences, especially the heels and sacrum. Skin should be cleansed with warm water and a mild cleansing agent to minimize irritation and dryness. Ev-

ery effort should be made to minimize environmental factors leading to skin drying, such as low humidity (less than 40%) and exposure to cold. Decreased skin hydration can result in decreased pliability. Dry skin should be managed with moisturizers. Products with petroleum (e.g., Vaseline, Kerasol) are very effective over-the-counter products.

Contrary to what used to be taught in nursing school, massaging over bony prominences should be avoided. Previously, it was believed that this promoted circulation. However, postmortem biopsies found degenerated tissue in those areas exposed to massage but found no degenerated tissue on those areas that were not massaged. All efforts should be made to avoid exposing the skin to perspiration, wound drainage, or urine and fecal incontinence. When disposable briefs are used to manage incontinence, the resident must be checked and changed frequently since perineal dermatitis and/or cutaneous candidiasis can develop quickly. Using disposable underpads to control excessive moisture and perspiration may help wick moisture away from skin. Moisturizers and moisture barriers (e.g., Calmoseptine or CriticAid), should be used to protect the skin. After each incontinence episode, the perineal area should be cleaned gently, dried well, and have a moisture barrier applied.

Nutrition

Several studies identify the association between pressure ulcer development and malnutrition. Ensuring an adequate diet to prevent malnutrition that is compatible with an older adult's food preferences and the goals of care is a reasonable strategy to reduce the risk of ulcer formation. It is important to note that hydration is not separate from nutrition; a dehydrated or hypovolemic resident is also at greater risk for pressure ulcer development. The clinician may order lab work including such things as protein markers, pre-albumin, and/or albumin in order to track dietary interventions, usually initiated by a licensed dietician.

Mechanical Loading

Minimizing friction and shear is important and can be accomplished with proper repositioning, transferring, and turning techniques. The use of lubricants (e.g., cornstarch and creams), protective films (e.g., transparent film dressings and skin sealants), protective dressings (e.g., hydrocolloids), and protective padding may be used to reduce the possibility of friction and shear. Older adults at risk for developing pressure ulcers should be repositioned at least every 1–2 hours. Bed-positioning devices such as pillows or foam wedges should be used to keep bony prominences from direct contact with one another (e.g., ankles rubbing against each other). The head of the bed should be at the lowest degree of elevation (i.e., 30 degrees, preferably) consistent with medical conditions. Lifting devices, such as trapezes or bed linen to move the person in bed, will also decrease the potential for friction and shear forces. Studies suggest that approximately 20% of all pressure ulcer development occurs at the heels and is attributed to the limited amount of soft tissue over the heel. See Exhibit 33.1 for specific clinical interventions to prevent heel pressure ulcers.

Older adults seated in a chair should be assessed for postural alignment, weight distribution, and balance. They should be taught and/or reminded to shift or move the area that is currently experiencing the pressure (e.g., moving the hips/buttocks or the heels) every 15 minutes. Use of doughnuts as seating cushions

is contraindicated because they increase pressure over the area of contact and may actually cause pressure ulcers. Wheelchair/chair cushions are more appropriate. For example, a Roho cushion (information available at http://www.roho.com/) or Roho-type cushion is appropriate typically for residents with a stage II to IV pressure ulcer who want and need to be up in a chair or wheelchair. An occupational therapist can provide consultation on appropriate seating and positioning to decrease pressure and prevent breakdown or exacerbation of an existing wound.

Mobility

Maintaining or improving mobility is also extremely important. It is one of the most effective ways to decrease pressure on bony prominences. For bed-bound residents, there are benefits of both active and passive range-of-motion exercises. Those residents not confined to bed should be encouraged to move from bed to chair to standing to ambulating (with assistance as needed) in order to minimize the risk of developing pressure ulcers.

Support Surfaces

Any older adult identified as being at risk for developing pressure ulcers should be placed on a pressure-reducing device of which there are two types: *static* (foam, static air, gel or water, or a combination) and *dynamic* (alternating air, low air loss, or air fluidized). Most static devices are less expensive than dynamic surfaces. Table 33.1 provides details about the various types of support surfaces that can guide selection for particular situations. Most clinical experts agree that for pressure ulcer prevention, the use of static devices is appropriate. Three conditions warrant consideration of a dynamic surface:

(1) Bottoming-out has occurred (i.e., the static surface is compressed to less than 1 inch)
(2) The resident is at high risk for pressure ulcers; reactive hyperemia is noted on a bony prominence despite the use of a static support surface
(3) Urinary or fecal incontinence is present

Although effective at reducing pressure, dynamic airflow beds have several potential adverse effects, including dehydration (especially the fluidized beds), sensory deprivation, loss of muscle strength, and difficulty with mobilization. It is important to note that a special chuck or bed pad must be used with a dynamic

33.1 | Prevention of Heel Pressure Ulcers

- Assess the heels of residents at high risk for pressure ulcers, daily.
- Use moisturizer on the heels once or twice a day; do not massage.
- Never apply hydrocolloid dressing (either single or extra thick) to the heels of older persons with reactive hyperemia (pre-stage I) as progression may rapidly move to stage III or IV.
- Residents should wear cotton socks to help prevent friction; remove the socks at bedtime.
- Residents using wheelchairs should wear properly fitting padded sneakers or shoes. Check for pressure points between the person's feet/legs and the foot holders.
- To support heels off the bed surface: place a pillow vertically—not horizontally—under the resident's legs.
- Consider bilateral heel lift boots in compromised or acutely ill bedridden residents.
- Turn every 1–2 hours, repositioning heels.

33.1 | Support Surfaces for Persons at Risk for Pressure Ulcers

TYPE	EXAMPLES	SUPPORT AREA	LOW MOISTURE RETENTION	REDUCED HEAT ACCUMULATION	SHEAR REDUCTION	PRESSURE REDUCTION	COST PER DAY
Static surfaces	Foam	Yes	No	No	No	Yes	Low
	Standard mattress	No	No	No	No	No	Low
	Static flotation—air or water	Yes	No	No	Yes	Yes	Low
Dynamic surfaces	Air fluidized	Yes	Yes	Yes	Yes	Yes	High
	Low-air-loss	Yes	Yes	Yes	?	Yes	High
	Alternating air	Yes	No	No	Yes	Yes	Moderate

From *Treatment of Pressure Ulcers*. Clinical Practice Guideline No. 15 (p. 38), by N. Bergstrom, M. A. Bennett, C. E. Carlson, R. Allman, O. M. Alvarez, R. A. Frantz, et al., 1994, Rockville, MD: U.S. Department of Health and Human Services, Public Health Service, Agency for Health Care Policy and Research. Copyright ©1994 by National Library of Medicine. Adapted with permission.

surface to allow transport of air to the torso, where it is needed for incontinent residents. This is done to keep the area clean and dry but also to maintain the appropriate pressure-relieving environment.

MANAGEMENT

The AHRQ evidence-based guidelines on the management of pressure ulcers, *Treatment of Pressure Ulcers* (AHRQ, 1994), reviews the foundation for providing evidence-based pressure ulcer management. Management consists of assessment, treatment, monitoring, and control of infections.

Assessment

A pressure ulcer will not heal unless underlying causes are identified and effective interventions are implemented. When a pressure ulcer has developed, systematic evaluation is necessary. Table 33.2 presents an approach to assessment and documentation when a pressure ulcer develops. There is no universal agreement on a single system for classifying pressure ulcers. Most experts agree that the wound stage, amount of

exudates, and resident condition/status determine the appropriate treatment plan. However, it bears noting that stage alone does not determine the seriousness of the ulcer. Most systems use four stages to classify ulceration. Table 33.3 describes one staging system. When eschar, a thick brown or black devitalized tissue, is covering the ulcer, it cannot be staged.

The challenge for most staging systems occurs in the definition/description of a stage I pressure ulcer. There is more variability in attempts to classify the first stage of ulcer development than in any other stage. Most systems (i.e., AHRQ, minimum data set) define stage I pressure ulcer as nonblanchable erythema of intact skin. However, it is difficult to blanch darkly pigmented skin. To address this concern, the National Pressure Ulcer Advisory Panel (NPUAP) revised its definition of a stage I pressure ulcer to encompass the skin alterations that might be seen in stage I pressure ulcers regardless of skin pigmentation, that is, an observable pressure-related alteration of intact skin whose indicators, as compared with an adjacent or opposite area on the body, may include changes in one or more of the following: skin temperature (warmth or coolness), tissue consistency (firm or boggy feel), or sensation (pain, itching). The NPUAP definition further states that the

 | A Systematic Approach to the Management of Pressure Ulcers

EVALUATE AND DOCUMENT:	CONSIDER THESE STRATEGIES:
Location	■ Examine high-risk sites daily.
	■ Develop targeted pressure-relieving strategies (e.g., positioning and repositioning, padding, seat cushions, pressure-reducing or relieving mattress and heel elevation).
	■ Limit shearing forces by special attention to positioning when the head of bed is elevated. No more than 30 degrees head elevation unless medically contraindicated.
	■ Lift rather than slide the resident.
	■ Cleanse and dry regularly if frequently incontinent. Gently clean and pat dry skin—no rubbing or scrubbing.
Stage	■ Differentiate between stage I lesions (i.e., nonblanchable erythema related to extravasation of red blood cells into the interstitium) and deep tissue injuries that can progress to full-thickness lesions.
	■ Discuss with caregivers and families the possibility of significant pressure ulcer development, generally stage III or IV, when deep tissue injury is identified.
Area	■ Record diameter for circular lesions. The longest, farthest, and deepest measurements in cm.
	■ Record lengths of largest perpendiculars for irregular lesions.
Depth	■ Measure depth from plane of skin, usually with q-tip and finger tip method.
	■ Probe and measure extent of undermining or depth of sinus tracts. Use clock locations. For example, 1.5 cm at 9 o'clock undermining.
Drainage	■ Estimate amount (scant, minimal, moderate, heavy, or saturated).
	■ Identify color, consistency (serous or purulence), and odor.
	■ Monitor hematocrit if more than minor blood loss occurs with dressing changes.
	■ Monitor serum albumin if volume of ulcer drainage is large.
Necrosis	■ Consider simple blunt debridement of small amounts of necrotic tissue.
	■ Involve general or plastic surgeons for extensive debridement.
	■ Monitor damage to healthy tissue whenever using blunt, enzymatic, or wet-to-dry dressings for debridement.
	■ Monitor use of pressure dressings (which can cause necrosis) after blunt debridement.

(continued)

33.2 | A Systematic Approach to the Management of Pressure Ulcers *(continued)*

EVALUATE AND DOCUMENT:	CONSIDER THESE STRATEGIES:
Granulation	■ Identify red granulation as an indication that wound healing is occurring.
	■ Look for regression when other infections (e.g., urinary tract infection or pneumonia) occur. This is the time for greater vigilance and possible increase in interventions.
	■ Develop strategies to protect and enhance growth of granulation tissue (e.g., nourishment, vitamins, and minerals; use of proper dressings and frequency of changing to ensure moist and optimal wound environment).
	■ Avoid damage with dressing changes. Use a skin prep or barrier to periwound to prevent skin damage (e.g., maceration, dermatitis, fungal infections, denuding, etc.).
	■ Identify epithelial growth at edges of wound for evaluation of healing and protect with prep or barrier creams/ointments.
Cellulitis	■ Differentiate from a thin rim of erythema surrounding most healing wounds.
	■ Look for tender, warm, erythematic, edematous skin particularly if there is progression.
	■ Consider treatment with systemic antibiotics active against gram-positive cocci.

From *Geriatrics Review Syllabus: A Core Curriculum in Geriatric Medicine* (4th ed., p. 155), by E. L. Cobbs, E. H. Duthie, Jr., & J. B. Murphy, 1996, Dubuque, IA: Kendall Hunt Publishing Company for the American Geriatrics Society. Copyright ©1996 by American Geriatrics Society. Reprinted with permission.

pressure ulcer appears as a defined area of persistent redness in lightly pigmented skin, whereas in darker skin tones, the pressure ulcer may appear with persistent erythema, or blue or purple hues. Although this definition is cumbersome, it is the only definition that includes residents with darkly pigmented skin.

Treatment

Debridement

Debridement is necessary when there is necrotic (i.e., dead) tissue within the wound that is likely to support the growth of pathologic organisms that prevent healing. The four major types of debridement methods in the United States are: mechanical, enzymatic, autolytic, and sharp (Table 33.4). Biosurgery (i.e., maggot or larva therapy), widely used in Europe, is another potential debridement option. The debridement method selected should be on the basis of the resident's health condition, the ulcer presentation, the presence or absence of infection, and the resident's ability to tolerate the procedure.

Dressings

Numerous types of dressings are used to treat and heal pressure ulcers. The use of wet-to-dry gauze has been discouraged by clinical experts because it is, in effect, a debriding technique that can damage the tissue matrix and retard healing. Many experts advocate the use of hydrocolloid dressings, which, when compared with gauze, significantly speed the healing process. Hydrocolloids require fewer dressing changes (inflicting less trauma), block bacteria from penetrating the wound bed, and maintain a moist wound environment (facilitating increases in the growth factors needed in the healing process). Moreover, studies demonstrate that use of hydrocolloids, when compared with use of gauze, decreases direct and indirect institutional costs. It is essential to select an appropriate treatment/dressing on several factors: stage of the pressure ulcer, amount of wound exudate, potential for or actual presence of infection, and frequency of dressing change (availability of staff to change the dressing, etc.). Table 33.5 identifies some of the most common treatments and indications for their use.

33.3 | Staging System for Pressure Ulcers

Suspected deep tissue injury	Purple or maroon localized area of discolored intact skin or blood-filled blister due to damage of underlying soft tissue from pressure and/or shear. The area may be preceded by tissue that is painful, firm, mushy, boggy, warmer, or cooler as compared to adjacent tissue. Further description: Deep tissue injury may be difficult to detect in individuals with dark skin tones. Evolution may include a thin blister over a dark ulcer bed. The ulcer may further evolve and become covered with eschar. Evolution may be rapid, exposing additional layers of tissue even with optimal treatment.
Stage I	Persistent nonblanchable erythema of intact skin.[a]
Stage II	Partial-thickness skin loss involving epidermis or dermis, or both. The ulcer is superficial and presents clinically as an abrasion, blister, or shallow crater.
Stage III	Full-thickness skin loss involving damage or necrosis of subcutaneous tissue that may extend down to, but not through, underlying fascia.
Stage IV	Full-thickness skin loss with extensive destruction, tissue necrosis, or damage to muscle, bone, or supporting structures (e.g., tendon or joint capsule). Undermining and sinus tracts may also be associated with stage IV pressure ulcers.
Unstageable	Full thickness tissue loss in which the base of the ulcer is covered by slough (yellow, tan, gray, green, or brown) and/or eschar (tan, brown, or black) in the ulcer bed. Further description: Until enough slough and/or eschar is removed to expose the base of the ulcer, the true depth, and therefore stage, cannot be determined. Stable (dry, adherent, intact without erythema, flatulence, edema) eschar on the heels serves as the body's natural (biological) cover and *should not be removed*.

[a]The National Pressure Ulcer Advisory Panel further expands this definition as follows: A stage I pressure ulcer is an observable pressure-related alteration of intact skin whose indicators as compared to the adjacent or opposite area on the body may include changes in one or more of the following: skin temperature (warmth or coolness), tissue consistency (firm or boggy feel), and/or sensation (pain, itching). The ulcer appears as a defined area of persistent redness in lightly pigmented skin, whereas in darker skin tones, the ulcer may appear with persistent red, blue, or purple hues.

From *Treatment of Pressure Ulcers. Clinical Practice Guideline No. 15* (pp. 47–49), by N. Bergstrom, M. A. Bennett, C. E. Carlson, R. Allman, O. M. Alvarez, R. A. Frantz, et al., 1994, Rockville, MD: U.S. Department of Health and Human Services, Public Health Service, Agency for Health Care Policy and Research. Copyright ©1994 by National Library of Medicine. Adapted with permission.

Surgical Repair

Surgical repair of a pressure ulcer is a viable option for stage III and stage IV pressure ulcers. Given that many stage III and stage IV pressure ulcers eventually heal over a long period of time with the use of modern wound-healing principles, and the rate of recurrence of surgically closed pressure ulcers is high, the benefits of surgery must be carefully weighed. When the surgical option is exercised, the most common type of surgical repairs are direct closure, skin grafting, skin flaps, musculocutaneous flaps, and free flaps.

Diet and Nutritional Supplements

The importance of diet and dietary supplements for a malnourished resident with a pressure ulcer is controversial. Evidence to support the use of supplemental vitamins and minerals is equally weak.

New or Unproven Therapies

Several treatments advocated for healing pressure ulcers lack sufficient data to support their various claims. The therapeutic efficacy of hyperbaric oxygen, low-

33.4 | Debridement Methods

TYPE	DESCRIPTION	ADVANTAGES, DISADVANTAGES
Mechanical	Use of physical forces to remove devitalized tissues. Methods include wet-to-dry irrigation (using 19-gauge needle with 35-cc syringe), hydrotherapy, and dextranomer	This approach is a nonselective removal of both devitalized and vitalized tissues; typically painful and does not provide optimal wound environment
Surgical, sharp	Use of scalpel, scissors, and forceps to remove devitalized tissue; laser debridement is also in this category	Quick, effective if performed by skilled professional; should be used when infection is suspected; pain management is needed
Enzymatic	Use of topical debriding agent to dissolve the devitalized tissue (by chemical force)	Appropriate when there are no signs or symptoms of local infection. Does not damage surrounding skin, although there may be some sensitivities
Autolytic	Use of dressings to allow the devitalized tissue to self-digest from the enzymes found in the ulcer fluids (by natural force)	Recommended when the older person cannot tolerate other forms of debridement and when infection is not suspected; may take a long time to be effective
Biosurgery	Use of larvae to digest devitalized tissue	Quick, effective; good option when older person cannot tolerate surgical debridement

energy laser irradiation, and therapeutic ultrasound has not been established. However, areas of great promise include the use of recombinant platelet-derived growth factors to stimulate healing and skin equivalents that may heal stage III and stage IV pressure ulcers. Preliminary data on the uses of electrical stimulation, vacuum-assisted closures, and warm-up therapy (which increases the basal temperature of the ulcer to promote healing) are promising.

Monitoring Healing

Monitoring the healing of pressure ulcers is challenging. Accurate measurements of a pressure ulcer can inform the clinician about treatment effectiveness. However, traditional measurements (using rulers and tracing paper) produce highly variable results among raters. Recently, two instruments to measure healing of pressure ulcers have been developed with some level of validity and reliability. The Pressure Sore Status Tool and the Pressure Ulcer Scale for Healing (PUSH) tool (National Pressure Ulcer Advisory Panel, 1998) are both excellent tools for monitoring pressure-ulcer healing. The PUSH tool helps categorize the ulcer with respect to surface area, exudate, and type of wound tissue. The nurse using this tool records a subscore for each of these ulcer characteristics and then adds the subscores to obtain the total score. A comparison of total scores measured over time is an indication of the ulcer's improvement or deterioration. High-frequency portable ultrasound to measure wound healing provides three-dimensional measurement data and is quite effective in objectively monitoring healing. Moreover, because ultrasound is color blind, it can detect stage I pressure ulcers in darkly pigmented skin.

Reverse staging of pressure ulcers to monitor healing has generated considerable debate. Staging is appropriate only for defining the maximum anatomic depth of tissue damage—when the etiology is pressure. A stage IV pressure ulcer cannot become a stage III, stage II, and then stage I ulcer; reverse staging does not accurately characterize what is physiologically occurring as

33.5 | Common Dressings for Treating Pressure Ulcers

DRESSING	INDICATIONS	CONTRAINDICATIONS	EXAMPLE	COMMENTS
Transparent film	Stage I, II, simple skin tear Protection from friction Superficial scrape	Highly draining ulcers Suspected skin infection or fungus	Bioclusive Tegaderm Op-site	Apply skin prep to intact skin to protect from adhesive
Foam island	Stage II, III Low to moderate exudate Can apply as window to secure transparent film	Excessive exudate Dry, crusted wound	Allevyn Lyofoam	May also use for protection of the wound (e.g., newly healed wound or open wounds at risk for trauma, like on the legs or feet)
Hydrocolloids	Stage II, III Low to moderate drainage Good periwound skin integrity Occlusive dressing Autolytic debridement of necrotic tissue	Poor skin integrity Infected ulcers Heel ulcers	DuoDERM Extra thin film DuoDERM Tegasorb RepliCare Comfeel Nu-derm	Left in place 3–5 days Can apply as window to secure transparent film Can apply over alginate to control drainage Must control maceration Apply skin prep to intact skin to protect from adhesive
Alginate (seaweed)	Stage III, IV Excessive drainage	Dry or minimally draining wound Tunneling, may not retrieve all Superficial wounds with maceration	Sorbsan Kaltostat Algosteril AlgiDERM	Apply dressing within wound borders Requires secondary dressing Must use skin prep or barriers Must control for maceration
Hydrogel				
Amorphous gels	Stage II, III, IV	Macerated areas Wounds with moderate exudate	IntraSite gel SoloSite gel Restore gel	Needs to be combined with gauze dressing Stays moist longer than saline gauze Changed once daily Used as alternative to saline gauze for packing deep wounds with tunnels, undermining Reduces adherence of gauze, hydrofiber or alginate to wound Must control for maceration
Gel sheet	Stage II	Macerated areas Wounds with moderate to heavy exudate	Vigilon Restore Impregnated Gauze	Needs to be held in place with topper dressing, unless with adhesive border Must control for maceration

(continued)

33.5 | Common Dressings for Treating Pressure Ulcers *(continued)*

DRESSING	INDICATIONS	CONTRAINDICATIONS	EXAMPLE	COMMENTS
Gauze packing (moistened with saline, wet-moist)	Stage III, IV Wounds with depth, especially those with tunnels, undermining	Highly draining ulcers Suspected skin infection or fungus	2" × 2", 4" × 4" Fluffed Kerlix Plain NuGauze	Must use a semipermeable membrane (transparent film) to maintain moist wound environment or dressing is considered wet-dry
Silver (Ag) dressings (silver with alginates, gels, charcoal)	Stage II, III, IV Malodorous wounds High level of exudates Wound highly suspicious for critical bacterial load Periwound with signs of inflammation Slow-healing wound	Sensitivity to Ag products Signs of systemic side effects, esp. erythema multiforme Interstitial nephritis Leukopenia Skin necrosis Concurrent use with proteolytic enzyme debridement (Santyl, Accuzyme)	SilvaSorb gel Silverlon Aquacel Ag Hydrofiber Mepilex Ag Foam Acticoat	Used for infected and/or highly colonized wounds Have different percentages of silver Good for diabetic and PVD wounds
VAC (vacuum-assisted closure)	Stage III, IV Nonhealing wounds Surgical debridement	Untreated osteomyelitis Fistula Bleeding Cancer	VAC	Stimulates cell growth with negative pressure therapy Different levels of pressure Different types of foams (moist, silver, plain)
Hydrofibers	Stage II, III, IV Moderate exudating wounds	Dry or minimally draining wound Tunneling, may not retrieve all	Aquacel Aquacel Ag	Better for superficial wounds, as generally prevents less maceration to periwound than alginates Requires secondary dressing Must use skin prep or barriers

the pressure ulcer heals. When a stage IV pressure ulcer has healed, it should be classified as a healed stage IV pressure ulcer, not a stage 0. When pressure ulcers heal, the ulcer moves to a progressively more shallow depth; healing does not replace lost muscle, subcutaneous fat, or dermis before they re-epithelialize. Instead, pressure ulcers are filled with granulation (scar) tissue composed primarily of endothelial cells, fibroblasts, collagen, and extracellular matrix. The scar tissue's tensile strength is typically less than 80% of normal, atraumatic skin. Thus, residents and caregivers need to continue to be vigilant with protection and pressure reduction at that area. The progress of healing can be documented only by describing ulcer characteristics or measuring wound characteristics with a validated tool.

Ulcer treatment/care should be evaluated for healing progress on a weekly basis. There are no standard healing rates for pressure ulcers. However, a wound that does not close within 3 months time is considered a chronic, nonhealing wound that requires consult with a certified wound specialist. Most stage I pressure ulcers heal within 1 day to 1 week; stage II, within 5 days to 3 months; stage III, within 1 month to 6 months; and stage IV, within 6 months to 1 year. Clearly, some full-thickness pressure ulcers may never heal, depending on comorbidity. However, no clear guidelines exist to determine when a pressure ulcer can be truly defined as recalcitrant (never healing) or what characteristics must be present to predict that an ulcer will never heal.

Infection Control

All pressure ulcers become colonized with both aerobic (i.e., requiring oxygen to grow) and anaerobic (i.e., not requiring oxygen) bacteria. However, superficial swab cultures of the wounds are not helpful in determining which organism may be causing the infection. Therefore, routine swab cultures are not recommended. However, evidence suggests that quantitative tissue swab cultures can be used to determine the wound's *bioburden*. Wound cleansing and dressing changes are two of the most important methods for minimizing the amount of bacterial colonization. Increasing the frequency of wound cleansing and dressing changes is an important first step when purulent or foul-smelling drainage is observed on the ulcer. Many clinicians use vacuum-assisted closure (VAC) to help continuously remove exudates from infected wounds. In these cases, the foam dressing is not changed typically every 3 days, but daily. When ulcers are not healing or have persistent exudate after 2 weeks of optimal cleansing and dressing changes, it is reasonable to consider the use of antimicrobials.

Topical antimicrobials can decrease the bioburden in pressure ulcers. Antimicrobials such as silver sulfadiazine and mupirocin (Bactroban) ointment can be used daily or every other day for 1 to 2 weeks, depending on exudates, with careful monitoring for sensitivities. Because prolonged use of these antimicrobials may result in resistant organisms, they should not be used indefinitely. Silver-impregnated dressings to decrease bioburden are increasingly being used. Although the exact mechanism of how silver kills the infection remains unknown, it is hypothesized that it stops the enzyme that feeds the proliferation of bacteria, viruses, and fungi. Dressings such as Aquacel Ag, Acticoat, Actisorb, and Arglaes control bacterial load and the odor caused by bacteria. The dressing that is selected will determine how the silver is delivered, percentage delivered, length of treatment, amount of exudate absorption, incidence of maceration, ease of dressing removal, and pain intensity at dressing changes. It is important to select a dressing that meets the resident's needs and staff availability to apply the dressing.

Because most topical antibiotics do not penetrate the wound bed, they are not effective for control of infections. When ulcers fail to heal despite the treatments described previously, it is time to consider the possibility of cellulitis or osteomyelitis. Biopsy of the ulcer for quantitative bacterial cultures or of the underlying bone can be used to establish these diagnoses. An MRI or three-phase bone scan can also provide a definitive diagnosis of osteomyelitis. Cellulitis, osteomyelitis, bacteremia, and sepsis are all indications for the use of systemic antibiotics.

The use of topical antiseptics (e.g., povidone iodine, iodophor, sodium hypochlorite, hydrogen peroxide, and acetic acid) is not recommended because of their tissue toxicity. However, recent studies suggest that diluted povidone iodine ($< 5\%$) is not cytotoxic to healthy granulation tissue.

COMPLICATIONS FROM PRESSURE ULCERS

The development of pressure ulcers can lead to several complications, probably the most serious of which is sepsis. When a pressure ulcer is present and there is aerobic or anaerobic bacteremia, or both, the pressure ulcer is most often the primary source of the infection. Additional complications of pressure ulcers include localized infection, cellulitis, and osteomyelitis. Quite often, a nonhealing pressure ulcer may indicate underlying osteomyelitis. Mortality can also be associated with pressure ulcer development. Several studies report the association of pressure ulcer development and mortality in both hospital and nursing home settings. In fact, mortality rate is reportedly as high as 60% for older adults who develop a pressure ulcer within 1 year of hospital discharge. Other complications of pressure ulcers include pain, depression, isolation, and altered body image. All of these complications have been associated with decreased healing in the pressure ulcer.

SETTING GOALS

Many pressure ulcers in older adults may not be healable because of acuity, other underlying medical illnesses, or inability to tolerate certain treatment regimens. Maintaining quality of life and dignity at end of life should always take priority. Discussion with the resident (if possible) and/or family members regarding the inability to heal a pressure ulcer—and that the goals of care have now focused on prevention of worsening of the wound and minimizing the risk of sepsis—may be the best standard of care that a clinician can provide.

RESOURCES

Agency for Health Care Policy and Research. (1992). *Pressure ulcers in adults: Prediction and prevention*. Retrieved December 1, 2008, from http://www.guideline.gov/summary/summary. aspx?doc_id = 2601&nbr = 1827&string = pressure + ulcers

Agency for Healthcare Research and Quality. (1994). *Treatment of pressure ulcers*. Retrieved December 1, 2008, from http://www.guideline.gov/summary/summary.aspx?doc_id = 810&nbr = 8&string = pressure + ulcer

American Medical Directors Association. (2008). *Pressure ulcers in the long-term care setting clinical practice guideline*. Columbia, MD: Author.

Braden, B., & Bergstrom, N. (2001). *The Braden Scale*. Retrieved December 1, 2008, from http://www.bradenscale.com/bradenscale.htm

Lyder, C. H., Shannon, R., Empleo-Frazier, O., McGeHee, D., & White, C. (2002). A comprehensive program to prevent pressure ulcers in long-term care: Exploring costs and outcomes. *Ostomy Wound Management, 48*(4), 52–62

Madhuri, R. (2008). Skin and wound care: Important considerations in the older adult. *Advances in Skin and Wound Care, 21*, 424–436.

National Pressure Ulcer Advisory Panel. (1998). *Pressure Ulcer Scale for Healing (PUSH)*. Retrieved December 1, 2008, from http://www.npuap.org/PDF/push3.pdf

Norton, D., McLaren, R., & Exton-Smith, A. N. (1962). *An investigation of geriatric nursing problems in the hospital*. Retrieved December 1, 2008. http://www.woundcarehelpline.com/Norton Scale.pdf

Psychological Health

Mental health is a critical aspect of aging well and is particularly important to address in community settings, such as assisted living. Some older adults have had lifelong mental health problems such as manic depression, bipolar disorders, schizophrenia, or generalized personality disorders. Aging may place some additional challenges on their ability to cope, and, as such, these problems may require new and innovative treatment approaches. Conversely, there are some older adults who acquire mental health problems in old age including such things as depression and dementia. This section will review these disorders and provide appropriate treatment options including both pharmacological and behavioral interventions.

34

Depression and Other Mood Disorders

Gary J. Kennedy and Maureen Kilby

Depression in older adults is a common, persistent, and sometimes recurrent disorder resulting from psychosocial stress or the physiologic effects of disease. This psychological problem can lead to disability, cognitive impairment, exacerbation of medical problems, increased use of health care services, and increased suicide. Unfortunately, the signs and symptoms of depression are easily missed in older adults or are assumed to be due to normal age changes. Specifically, these individuals do not present with the typical symptoms of depression, such as depressed mood or sadness. Sorting out the complex interrelationships between symptoms and signs of depression caused by physical illnesses and those caused primarily by an affective disorder or related psychiatric diagnosis is challenging for health care providers. Recognition is critical so that appropriate behavioral and pharmacological interventions can be implemented. In so doing, nurses and others in assisted living communities can help older adults maintain function and quality of life, reduce the need for health care resources, and prevent further morbidity and even mortality.

EPIDEMIOLOGY

The prevalence of major depression among older adults actually decreases with age. Among community-dwelling older adults, prevalence is 6.5% to 9%, but an additional 2% experience *dysthymia* (i.e., a chronic depressive disorder characterized by functional impairment and at least 2 years of depressive symptoms that also consistently decreases with age). Major depression, however, is found in 16% to 50% of older adults in institutional settings. The lower reported rate of major depression among older adults may be due to the challenges of diagnosing depression among older individuals and the fact that many cases might be missed. The prevalence of *subsyndromal depression* (i.e., symptoms of depression that do not meet standard criteria for major clinical depression) steadily increases with age, however, ranging from 10% to 25% among community-dwelling older adults and increasing to 50% among those in residential long-term care. Depression is implicated with increased mortality and morbidity including increased incidences of cardiovascular disease, weight change, functional decline, and impaired cognition. When depression is associated with other medical problems (e.g., hip fracture or osteoarthritis), there is often exacerbation of pain, poor compliance and motivation, and impaired recovery and function. Older adults account for 25% of all suicides; as many as 75% of older adults who committed suicide were suffering from depression.

CLINICAL PRESENTATION AND DIAGNOSIS

The Geriatric Syndrome of Late-Life Depression

Symptoms and criteria of major depression, listed in Exhibit 34.1, are drawn from the fourth edition of the *Diagnostic and Statistical Manual of Mental Disorders* (*DSM-IV*). There are some differences in signs and symptoms expressed by younger and older depressed patients. Older patients are more preoccupied with somatic symptoms and less frequently report depressed mood and guilty preoccupations. It is not unusual for an older adult with depression to express a persistent loss of pleasure and interest in previously enjoyable activities (*anhedonia*) rather than the more traditional symptom of sustained feelings of sadness. Thus, one need not exhibit depressed mood in order to meet criteria for major depressive disorder.

34.1 | *DSM-IV* Diagnostic Criteria for Major Depression

Depressed mood[a]

Loss of interest or pleasure[a]

Appetite change or weight loss

Insomnia or hypersomnia

Psychomotor agitation or retardation

Loss of energy

Feelings of worthlessness or guilt

Difficulties with concentration or decision making

Recurrent thoughts of death or suicide

---

[a]At least one of which must be present for a diagnosis of major depression.
From *Diagnostic and Statistical Manual of Mental Disorders* (4th ed.), by American Psychiatric Association, 1994, Washington, DC: Author. Copyright ©1994 by American Psychiatric Association. Reprinted with permission.

Diagnosis of major depression in older adults is often complicated by the overlap among symptoms of major depression with the symptoms of physical illness. Coexisting problems such as pain, cognitive impairment, chronic medical problems (arthritis, diabetes, heart failure), alcohol or substance abuse can complicate diagnosis and treatment of major depression. Patients with serious medical illness may be preoccupied with thoughts about death or feel worthless because of concomitant disability. If symptoms of major depression persist following a loss (e.g., loss of a spouse, home, pet) then treatment should be considered. The *DSM-IV* criteria indicate that true depressive symptoms should not be considered those that are directly associated with a medical condition or medication used to treat it. For example, an individual who is believed to be depressed secondary to new onset hypothyroidism should not be diagnosed with a depression. Rather, that individual should have the diagnosis of hypothyroidism added to his or her problem list. This distinction in older adults is extremely difficult to make and results in clinicians often diagnosing depression in situations that do not meet the traditional *DSM-IV* guidelines.

Screening for mood symptoms is an important part of a comprehensive assessment of all older adults regardless of socioeconomic or ethnic status, although cultural variation may influence how emotional states are expressed. The Patient Health Questionaire-2 (Exhibit 34.2) consists of two questions that assess the frequency of depressed mood and anhedonia during the preceding 2-week period. This is a useful first-step depression screen and is easily administered in the assisted living setting. If the screen is positive, it should be followed by additional testing and referral to the primary health care provider. Since the diagnosis of depression hinges on a qualitative change from a patient's normal mood state, it is essential to obtain information from involved family members or caregivers to determine whether or not there is evidence of a change in mood.

Bipolar Depression

Diagnosis of a bipolar depression requires that the individual exhibit a distinct period of persistently elevated mood lasting for 1 or more weeks and three additional symptoms, among which are inflated self-esteem or grandiosity, hypersexuality, increased activity, decreased need for sleep, pressured speech, racing thoughts, spending sprees or flight of ideas, and distractibility. Grandiose or paranoid delusions may be present. Although the criteria for diagnosing bipolar disorder in

34.2 | The Patient Health Questionaire-2 (PHQ-2)

Over the past 2 weeks, how often have you been bothered by any of the following problems	Not at all	Several days	More than half the days	Nearly every day
1. Little interest or pleasure in doing things	0	1	2	3
2. Feeling down, depressed, or hopeless	0	1	2	3

From "The Patient Health Questionnaire-2: Validity of a Two-Item Depression Screener," by K. Kroenke, R. L. Spitzer, and J. B. Williams, 2003, *Medical Care, 41*(11), p. 1285. Copyright ©2003 by Lippincott Williams & Wilkins, Inc. Reprinted with permission.

younger and older patients are identical, some differences have been noted. Elderly patients with bipolar disorder are more likely to have a mixture of depression and marked irritability. In conversation, they may tend to go off on tangents. Hypersexuality and grandiosity are less common in older adults. Maniclike syndromes in late life are also distinguished by a greater likelihood of confusion, often a reflection of an underlying cognitive disturbance.

Depression Associated With Structural Brain Disease

Major depression is commonly associated with cognitive impairment and individuals who have been diagnosed with Alzheimer's disease. It is sometimes difficult to tell, however, which disease is the problem: depression can cause some memory and behavior problems such as impaired concentration, indecisiveness, and lack of motivation, which are also associated with dementia. An older person with depression may report both memory loss and poor concentration and be unable to perform simple cognitive tests without being demented. Conversely, residents with true dementia may have symptoms that imitate depression, such as loss of interest, apathy, psychomotor retardation (i.e., slowness when doing tasks such as bathing, dressing, or walking), and disrupted sleep (i.e., may sleep too much or too little).

Bereavement

Bereavement is likely among older adults. Feelings of sadness, disturbed sleep, and diminished appetite are common among bereaved persons but are generally time limited and resolve within a few months. Older adults who experience a loss, however, are less likely to progress to the point of being diagnosed with a major depression when compared to younger individuals. Bereavement that has evolved into a major depression is characterized by morbid preoccupations with guilt or suicidal ideas beyond transient thoughts of joining the deceased that would be expected in association with the loss.

THE PROGRESSION OF DEPRESSION

Major depression is often a recurrent disorder in both younger and older adults. Generally, about one-third of individuals with major depression will continue to remain depressed over time, and another third will have partial recovery with residual disability (i.e., they may have days in which they are not willing to participate in routine activities, won't eat, dress, or take medications). Patients who suffer their first episode of major depression in later life take longer to recover. Depressed older adults also tend to visit health care providers more than nondepressed older adults. Depressed older adults tend not to do as well in the management of comorbid chronic illness and have increased mortality from cardiovascular disease (e.g., hypertension, atrial fibrillation, or heart failure) when compared to older adults who are not depressed.

Old age is associated with an increased risk for suicide, particularly among those who are depressed. Persons aged 65 and over represent less than 13% of the population but account for 25% of suicides. The likelihood that an attempt will be lethal (i.e., that they will actually kill themselves) is also higher among older adults when compared to young adults. The specific risk factors for late-life suicide include having some type of physical illness, living alone, being male, and alcoholism. Older men and women tend toward violent suicide, with use of firearms and hanging being the most commonly used methods.

TREATMENT OF DEPRESSION

Overview

Several treatment modalities are available to manage depression in older persons (Exhibit 34.3). Pharmacological, behavioral interventions, and psychotherapy are somewhat effective in mild to moderate depression in the outpatient geriatric population. Medications most commonly include selective serotonin reuptake inhibitors (SSRIs) and tricyclic antidepressants (TCAs); they are equally effective. However, there are more side effects and risks associated with TCAs when compared to the SSRIs; hence, SSRIs are more commonly prescribed. Behavioral interventions, such as exercise and cognitive behavioral therapy, are also reported to be effective. Choice of treatment(s) depends on many factors, including the primary disorder causing the depression, severity of symptoms, availability and practicality of the various treatment modalities, and underlying conditions that might contraindicate a specific form of treatment (e.g., cognitive issues that may make psychotherapy more difficult or underlying medical problems that increase the risk of medication management). Electroconvulsive therapy (ECT) is also effective when other treatment options (e.g., behavioral interventions and medications) are not successful.

The course of treatment for major depression is conceptualized as: acute treatment to reverse the current episode, continuation treatment to prevent relapse, and maintenance treatment to prevent recurrence. Continuation treatment to stabilize recovery involves ongoing antidepressant therapy for an additional 6 to 12 months to reduce the possibility of relapse. Maintenance treatment (3 years or longer) is provided to patients with a history of recurrent depression. Duration of maintenance therapy should be based on the frequency and severity of previous episodes. Recurrent episodes complicated by suicidal ideas or attempts warrant lifelong treatment.

Psychotherapy

Exhibit 34.3 lists the variety and characteristics of behavioral interventions (i.e., psychotherapies) recommended for older adults. These include cognitive-behavioral therapy, interpersonal psychotherapy, and problem-solving therapy. Problem-solving therapy involves working with the patient to identify practical life difficulties that are causing distress and providing guidance to help the patient identify solutions. The treatment is delivered generally in six to eight meetings spaced 1 to 2 weeks apart. Cognitive and interpersonal psychotherapy are also time-limited but less highly structured. Psychotherapy combined with antidepressant medication is recommended for all patients with severe or suicidal depression. Generally this treatment is covered by secondary insurers including Medicare.

Exercise Programs

A supervised physical exercise program consisting of walking or an aerobic exercise can reduce mild to moderate depression in older adults. It may be difficult to get depressed residents to participate in an exercise program. Persistent encouragement will show the individual how much you care about him or her and may ultimately get him or her to start a class or an activity. Reinforcing this behavior and providing continued encouragement to adhere to the class or activity can be very effective. In some individuals, however, treatment with an antidepressant medication may be needed before he or she will even consider attending the class or engaging in, for example, a walking program.

Choice of Antidepressants: First Considerations

Among the many antidepressant medications that clinicians can use, the choice of agent depends on the patient's comorbid medical conditions, the side effect profile of the antidepressant, and the individual's sensitivity to these effects. Potential interactions with other medications have to be considered. Complaints of sleep disturbance, anxiety, or psychomotor retardation will direct the practitioner toward agents that are,

34.3 | Behavioral Interventions for Depression in Older Adults

THERAPY	DISTINGUISHING CHARACTERISTICS
Short-term psychodynamic	Problem focused Transference not examined
Life review, reminiscence	Recall of personal history to master one's present and future
Supportive	Meant to maintain present level of function or symptom control
Dementia caregiver counseling	Focused on the caregiver role and activities Combines elements of cognitive-behavioral, problem-solving, and interpersonal therapy
Bereavement therapy	Restructuring (not restoration) the experience of the lost loved one though review of both positive and negative aspects of the relationship
Behavioral	Educational, pragmatic Directed at reducing negative and increasing positive experiences
Dialectical-behavioral therapy	Focused on reduction of counterproductive behaviors Emphasis on acceptance of affect and the inevitability of conflict
Cognitive-behavioral therapy	Active time limited therapy that aims to change individuals' thinking and behavior that influence their depression Based on the assumption that irrational thoughts and beliefs, overgeneralization of negative events, a pessimistic outlook on life, a tendency to focus on problems and failures, and negative self-assessment, as well as other cognitive distortions, promote the development of psychological problems, especially depression. Focus is to help the resident identify and understand how these cognitive distortions affect his or her life Interventions thus focus on helping the individual reinterpret his or her situation
Problem-solving therapy	Problem-solving therapy shifts the focus of therapy from the individual to the social context in which he or she lives (e.g., family, institution) This approach differs from other therapies by emphasizing the *social context*, or social situation, of human problems The therapist approaches each problem with techniques specific to the situation. The *goals* of this therapy are to solve problems, achieve goals, and change the patient's behavior. Examples of interventions would involve having the resident call someone for dinner if the depression was associated with loneliness.
Interpersonal therapy	Interpersonal therapy focuses on the interactions between people and the development of a person's psychiatric symptoms. Interpersonal therapists focus on the functional role of depression rather than its cause. The focus is more on the symptoms of depression than the causes. For example, the therapist would work with the individual to have him or her attend a class, go to the dining room, or visit with friends

respectively, more sedative or more activating. Sertraline and citalopram are often preferred because adverse effects and drug interactions are less likely than with some other SSRIs, such as fluoxetine and paroxetine. It is important for nurses to understand the utility of these medications as well as their potential side effects.

Selective Serotonin Reuptake Inhibitors

Information about commonly used SSRIs is shown in Table 34.1. Although SSRIs are generally free of severe side effects, a small proportion of older adult patients develop hyponatremia (i.e., low blood sodium levels).

This can result in some confusion, and, if the sodium level drops low enough (below 112), it can cause seizures and death. Some individuals are unable to tolerate SSRIs because of individual responses to the medications including such things as anxiety, sleep disturbances, or agitation. Decreased sexual desire commonly occurs with all SSRIs; inquiring about sexual function and desire is an important part of monitoring residents. SSRIs may cause either weight loss or weight gain. Long-term use, particularly, seems to result in weight gain. As with all medications, there is the potential for the SSRIs to interact with other drugs the individual may be taking on a regular basis.

34.1 | Selective Serotonin-Reuptake Inhibitors for Older Adults

GENERIC (TRADE) NAME	INITIAL DOSAGE	FINAL DOSAGE	SEDATIVE POTENTIAL	PRECAUTIONS	ADVANTAGES
Citalopram (Celexa)	10 mg A.M.	20–40 mg A.M.	Low	Side effects include nausea, tremor, dizziness, sweating, agitation	Few drug interactions, well tolerated
Escitalopram (Lexapro)	10 mg A.M.	10–20 mg A.M.	Low	Nausea, tremor, dizziness, sweating, agitation	May have fewer side effects than citalopram, well tolerated
Fluoxetine (Prozac)	10 mg A.M.	20–40 mg A.M.	Low	Nausea, tremor, dizziness, sweating, agitation, prolonged half-life, insomnia, drug interactions	Liquid preparation available
Fluvoxamine (Luvox)	50 mg or less	50–300 mg Divide dose > 100 mg	Mild	Headache, nausea, dizziness, sleep disturbance, abnormal ejaculation	Effective for OCD treatment
Paroxetine (Paxil)	10 mg hs	20–40 mg hs	Low	Nausea, tremor, dizziness, sweating, agitation, drug interactions, anticholinergic effects	Mild sedative effect
Sertraline (Zoloft)	25 mg A.M.	100–200 mg A.M.	Low	Nausea, tremor, dizziness, sweating, agitation	Few drug interactions, well tolerated

Note: hs = *hora somni* (at bedtime); OCD = obsessive-compulsive disorder.

SSRIs are considered particularly safe for older adults, however, because unlike the TCAs they do not cause orthostatic hypotension (i.e., a 20 mm drop in either systolic or diastolic blood pressure when the individual comes to a standing position), arrhythmias, or marked sedation.

Serotonin syndrome is a specific drug reaction experienced by older adults on SSRIs. It results from overstimulation of the serotonin receptors in the brain when SSRIs are used in combination with certain medications (see Exhibit 34.4). Symptoms include hyperactivity, elevated heart rate, mental confusion, agitation, shivering, sweating, uncoordination, seizures, and diarrhea. If these signs and symptoms are noted in a resident who is on an SSRI, they should be immediately reported to the individual's primary health care provider.

Older adults can experience a withdrawal syndrome following immediate discontinuation of an SSRI. Symptoms include lightheadedness, insomnia, agitation, nausea, headache, and sensory disturbances. Mood disturbance may also occur. A resident who abruptly stops taking the SSRI for any reason (e.g., prescription was not filled in a timely fashion; didn't think he/she needed it; etc.), should be monitored for symptoms of withdrawal. It is altogether possible that the withdrawal symptoms appear first—that is, before the reason for not taking the SSRI is known!

34.4 | Drugs That May Induce Serotonin Syndrome When Taken With an Antidepressant

Ecstasy

Cocaine

Lithium

St John's wort (herbal antidepressant)

Diethylproprion

Dextromethorphan (found in cough suppressants)

Buspar

Selgene

Tegretol, carbium, carbamazepine

Pethidine, fortral, tramadol

Triptans-naramig, imigran, zomig

Phentermine, fenfluramine

Tryptophan

Tricyclic Antidepressants

The TCAs nortriptyline and desipramine are the most appropriate for use in older adults. See Table 34.2 for a detailed summary of dosing, formulations, precautions, and advantages of these agents. They are effective in the most severe forms of depression but are associated with anticholinergic side effects that result in any number of symptoms including confusion, dizziness, dry mouth, urinary retention, and constipation (see Chapter 20, "Pharmacotherapy"). As noted previously, TCAs are associated with the risk of cardiac problems including heart block.

Other Antidepressants

Other antidepressants, including stimulants, are listed in Table 34.3 with information regarding dosing, formulations, precautions, and advantages. Bupropion is generally safe, free of sexual side effects, and well tolerated when used at recommended doses. There is an increased risk of seizure, however, particularly at higher dosages. Bupropion does tend to be activating (i.e., may cause insomnia as well) and thus should be given in the morning.

Venlafaxine is effective in the management of depression and anxiety, although it may result in hypertension when used at high dosages. Duloxetine is a new antidepressant medication that has been approved for the treatment of both depression and management of pain due to peripheral neuropathy (i.e., a condition of the nervous system that usually begins in the hands and/or feet with symptoms of numbness, tingling, and burning). Mirtazapine, another antidepressant, has sedating side effects thus are generally given as a single bedtime dose to individuals who have depression and difficulty sleeping. This drug is also associated with increased appetite and weight gain.

The group of antidepressants referred to as monoamine oxidase inhibitors (MAOIs) are older antidepressants that are generally not used unless all other treatment options are not effective. This group of medications can result in orthostatic hypotension. In addition, the individual has to avoid eating foods rich in tyramine (e.g., cheeses, wine) because of the danger of precipitating a life-threatening hypertensive crisis. The combined use of MAOIs with an SSRI or meperidine can cause a fatal serotonin syndrome associated with delirium and hyperthermia and thus should be avoided. Last, methylphenidate and other stimulants have been used to treat major depression to reverse the apathy (the absence of emotion or energy noted in many individuals

34.2 | Tricyclic Antidepressants Commonly Used for Depression in Older Adults

GENERIC (TRADE) NAME	INITIAL DOSAGE	FINAL DOSAGE	SEDATIVE POTENTIAL	PRECAUTIONS	ADVANTAGES
Desipramine (Norpramin)	10–25 mg hs	25–150 mg hs	Low	May be fatal in overdose May exacerbate glaucoma, anticholinergic effects	Therapeutic plasma level 115–200 ng/mL May have stimulant properties
Nortriptyline (Pamelor, Aventyl)	10–25 mg hs	25–100 mg hs	Moderate	Lower final dose May be fatal in overdose May exacerbate glaucoma, anticholinergic effects	Therapeutic window for plasma levels of 50–150 ng/mL

Note: hs = *hora somni* (at bedtime).

34.3 | Other Antidepressants, Including Stimulants, for Older Adults

GENERIC (TRADE) NAME	INITIAL DOSAGE	FINAL DOSAGE	SEDATIVE POTENTIAL	PRECAUTIONS	ADVANTAGES
Other antidepressants					
Bupropion (Wellbutrin SR)	SR: 75 mg qd	SR: 150–300 mg qd	Low	Dopaminergic, nor-adrenergic, agitation, insomnia, seizures Dose should be divided	May help apathetic depression Sustained-release form available
Duloxetine (Cymbalta)	20 mg	30–60 mg	Low	Drug interactions (CYP 1A2, 2D6 substrate)	Equally SSRI and SNRI, narrow dose range FDA approved for neuropathic pain
Hypericum perforatum, or St. John's wort	300 mg bid	900 mg tid	Low	Use standardized, freeze-dried extract, 0.3% hypericin Drug interactions with other antidepressants	Low side effect profile, OTC

(continued)

34.3 | Other Antidepressants, Including Stimulants, for Older Adults *(continued)*

GENERIC (TRADE) NAME	INITIAL DOSAGE	FINAL DOSAGE	SEDATIVE POTENTIAL	PRECAUTIONS	ADVANTAGES
Mirtazapine (Remeron, Sol-tabs)	7.5 mg hs	15–45 mg hs	Moderate	Prolonged half-life, renal clearance Dry mouth, weight gain Serotonergic and noradrenergic	Sedative effects may improve sleep
Trazodone (Desyrel)	25–50 mg hs	100–200 mg hs	High	Very sedative	For sleep disturbance
Venlafaxine (Effexor, Effexor XR)	37.5 mg bid XR: 75 mg qd	75–225 mg qd	Low	Headache, nausea, vomiting Hypertension, withdrawal syndrome	Fewer drug interactions Extended-release preparation available, may be more effective than SSRIs
Stimulants					
Methylphenidate (Ritalin)	5 mg A.M.	20 mg bid	Low	Side effects include anorexia, insomnia Daytime use only	Quick results For frail and apathetic patients
Modafinil (Provigil)	200 mg A.M.	400 mg A.M.	Low	Little used in elderly patients	Once-daily dosing, reverses daytime sedation sometimes observed with SSRIs

Note: bid = *bis in die* (twice a day); FDA = U.S. Food and Drug Administration; hs = *hora somni* (at bedtime); OTC = over-the-counter; qd = *quaque die* (every day); SR = sustained release; SNRI = serotonin norepinephrine reuptake inhibitor; SSRI = selective serotonin reuptake inhibitor; tid = *ter in die* (three times a day); XR = extended release.

with depression). Benzodiazepines may also be useful for treating the anxiety and sleep disturbance associated with a major depression. Careful monitoring is needed to watch for changes in memory, gait, and increased sleeping when using these drugs.

MANAGEMENT OF BIPOLAR DISORDER

Most persons with bipolar disorder have been previously diagnosed during adulthood and often receive long-term treatment with an antimanic medication. Many medications are effective for this type of depression. Lithium carbonate is highly effective for the acute and maintenance treatment of classical manic episodes. Older individuals, particularly those who have been treated with lithium for many years, may develop side effects that include a tremor, diarrhea, pseudo-parkinsonism (Parkinson's disease symptoms that are due to medications) or hypothyroid disorders. Antiseizure medications such as valproic acid (Valproate, divalproex) and carbamazepine have been approved for the treatment of bipolar disorder. These are generally used at low dosages in older adults and are well tolerated. Likewise, antipsychotic medications can be used to treat the mania associated with manic depression. Monitoring residents on these medications should include observations for weight gain, confusion, sleepiness, and changes in physical function (e.g., decreased ability to walk).

Electroconvulsive Therapy for the Treatment of Depression

In some individuals, behavioral and medication management of depression is not effective. In these cases, ECT may be effective. Usually done on an outpatient basis, ECT can continue at intervals over time (e.g., starting with several times weekly and then once a month, indefinitely). There are generally no immediate side effects with treatment, although, particularly if the resident undergoes repeated treatment over time, there may be evidence of confusion or worsening of an underlying dementia.

RESOURCES

Ayers, C.R., Sorrell, J.T., Thorp, S.R., & Wetherell, J.L. (2007). Evidence-based psychological treatments for late-life anxiety. *Psychology and Aging, 22*(1), 8–17.

Frazer, C.J., Christensen, H., & Griffiths, K.M. (2005). Effectiveness of treatments for depression in older people. *Medical Journal of Australia, 182*(12), 627–632.

Gatz, M. (2007). Commentary on evidence-based psychological treatments for older adults. *Psychology and Aging, 22*(1), 52–55.

Kotlyar, M., Dysken, M., & Adson, D.E. (2005). Update on drug-induced depression in the elderly. *American Journal of Geriatric Pharmacotherapy, 3*(4), 288–300.

Kroenke, K., Spitzer, R.L., & Williams, J.B. (2003). The patient health questionnaire-2: Validity of a two-item depression screener. *Medical Care 41*(11), 1284–1292.

35

Anxiety Disorders

Erin L. Cassidy, Javaid I. Sheikh,
and Elizabeth Galik

Older adults suffer from the entire range of anxiety disorders. The published literature on anxiety in older adults, however, is relatively sparse. As a result, some characterizations and treatment strategies described in this chapter are based on research carried out in younger populations but have been modified and take into account the physiologic and psychological differences between older and younger adults. The challenges to proper assessment of geriatric anxiety include medical comorbidity, the difficulty of differentiating anxiety from depression, false high scores on anxiety rating scales resulting from overemphasis of cardiac and respiratory problems, and the tendency of older adults to resist psychiatric evaluation.

Anxiety assessment begins with an interview to assess the course and nature of symptoms, as well as assessment of the older adult's mental status and social support. Although discrete anxiety disorders such as panic disorders are less prevalent among older than among younger adults, anxiety as a symptom is a common problem. The ability to recognize and effectively treat anxiety in older adults is important, given the debilitating effects that an unhealthy level of anxiety can have in this population.

CLASSES OF ANXIETY DISORDERS

The types of anxiety disorders as currently defined in the fourth edition of the *Diagnostic and Statistical Manual of Mental Disorders* (*DSM-IV*) are listed in Table 35.1.

Panic Disorder

Panic attacks are acute, discrete episodes of intense anxiety that are a reaction to some perceived threat (e.g., emotional, environmental). The term *panic attack* is used when a person experiences an intense and acute reaction to an internal or external cue lasting from a few minutes to a half hour. Physiologic symptoms may include trembling, rapid heart rate, sweating, shortness of breath, chest pain, dizziness, nausea, and the sense that one is somehow detached from one's surroundings. For example, a resident might have a fear of being trapped on an elevator and report feeling dizzy and nauseated when entering one. Another might report high levels of acute anxiety at the mere sight of elevator doors. Sometimes, symptoms can be severe enough that a resident feels like he or she might be dying. A clinically significant degree of panic symptoms exists if a review of the resident's history reveals that recurrent and unpredictable panic attacks have occurred for at least 1 month and time is being spent in worried anticipation of possible reoccurrence. *Agoraphobia* is a persistent fear of situations that result in a panic attack, as when a resident reports remaining at home or in the assisted living community (ALC) in order to avoid a panic attack. Comparison of young and older adults with panic disorder indicates that age of onset can affect the clinical presentation. Individuals with late-onset panic disorder (i.e., at or after age 55) report fewer panic symptoms and less avoidance, and they score lower on somatization measures than do those with early-onset panic

35.1 | Types of Anxiety Disorders Defined in *DSM-IV*

Panic disorder without agoraphobia

Panic disorder with agoraphobia

Agoraphobia without history of panic disorder

Specific phobias

   Animal type
   Natural environment type
   Blood-injection-injury type
   Situational type
   Other type

Social phobia

Obsessive-compulsive disorder

Posttraumatic stress disorder

Acute stress disorder

Generalized anxiety disorder

Anxiety disorder due to a general medical condition

Substance-induced anxiety disorder

Anxiety disorder not otherwise specified

disorder. Also, earlier-onset panic disorder more commonly persists into old age.

Phobic Disorders

Phobias include several distinct disorders, categorized as *specific phobia* and *social phobia*. A specific phobia involves a distinct trigger, such as a specific person, animal, place, object, event, or situation that causes anxiety. Typically, the anxiety level increases instantly when the feared trigger is encountered. Interestingly, the sufferer is able to identify this fear as unrealistic and unsupported, even though the fear and physiologic responses persist. Specific phobias often involve a great amount of anticipatory anxiety (i.e., thoughts of just the possibility of encountering the feared stimulus); avoidance behaviors are likely. The consequence of such a clinical profile is that the older adult experiences a variety of personal

difficulties as a result of the anxiety. These behaviors interfere with daily routines and relationships and decrease the person's opportunities to experience pleasurable situations (for fear that a trigger might be present). The anxiety experienced by the older individual may also contribute to secondary symptoms, such as frustration, hopelessness, and a sense that one lacks control in one's life. The level of anxiety or fear usually varies as a function of both the degree of proximity to the phobic stimuli and the degree to which escape is perceived to be limited. Examples of common phobias include fear of specific animals, closed spaces, flying, or heights. Phobic disorders tend to be chronic and persist into old age. However, fear of falling is a specific phobia that is increasingly recognized to have an onset in later life.

Persons with social phobia suffer from fears that they will behave in a manner that is inept or embarrassing. Commonly, the fear is that of trembling, blushing, or sweating profusely in social situations. Again, as with specific phobias, social phobia is often accompanied with a significant degree of anticipatory anxiety or avoidance, or both. Though systematic studies of this disorder in elderly persons are lacking, epidemiologic data indicate that this disorder is chronic and persistent in old age.

Obsessive-Compulsive Disorder

Obsessive-compulsive disorder involves persistent thoughts (i.e., obsessions) and behaviors (i.e., compulsions) performed in an effort to decrease the anxiety experienced as a result of the thoughts. Obsessions are thoughts or ideas that come to a person's mind, commonly while completing a specific task or during a particular type of situation. For example, a resident may wash his hands repeatedly, for hours at a time, after shaking a stranger's hand; the unwanted thought is that he may have exposed himself to a serious disease. The act of washing in this example is the compulsion. Obsessive-compulsive disorder is chronic and often disabling. Depression and other symptoms of anxiety may also be present in addition to the obsessive-compulsive symptoms. A new occurrence of obsessive-compulsive disorder in late life is unlikely. More commonly, symptoms of obsessions occur along with a depressive syndrome or early dementia. For example, obsessions about paying bills on time may occur in the context of difficulty in estimating time and planning.

Posttraumatic Stress Disorder

The distinctive feature of posttraumatic stress disorder is that the person has experienced, either as a witness or a victim, a traumatic event to which he or she has reacted with feelings of fear and helplessness. Examples of such events include those that involve actual or threatened death or serious injury, other threats to one's integrity, witnessing an event that involves death or serious injury of another, or even hearing about death or serious injury to a family member or close associate. Commonly observed symptoms include the re-experiencing of the traumatic event, avoidance (both cognitively and behaviorally) of stimuli associated with the event, psychological numbing, and increased physiologic arousal. Symptoms of hyperarousal include difficulty falling or staying asleep, hypervigilance, and exaggerated startle response. Disorders often found to occur with posttraumatic stress disorder include depression, panic disorder, and substance-use disorders. Symptoms must be present for at least 1 month and cause clinically significant distress or impairment in social, occupational, or other important areas of functioning.

Generalized Anxiety Disorder

The distinctive symptoms of generalized anxiety disorder include feeling easily tired and experiencing other physical symptoms, such as muscle tension, having trouble sleeping through the night, difficulty concentrating on a task, and feeling irritable or on edge. These symptoms need to have occurred for at least 6 months and must be accompanied by the sense that one cannot control the feelings of anxiety. In addition, these feelings of intense worry must be a result of more than one stressor. For example, intense worry over financial matters or a medical illness alone, even with all the associated symptoms, in and of itself does not qualify a person for a diagnosis of generalized anxiety disorder. Because many older adults with this disorder also present with features of depression, the clinician may try to distinguish between the two diagnoses. Commonly the overlap is sufficiently extensive to preclude this distinction, as described later in the following section.

COMORBIDITY

Mixed Anxiety and Depression

Mixed anxiety and depression is a presentation that is included in the *DSM-IV* "Criteria for Further Study." The essential features of this proposed disorder are dysphoric mood (i.e., feeling sad or depressed) for at least 1 month and at least four specific anxious or depressive symptoms, such as irritability, worry, sleep distur-

bance, anticipating the worst, concentration or memory difficulties, and hopelessness. Clinicians working with older adults have long observed the significant overlap in symptoms of anxiety and depression.

Anxiety and Agitation in Dementia

Residents with dementia, living in ALCs or other long-term-care institutions, commonly display behaviors described as agitation. Agitation takes the form of verbal or motor activity that is either appropriate behavior but repeated frequently or inappropriate behavior that suggests lack of judgment. As many as 85% of dementia patients eventually develop disruptive, agitated behavior at some point during the course of their disease. Early identification of triggers, including environmental stimuli, medication side effects, and uncommunicated internal needs, can result in effective treatment and relief for caregivers. See Chapter 30, "Behavior Problems in Dementia," and Chapter 14, "Resident Assessment and Service Plan Construction," for details on diagnosing and managing disruptive, agitated behavior.

Anxiety and Medical Disorders

It is common to encounter residents with comorbid anxiety and medical disorders. This could be due to a longstanding anxiety disorder that coincidentally occurs alongside a medical illness, or there could be interplay between the two. Some conditions are exacerbated by anxiety, such as the common cold or influenza; others are precipitated by high levels of anxiety, such as angina pectoris or myocardial infarction. Other medical illnesses that commonly accompany an anxiety disorder include cardiovascular illnesses, pulmonary disorders, hyperthyroidism, and drug side effects (e.g., thyroid hormone replacements, antipsychotics, caffeine, theophylline, selective serotonin reuptake inhibitors [SSRIs]) or interactions. Given the complicated clinical picture that results when anxiety and medical disorders coexist, a thorough assessment, including a clinical history, is imperative before treatment begins.

PHARMACOLOGIC MANAGEMENT

Numerous compounds have been used over the years as anti-anxiety agents: alcohol, barbiturates, antihistamines, benzodiazepines, antipsychotic medications, and β-blockers. Although empirical studies of the use of anxiolytics in treating older adults are lacking, the efficacy of these medications is inferred from clinical practice with younger adults, and their use is modified by age-appropriate dosing. A brief description of the various classes of compounds currently favored as anxiolytics follows. Table 35.2 summarizes the treatment strategies for anxiety disorders in older adults.

Antidepressants

Antidepressants are efficacious in the treatment of panic disorder, obsessive-compulsive disorder, generalized anxiety disorder, and posttraumatic stress disorder. Given their relatively favorable side effect profile, the SSRIs or serotonin norepinephrine reuptake inhibitors (SNRIs) (e.g., venlafaxine) should be considered the drugs of choice for these disorders. Furthermore,

SSRIs should also be considered treatments of choice for treating mixed anxiety and depression. SNRIs, such as venlafaxine, should be considered as alternatives for those individuals who do not respond to SSRIs or who develop adverse effects. The SNRIs affect two neurotransmitter systems—serotonin and norepinephrine—and may be effective when a previous trial of an SSRI has failed. Case reports, open-label trials, and, more recently, controlled trials of serotonergic antidepressants like trazodone and SSRIs suggest a modest degree of efficacy in the management of anxiety and agitation in dementia, particularly when residents are not psychotic and comorbid depression is a strong possibility (see also Chapter 30, "Behavior Problems in Dementia").

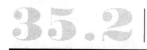 | Treatment Strategies for Anxiety Disorders in Older Adults

DISORDER	FIRST-LINE TREATMENTS	SECOND-LINE TREATMENTS
Panic disorder with or without agoraphobia	SSRIs,[a] SNRIs,[a] CBT	Newer antidepressants, benzodiazepines[b]
Social phobia		
Generalized	SSRIs[a] or phenelzine[OL] plus CBT	Benzodiazepines[b]
Specific	β-blockers plus CBT	Buspirone
Simple (specific) phobia	CBT or benzodiazepines[b]	β-blockers
Obsessive-compulsive disorder	SSRIs[a] plus CBT	Clomipramine, combination pharmacotherapy
Posttraumatic stress disorder	SSRIs[a] or SNRIs[a]	CBT, newer antidepressants
Generalized anxiety disorder	SNRIs,[a] SSRIs,[a] CBT	TCAs, benzodiazepines,[b] newer antidepressants
Anxiety and medical disorders	Identify and treat underlying cause, use SSRIs[a] or SNRIs[a] in primary anxiety disorder	Benzodiazepines[b]
Mixed anxiety depression	SSRIs[a] or SNRIs[a]	Buspirone, benzodiazepines,[b] CBT
Anxiety and agitation in dementia	Atypical antipsychotics[OL] or trazodone[OL]	Benzodiazepines,[b] anticonvulsants

Note: CBT = cognitive-behavioral therapy; [OL] = off label, not approved by the U.S. Food and Drug Administration for this use; SNRIs = serotonin norepinephrine reuptake inhibitors (e.g., venlafaxine); SSRIs = selective serotonin reuptake inhibitors (e.g., sertraline); TCAs = tricyclic antidepressants.
[a]Not all SSRIs and SNRIs are approved for anxiety disorders or all types of anxiety disorders. For example, the SSRI escitalopram is not approved for anxiety; nor is the SNRI duloxetine.
[b]Preferably, benzodiazepines with a short half-life and no active metabolites (e.g., lorazepam).

Benzodiazepines

Since the 1980s, benzodiazepines have been the most commonly prescribed anxiolytics for both young and older adults, but their use is now discouraged. When anxiety symptoms are severe, benzodiazepines with a short half-life, such as lorazepam and oxazepam, are preferable in treating older adults because they are metabolized by direct conjugation, a process relatively unaffected by aging. However, it is preferable to limit the use of even short-acting benzodiazepines to less than 6 months because long-term use is fraught with multiple complications, such as motor incoordination and falls, cognitive impairment, depression, and the potential for abuse and dependence.

Buspirone, Antihistamines, and Atypical Antipsychotics

Several studies suggest that buspirone, an anxiolytic medication with some serotonin-agonist properties, is effective in the treatment of individuals with generalized anxiety disorder, although clinical experience is less positive. Buspirone appears to be a safer choice than benzodiazepines for residents taking several other medications or needing to be treated for longer periods of time. One drawback of buspirone is the amount of time required to see a clinical response (approximately 4 weeks). This suggests that concomitant use of a short-acting benzodiazepine in the initial stage of treatment would be useful for some residents. Buspirone may also be efficacious in reducing symptoms of anxiety and agitation in residents with dementia. Antihistamines such as hydroxyzine and diphenhydramine[OL] are sometimes used to manage mild anxiety, but there are few data that demonstrate efficacy, and the anticholinergic properties of these agents can cause serious problems, such as sedation and confusion. To manage severe anxiety and agitation associated with dementia that has not responded to other forms of treatment, atypical antipsychotics, such as risperidone[OL], olanzapine[OL], and quetiapine[OL], may be used. The antipsychotics are more effective in the presence of an underlying psychosis. Clinicians must use caution when prescribing antipsychotics given their side effect profile and the increased risk of death from cerebrovascular complications when given to older adults with dementia.

PSYCHOLOGICAL MANAGEMENT

Although pharmacotherapy is commonly the first-line treatment for late-life anxiety disorders, psychological treatments are often adequate, either alone or in combination with medication. Techniques generally fall into three categories: relaxation training, cognitive restructuring, and exposure with response prevention. Relaxation training can be employed with the use of music, visual imagery, aromatherapy, or instruction in relaxation techniques. Cognitive restructuring helps the older adult identify triggers and stimuli that maintain anxiety and helps him or her to slowly gain more control over the effect of such stimuli and develop a range of coping strategies and tools. Exposure with response prevention is particularly effective with both panic disorder and obsessive-compulsive disorder. Treatment typically includes a combination of behavioral approaches. Success depends on appropriateness of the older adult for psychotherapy; his or her support system, intellectual functioning, and motivation level; the degree of coordination of care with medical professionals; and the nature of the disorder.

RESOURCES

Ayres, C. R. (2007). Evidence-based psychological treatments for late-life anxiety. *Psychology and Aging, 22*(1), 8–17.

Cairney, J., & Streiner, D. L. (2008). Comorbid depression and anxiety in later life: Patterns of association, subjective well-being, and impairment. *American Journal of Geriatric Psychiatry, 16*(3), 201–208.

De Beurs, E., Beekman, A. T., Deeg, D. J., Van Dyck, R., & Van Tilburg, W. (2000). Predictors of change in anxiety symptoms of older persons: Results from the Longitudinal Aging Study Amsterdam. *Psychological Medicine, 30*(3), 515–527.

Kogan, J. N., Edelstein, B. A., & McKee, D. R. (2000). Assessment of anxiety in older adults. *Journal of Anxiety Disorders, 14*(2), 109–132.

Mostofsky, D. I., & Barlow, D. H. (Eds.) (2000). *The management of stress and anxiety in medical disorders.* Needham Heights, MA: Allyn & Bacon.

Sheikh, J. I. (2003). Anxiety in older adults: Assessment and management of three common presentations. *Geriatrics, 58*(5), 44–45.

Smith, M., & Rosenblatt, A. (2008). Anxiety symptoms among assisted living residents: Implications of the "no difference" finding for participants with and without dementia. *Research in Gerontological Nursing, 1*(2), 97–104.

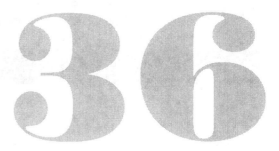

Personality and Somatoform Disorders

Marc Edward Agronin and Elizabeth Galik

Personality disorders are defined by the presence of chronic and pervasive patterns of inflexible and maladaptive inner experiences and behaviors. These patterns lead to significant disruptions in several spheres of function, including cognitive perception and interpretation, emotional expression, interpersonal relations, and impulse control. People with personality disorders are often distinguished by repeated episodes of disruptive or noxious behaviors, and as a result they often are perceived negatively. Descriptive terms applied to those with personality disorders include "difficult," "dramatic," and "overbearing," to name just a few. The developmental roots of personality disorders are believed to lie in childhood and adolescence, but their features can present clinically at any age. These features represent the influence of both genetic and environmental factors.

The *Diagnostic and Statistical Manual of Mental Disorders, Text Revision* (*DSM-IV-TR*) describes 10 personality disorders, grouped into three broad clusters based on common phenomenology. Depressive and passive-aggressive personality disorders are two additional categories but are considered provisional since they lack the empirical support of the other 10 diagnoses. Brief definitions and late-life features of all 12 personality disorders are provided in Table 36.1.

Many older adults with personality disorders can easily become overwhelmed by age-associated losses and stresses, largely because they lack appropriate coping skills and the personal, social, or financial resources to buffer their losses. In particular, admission to a hospital or long-term care setting poses a unique stress on all older adults with personality disorders in late life. The loss of a familiar environment, personal items, privacy, and control over one's schedule can lead to a sense of disorganization and displacement. Conflict in an assisted living (AL) setting begins when residents with personality disorders try to cope with the stresses imposed by the new environment; this exaggerates their maladaptive behaviors. For example, an obsessive-compulsive person may attempt to maintain a sense of control by demanding rigid adherence to schedules and rules of hygiene. Dependent residents may feel helpless and panicked if they feel they are not receiving sufficient attention to their needs, and they may respond with clinging behaviors and excessive questions or requests for assistance. Paranoid, antisocial, and borderline personality disorder individuals (see Table 36.1) may repeatedly refuse to cooperate with treatment plans or facility rules.

EPIDEMIOLOGY

Prevalence rates of personality disorders among community-residing older adults range from 5% to 10%, a

36.1 | Features of Personality Disorders

CLUSTER, DISORDER	GENERAL FEATURES[a]	FEATURES SPECIFIC TO OLDER ADULTS
Cluster A: Odd or eccentric behaviors		
Paranoid	Pervasive suspiciousness of the motives of others, which often leads to irritability and hostility	Episodes of paranoid psychosis, agitation, and assaultiveness
Schizoid	Disinterest in social relationships, coupled with isolative and sometimes odd behaviors	Poor, strained, or absent relationships with caregivers
Schizotypal	Characteristic appearance, behaviors, and beliefs that are strange, unusual, or inappropriate	Beliefs that may become delusional and that may lead to conflicts with others; relationships with caregivers that may be strained or absent
Cluster B: Dramatic, emotional, or erratic behaviors		
Antisocial	Poor regard for social norms and laws; lack of conscience and empathy for others; frequent reckless and criminal behaviors	Frequent remission of antisocial behaviors with less aggression and impulsivity
Borderline	Impaired control of emotional expression and impulses associated with unstable interpersonal relations, poor self-identity, and self-injurious behaviors	Persistent emotional lability and unstable relationships, but fewer self-injurious and impulsive behaviors
Histrionic	Excessive emotionality and attention-seeking behaviors, sometimes appearing overly seductive or provocative	Behaviors that may become excessively disinhibited and disorganized, appearing manic
Narcissistic	Pervasive sense of entitlement, grandiosity, and arrogance, coupled with lack of empathy	May present as hostile, full of rage, paranoid, or depressed
Cluster C: Anxious or fearful behaviors		
Avoidant	Excessive sensitivity to rejection and social scrutiny; social demeanor that may be timid and inhibited	Social contacts that may be extremely limited, providing for inadequate support
Dependent	Excessive dependence on others to help make decisions and provide support	Commonly, comorbid depression; clinical appearance often with demanding or clinging behaviors if dependency needs not met
Obsessive-compulsive	Pervasive preoccupation with orderliness and cleanliness; a perfectionist, rigid, and controlling approach that may become more inflexible and indecisive under stress	Obsessive-compulsive traits that may become exaggerated in efforts to maintain control over somatic and environmental changes

(continued)

36.1 | Features of Personality Disorders *(continued)*

CLUSTER, DISORDER	GENERAL FEATURES[a]	FEATURES SPECIFIC TO OLDER ADULTS
Provisional personality disorders		
Passive-aggressive	Pervasive pattern of passive resistance to demands and authority, such as through procrastination; attitudes toward others and responsibilities that are often critical and resentful	No clear changes in late life
Depressive	Outlook on life that is pervasively gloomy and pessimistic; excessively guilt prone with poor self-esteem	Commonly seen with comorbid depression in late life

[a]From *Diagnostic and Statistical Manual of Mental Disorders* (4th ed., text revision), by American Psychiatric Association, 2000, Washington, DC: Author. Copyright ©2000 by American Psychiatric Association. Reprinted with permission.

slightly lower range than the 10% to 18% prevalence estimates for community-residing persons of all ages. In institutional settings, prevalence rates in combination with comorbid depression are much higher, ranging from 10% to over 50%, depending on the method of diagnosis. The most common personality disorders in late life are dependent, obsessive-compulsive, and paranoid. Although most research has demonstrated fewer diagnoses in older age groups, it is unclear whether this represents an actual difference in prevalence or merely reflects the fact that it is more difficult to make a diagnosis in older adults.

CHALLENGES IN ASSESSMENT AND DIAGNOSIS

Establishing a diagnosis of personality disorder in the older adult can be especially challenging because it requires a detailed, longitudinal psychiatric and psychosocial history. Residents and their informants are not always able to provide sufficient history, especially when it may span 50 years or more. History may be distorted by recall bias (i.e., the tendency to present more socially desirable traits) or memory impairment. Common personality disorders are described in Table 36.1. Schizotypal and paranoid persons may be reluctant to engage in clinical interviews and share personal history;

antisocial and narcissistic persons who lack insight into their problems may refuse to divulge relevant experiences. Records often do not provide sufficient information to determine prior personality dynamics. Remote diagnoses from previous decades cannot be easily correlated with current ones because the diagnostic criteria for personality disorders have changed significantly in the past 50 years. Given all these limitations, clinicians often are reluctant to make a diagnosis or to make judgments based on insufficient information.

A further diagnostic challenge is the need to isolate lifelong personality characteristics from a multitude of comorbid problems. Acute and chronic episodes of major depression, psychosis, and other major psychiatric disorders can considerably distort personality features. In addition, current diagnostic nomenclature might handicap late-life diagnosis since it is not age adjusted; many criteria fail to apply in late life. In addition to the many barriers to diagnosis of personality disorders in older adults, the uninformed clinician may assume that all older adults have disruptive personality features as a normal function of age.

ASSESSMENT AND DIAGNOSIS

Not every older person with prominent or troubling personality features has a personality disorder. Those who demonstrate rigid and maladaptive personality traits, but without the pervasiveness or severity as represented by *DSM-IV-TR* criteria (see Table 36.1), are better described as suffering from *personality dysfunction* or an *adjustment disorder*. An adjustment disorder might best characterize previously healthy and well-adjusted persons who demonstrate acute changes in personality as a result of severe stresses. For example, physical pain and disability can lead to dependent or avoidant behaviors that resemble those seen in personality disorders but without the pervasive pattern and degree of maladaptiveness. There is also considerable overlap between symptoms of major psychiatric disorders and those of personality disorders; without longitudinal history, it can be difficult to distinguish between them. For example, the odd thinking and unusual perceptual experiences seen in psychotic disorders may resemble behaviors seen in schizotypal personality disorder. Diagnosis of a personality disorder becomes more certain when seemingly acute behaviors emerge as enduring and pervasive personality traits. This diagnostic process depends on the opportunity to observe a person over time and in multiple settings or situations.

Personality disorders as described in *DSM-IV-TR* must also be differentiated from the diagnosis of *personality change* due to a specific medical condition, such as dementia, traumatic brain injury, or some seizure disorders. When personality change is a direct result of brain damage, it has classically been described within the context of an organic personality disorder, although this term is no longer used in *DSM* nomenclature. Most often, personality changes with an organic source involve impairments in executive functioning, consisting of poor impulse control, poor planning, and greater vulnerability to irritability or agitation. Along these lines, Alzheimer's disease and other dementias are often associated with personality changes, including apathy, egocentricity, and impulsivity. Frontal lobe brain injury may result in a disinhibited impulsive syndrome, or, conversely, an apathetic syndrome may result.

Long-Term Course

Personality disorders generally follow one of four possible courses: (a) they continue unchanged, (b) evolve into a different form or major psychiatric disorder (e.g., depression), (c) improve, or (d) remit. Few disorders have actually been studied over time, and rarely into late life. Several studies suggest that personality disorders may enter a period of relative quiescence in middle age, with fewer and less intense symptoms and increased adaptation. However, this period may precede their re-emergence in late life. Other researchers propose that personality disorders characterized by emotional and behavioral lability, including antisocial, borderline, histrionic, narcissistic, and dependent behaviors, tend to improve over time, although individuals remain vulnerable to depression. Paranoid, schizoid, schizotypal, and obsessive-compulsive personality disorders are thought to either remain stable or to worsen in late life.

Only antisocial and borderline personality disorders have been looked at longitudinally, and both show symptom improvement and even remission into middle and later life for a significant percentage of adults. At the same time, there can be persistent psychopathology that is not recognized within the context of existing antisocial or borderline diagnostic criteria. In other words, longstanding personality dynamics may manifest in new behaviors. For example, those with antisocial personality disorders demonstrate less aggressiveness, violence, and criminal acts as they age, but they still have antisocial tendencies expressed through substance abuse, disregard for safety, and noncompliance with institutional rules. Older borderline residents display less impulsivity, self-mutilation, and risk-taking, but more age-appropriate symptoms, such as the use of multiple medications and nonadherence with treatment and facility rules.

TREATMENT

The treatment of personality disorders in older adults is complicated and often has limited success. Given the chronic and pervasive nature of personality disorders, the overall goal of treatment is not to cure the disorder but to decrease the frequency and intensity of disruptive behaviors. The first step should always be to clarify the diagnosis and then to identify recent stressors that may account for the current presentation. This will guide the selection of *realistic target symptoms* and therapeutic approaches and will allow a treatment team to anticipate future stressors. Treatment of personality disorders in older adults uses the same basic approaches as with younger adults, but clinicians must incorporate a much broader understanding of the impact of age-related stressors and comorbid disorders. Psychotherapy has been used to treat personality disorders in older adults. However, there may be more limitations on time and intensity of therapy, and as a result treatment must focus more on short-term, cognitive-behavioral, and pharmacologic approaches.

In outpatient settings such as an assisted living community (ALC), clinicians have limited control over a person's environment and must therefore rely on one-to-one interventions if the individual is willing to participate in this type of treatment. Table 36.2 suggests therapeutic approaches that clinicians can employ with various personality disorders. AL and nursing home settings are opportunities for intervention. A staff meeting or case conference often provides the best forum to discuss disruptive persons and to coordinate a consistent treatment plan. Disruptive behaviors can sometimes be traced to particular activities or staff interactions that can be adapted as part of an overall treatment strategy. Sometimes, disengagement from residents reduces the intensity of disruptive interactions. In other situations, continuity of staffing and routinization of daily schedules is critical. In all situations, a treatment plan should be well documented and conveyed to the resident and family, as well as to all involved staff and caregivers. All plans must provide appropriate limits to ensure the safety of residents and staff. A written contract, signed by all parties, may be needed with nonadherent residents in order to eliminate misinterpretation and confusion. Although it is important to involve family members in the treatment plan, clinicians must recognize that residents with personality disorders often have conflictual relationships with their families. Attention should also be given to individual staff members who must work with residents displaying challenging behavior. Staff need opportunities to vent feelings of anxiety and frustration, and to feel acknowledged and supported by administration.

No reported studies look specifically at pharmacologic strategies for personality disorders in older adults; clinicians must instead extrapolate from guidelines used for younger persons. Psychotropic medications can be targeted at a particular personality disorder, specific symptoms or symptom clusters, or comorbid depression, anxiety, or psychosis. The goal is not to cure the disorder but to reduce the frequency and intensity of targeted symptoms. Antidepressant medication may be helpful for the target symptoms of depression and anxiety found in most personality disorders. Mood stabilizers (e.g., lithium carbonate[OL] and divalproex sodium[OL]) and antipsychotic medications reduce mood lability and impulsivity in borderline adults, and they may be useful with similar symptoms in antisocial personality disorder. Anti-anxiety agents are commonly used for transient agitation seen in borderline, antisocial, narcissistic, and paranoid disorders, and they may reduce social anxiety and panic in avoidant and dependent residents. Antidepressants are used commonly to treat the symptoms associated with obsessive-compulsive disorders (Table 36.1). Antipsychotic agents can treat the transient psychosis, agitation, and impulsivity seen in dramatic cluster and paranoid disorders, as well as the borderline psychosis and paranoia seen in odd cluster disorders (see Table 36.2).

Psychotropic medications are sometimes used as adjuncts to psychotherapy. In older adults, however, multiple medications, personality disorders, and the associated symptoms should be avoided in general, and particularly when there is a history of nonadherence, confusion, or impulsivity. Attention must be given to potential interactions with multiple other medications used to treat medical disorders.

SOMATOFORM DISORDERS

Somatoform disorders encompass a heterogeneous group of seven diagnoses that have in common the presence of physical symptoms or complaints without objective organic causes, and are strongly associated with psychological factors. Clinical characteristics of each diagnosis are summarized in Exhibit 36.1. These disorders are especially relevant to geriatric care because affected older adults are seen in all health care settings. However, somatoform disorders in older adults have not been well studied; research has usually focused on select diagnoses, such as hypochondriasis, in limited or biased samples.

Research also has looked at somatic symptom reporting rather than at specific diagnoses. Prevalence rate is not strongly associated with age, although there is weak evidence for a slight increase in hypochondriasis with age. Increased somatic preoccupation and symptoms are, however, associated with depression in late life. In addition to depression, increased somatic preoccupation is associated with the presence of the personality trait of *neuroticism*. Somatoform disorders are found more commonly in women and in lower socioeconomic groups.

Clinical Characteristics and Causes

It is important to understand that somatoform disorders do not represent intentional, conscious attempts by older adults to present factitious (i.e., contrived, made up) physical symptoms. Somatoform symptoms are experienced by the affected person as real physical pain and discomfort, usually without insight into associated psychological factors. Somatoform disorders do not represent delusional thinking as found in psychotic states, and they differ from psychosomatic disorders that are characterized by actual disease states with presumed

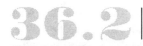 | Therapeutic Strategies for Personality Disorders in Late Life

CLUSTER A—PARANOID, SCHIZOID, SCHIZOTYPAL PERSONALITY DISORDERS

■ Always assess for and treat comorbid psychosis.

■ Do not force social interactions, but offer support and problem-solving assistance in a professional and consistent manner.

■ Do not challenge paranoid ideation; instead, solicit and empathize with emotional responses to the inner turmoil and fear of paranoid states.

CLUSTER B—ANTISOCIAL, BORDERLINE, HISTRIONIC, AND NARCISSISTIC PERSONALITY DISORDERS

■ Assess for and treat underlying mood lability, depression, anxiety, and substance abuse.

■ Adopt a consistent, structured, and predictable approach with strict boundaries to contain disruptive behaviors.

■ Adopt a team approach with all involved clinicians to devise a common plan; avoid staff splits between supporters and detractors of the resident.

■ Use written behavioral contracts and authority figures when necessary to address recurrent disruptive behaviors.

■ Do not personalize belligerent behaviors directed toward staff members; instead, provide opportunities for staff to ventilate frustration and negative thoughts and emotions with professional colleagues.

CLUSTER C—AVOIDANT, DEPENDENT, AND OBSESSIVE-COMPULSIVE PERSONALITY DISORDERS

■ Assess for and treat underlying anxiety, panic, and depression.

■ Provide regularly scheduled clinical contacts rather than on an as-needed basis.

■ When possible, provide case managers to solicit the needs of avoidant residents and to provide extra reassurance and attention to the needs of dependent and obsessive-compulsive residents.

DEPRESSIVE AND PASSIVE-AGGRESSIVE PERSONALITY DISORDERS

■ Differentiate between the depressive and negative attitudes and the actual symptoms of major depression. Provide appropriate and adequate antidepressant treatment.

■ Avoid becoming too pessimistic or burnt-out with attempts at providing care; shift focus to a supportive and nonjudgmental therapeutic relationship, with minimal expectations as to outcome.

■ Encourage individual psychotherapy to identify underlying emotions and to redirect negative attitudes toward more constructive activities.

36.1 | Clinical Characteristics of Somatoform Disorders

SOMATIZATION DISORDER

Multiple physical complaints in excess of what would be expected, given history and examination, prior to the age of 30 and lasting several years; complaints not fully explained by medical workup; must include four different sites of pain, two gastrointestinal symptoms, one sexual symptom, one pseudoneurologic symptom (not pain).

UNDIFFERENTIATED SOMATOFORM DISORDER

One or more physical complaints, lasting at least 6 months, that cannot be fully explained by appropriate medical workup and that result in considerable social, occupational, or functional impairment.

CONVERSION DISORDER

One or more motor or sensory deficits that cannot be fully explained by appropriate medical workup and that appear to be causally related to psychological factors.

PAIN DISORDER

Pain is the major focus of clinical presentation, and psychological factors are believed to be playing a critical role in the onset, severity, exacerbation, and maintenance of the pain.

HYPOCHONDRIASIS

A preoccupation with fears of having a serious illness, based on misinterpretation of bodily symptoms and resistant to appropriate medical evaluation and reassurance.

BODY DYSMORPHIC DISORDER

Preoccupation with an imagined defect in appearance. If there is an actual physical defect, this preoccupation greatly exceeds what would be expected.

SOMATOFORM DISORDER, NOT OTHERWISE SPECIFIED

The presence of somatoform symptoms that do not meet the criteria for other categories.

From *Diagnostic and Statistical Manual of Mental Disorders* (4th ed., text revision), by American Psychiatric Association, 2000, Washington, DC: Author. Copyright ©2000 by American Psychiatric Association. Reprinted with permission.

psychological triggers. Rather, somatoform disorders represent a complex interaction between mind and brain in which an affected person is unknowingly expressing psychological stress or conflict through the body. It is not surprising, then, that depression and anxiety are associated with increased somatic expressions. In late life, somatoform disorders, in particular hypochondriasis, may be a way for a person to express anxiety and the attempt to cope with accumulating fears and losses. These may include fears of abandonment by family and caregivers, loss of beauty, libido, and strength, financial setbacks, loss of independence, loss of social role (e.g., through retirement, loss of spouse, change in residence), and loneliness. The psychological distress and anxiety over such losses may be less threatening and more controllable when shifted to somatic complaints or symptoms. In turn, the adoption of a sick role might be reinforced by increased social contacts and support.

Causes of somatoform disorders are usually multifactorial and often are rooted in early developmental experiences and personality traits. Psychodynamic approaches suggest that these disorders result from unconscious conflict in which intolerable impulses or affects are expressed through more tolerable somatic symptoms or complaints. One reason for this may be that the affected individual is unable to identify and express emotional states; the body becomes the mode of expression.

Although psychodynamic explanations can apply across the life span, these conflicts often begin early in life, perhaps accounting for the relatively young age of onset for most somatoform disorders. In late life, psychological conflicts that results in significant depression and anxiety are for the most part the same conflicts that can lead to somatization. In addition, the presence of so many comorbid medical problems and the use of multiple medications may provide readily available somatic symptoms around which psychological conflict can center. In long-term care, residents are faced with many overwhelming losses; their own bodies often serve as the last bastion of control. Somatic preoccupation thus serves as a means of coping with stress, even though it is maladaptive and can result in excessive and unnecessary disability.

Treatment

Persons with somatoform disorder usually present with what appears to be legitimate somatic complaints with an unknown physical cause. It is only after repeated but fruitless workups, multiple and persistent complaints and requests, and sometimes angry and inappropriate reactions to treatment that clinicians begin to suspect a somatoform disorder. It is important for the health care professional to remember that from the resident's perspective, the symptoms and complaints are quite real and disturbing. It is never wise to challenge the resident or to suggest that the symptoms are all in his or her mind, even after a workup has made it obvious that psychological factors are involved. The typical response to such a diagnostic pronouncement is that the resident will seek additional opinions and medical tests that in turn can perpetuate a cycle of somatization that never addresses the underlying issues.

Therapeutically, staff working with the resident should attempt to foster an ongoing, supportive, consistent, and professional relationship with the affected resident. Such a relationship will reassure as well as protect the resident from excessive and unnecessary medical visits and procedures. The ALC staff should focus on responding to the resident's complaints, perhaps with periodic but regularly scheduled appointments, and to set limits on workup and treatment in a firm but empathetic manner. This can be difficult to do when residents become demanding and consume excessive amounts of staff time. However, AL staff must endeavor to remain professional and not personalize the situation or feel that they are failing the resident. Overall, the role of the ALC staff is to focus on symptom reduction and rehabilitation and not to attempt to force the resident to have insight into the potential psychological nature of his or her symptoms. It would be hazardous to prematurely diagnose a somatoform disorder when there might actually be an underlying medical problem that has not been properly diagnosed. For example, disorders such as multiple sclerosis and systemic lupus commonly have complex presentations that elude initial diagnostic workup. Moreover, many somatoform disorders coexist with actual disease states; for example, many persons with pseudoseizures also have an actual seizure disorder. At the same time, it is important for the primary care clinician to set limits on what medical care can offer, and to make appropriate referrals to specialists and mental health clinicians.

The mental health clinician can play an active role in addressing the somatoform disorder. Unfortunately, no particular treatment for any somatoform disorder has been found to have good efficacy, and most disorders tend to be lifelong. As a result, the goal of treatment is not to cure but to control symptoms. The mental health clinician first forms a therapeutic alliance based on empathetic listening and acknowledgment of physical discomfort, without trivializing the somatic complaints. Sometimes, an offer to review all available medical records can be a tangible way of conveying one's seriousness to the resident. Underlying anxiety and depression must be identified and treated with psychotherapy and, when necessary, antidepressant or anti-anxiety medications, or both. Cognitive-behavioral therapy focuses on identifying distorted thought patterns and anxiety, and replacing them with more realistic and adaptive strategies. A mental health professional may assist in determining whether cognitive-behavioral therapy may be of benefit. In many cases, however, the supportive nature of regular visits to a primary care provider may be sufficient to meet the needs of residents with somatoform disorders as well as other personality disorders.

RESOURCES

Agronin, M.E. (2004). Somatoform disorders. In D.G. Blazer, D.C. Steffens, & E.W. Busse (Eds.), *Textbook of geriatric psychiatry* (3rd ed., pp. 295–302). Washington, DC: American Psychiatric Press.

Agronin, M.E., & Maletta, G. (2000). Personality disorders in late life: Understanding and overcoming the gap in research. *American Journal of Geriatric Psychiatry, 8*(1), 4–18.

Balsis, S., Gleason, M., Woods, C.M., & Oltmanns, T.F. (2007). An item response theory analysis of DSM-IV personality disorder criteria across younger and older age groups. *Psychology and Aging, 22*(1), 171–185.

Lynch, T.R., Cheavens, J.S., Cukrowicz, K.C., Thorp, S.R., Bronner, L., & Beyer, J. (2007). Treatment of older adults with co-morbid personality disorder and depression: A dialectical behavior therapy approach. *International Journal of Geriatric Psychiatry, 22,* 131–143.

Rabinowitz, T., Hirdes, J.P., & Desjardins, I. (2005). Somatoform disorders. In M.E. Agronin & G.J. Maletta (Eds.), *Principles and practice of geriatric psychiatry* (pp. 538–589). Philadelphia, PA: Lippincott Williams & Wilkins.

Zweig, R.A. (2007). Personality disorder in older adults: Assessment challenges and strategies. *Professional Psychology: Research and Practice, 39*(3), 298–305.

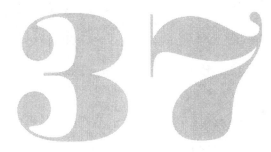

Substance Abuse

David W. Oslin and Ethel Mitty

The abuse and misuse of alcohol, psychoactive medications, illicit drugs, and nicotine have become significant public health concerns for the growing population of older adults. Substance abuse and dependence among older adults is common and renders them particularly vulnerable to the cognitive and physical effects of these substances. Typically, substance abuse problems are thought to occur only in those persons who use substances in high quantities and at regular intervals. Among older adults, however, negative health consequences have been demonstrated at consumption levels previously thought of as light to moderate, and certainly not in the amounts usually associated with a diagnosis of substance dependence. It is estimated that 4.4 million older adults will need substance abuse treatment in 2020; an increase from 1.7 million in 2001. A growing number of effective treatments lead not only to reductions in substance abuse but also to improvement in general health. Taken together, both the risks and the emergence of new treatments underscore the need to identify problems and provide appropriate treatment for those older adults suffering from the effects of substance misuse.

DEFINITIONS OF SUBSTANCE ABUSE

The first step in effective intervention is having valid criteria to determine which older adults would benefit from reducing or eliminating their substance abuse. Dependency is a maladaptive behavior. *Substance dependence* is defined as any use that imparts significant disability and warrants treatment. *Tolerance* is embedded in substance dependency and is defined as:

- Significant diminished effect from the same amount of the substance;
- Marked increase in need for the substance to achieve the desired effect (or intoxication);
- Desire to reduce substance use or lack of success in controlling it;
- Spending inordinate time and effort to obtain the substance or recover from its effect(s);
- Avoiding social or recreational activities because of substance misuse; and
- Continuing use even though aware of its negative consequences on physical and/or mental health.

Many older adults are not recognized as having problems related to their substance use, partly because the diagnostic criteria are difficult to interpret and apply consistently to older adults and, perhaps due to ageism, the *why bother* attitude of clinicians. It is a hidden epidemic: many older adults drink at home by themselves; thus, they are less likely than younger drinkers to be arrested, get into arguments, or have difficulties at work. Moreover, because many of the diseases caused or affected by substance misuse (e.g., hypertension, stroke, peptic ulcer disease) are common disorders in late life, clinicians may overlook the effects of substance use on the older patient who presents with these conditions. As such, older problem drinkers are less likely to be identified and referred for treatment than are their younger counterparts.

Given the difficulties assessing older adults for substance dependence, many experts advocate screening to identify those at risk for problem behaviors or who have at-risk or problem use. *At-risk use* is any use of a substance at a quantity or frequency greater than a recommended level often determined empirically on the basis of association with significant disability. The recommended upper limit of alcohol consumption for older adults is no more than seven standard drinks per week with no more than two episodes of binge drinking (i.e., four or more drinks in one day) during a 3-month period. *Problem substance use* is the consumption of any amount of an abusable substance that results in at least one problem related to this use, for example, use of benzodiazepines by a person with an unsteady gait.

On the other end of the spectrum, *abstinence* refers to drinking no alcohol in the previous 12 months. Approximately 60% to 70% of older adults are abstinent. It is useful to ascertain why alcohol is not used; some individuals are abstinent because of a previous history of alcohol problems. For this reason, it is particularly important to obtain a history of both current and past use. Some are abstinent because of recent illness; others have lifelong patterns of low-risk use or abstinence. Older adults with a previous history of alcohol problems may require preventive monitoring to determine if any new stresses could exacerbate an old pattern. In addition, a previous history of at-risk drinking or alcohol dependence increases the risk for developing other mental health problems in late life, such as depressive disorders or cognitive problems, and may limit treatment response because of brain damage.

Low-risk or moderate use of alcohol falls within the recommended guidelines for consumption and is not associated with problems. Older adults in this category are also able to employ reasonable limits on alcohol consumption, that is, they do not drink when driving a motor vehicle or boat, or when using contraindicated medications. It is important to note, however, that a change in physical health or in prescription medications may elevate even low-risk use to a problem level.

The most practical method for identifying persons who could benefit from intervention is to determine the quantity and frequency of their use of abusable substances. This method has advantages over formal diagnostic interviews because of its brevity, easily interpretable results, and absence of stigmatizing language, such as "addiction," "alcoholism," "alcoholic," or "alcohol dependence."

MAGNITUDE OF THE PROBLEM

Drug Use

Little is known about the epidemiology of substance-use disorders, other than alcoholism, in the older adult population. It is generally held that older drug addicts are only younger addicts grown old and that few older adults initiate drug use in their later years. A community-based study reported lifetime prevalence rates of drug abuse and dependence of 0.12% for elderly men and 0.06% for elderly women. The lifetime history of illicit drug use is 2.88% for men and 0.66% for women. No active cases were reported in either gender. In contrast, a more recent study of an elder-specific drug program in a veteran population found that one-quarter had either a primary drug problem or concurrent drug and alcohol problems. This study may be a reflection of the growing number of older adults who used drugs in the 1960s—a time of expanded drug experimentation in the United States and during the Vietnam War (1965–1973). The recent increase in hepatitis C among those age 60 and over may reflect both a history of intravenous drug use as well as increased risk of nosocomial infection with advanced age. Studies are needed to determine the prevalence and incidence of substance-use disorders involving nicotine, caffeine, benzodiazepines, marijuana, and opiates in later life.

Medication Use

Perhaps a unique problem among older adults is the misuse or inappropriate use of prescription and over-the-counter (OTC) medications. This problem includes the misuse of substances such as sedatives, hypnotics, narcotic and nonnarcotic analgesics, diet aids, and decongestants. Community surveys report that 60% of older adults take an analgesic, 22% take a central nervous system medication, and 11% take a benzodiazepine on a regular basis. Many medications used by older adults have the potential for inducing tolerance, withdrawal syndromes, and harmful medical consequences, such as cognitive changes, kidney disease, falls, and liver disease. In spite of a growing body of literature describing increases in morbidity and mortality associated with misuse of prescription and nonprescription medications, it is not considered a disorder by the *Diagnostic and Statistical Manual of Mental Disorders* (*DSM-IV*).

Medication use by all older adults needs to be monitored carefully to avoid potentially hazardous combinations of drugs, medications with a high risk for adverse effects, and ineffective or unnecessary medications (see Chapter 20, "Pharmacotherapy"). A practical approach is to reevaluate the older adult's medications every 3 to 6 months. Maintenance treatment should be continued only for those patients with specific target symptoms and a documented response to the treatment. The treatment regimen for those patients without a response or partial response needs reevaluation.

Alcohol Use

Alcohol abuse, defined clinically and also known as heavy drinking, is present in approximately 0.2% to 4% of the older adult population. Community-based epidemiologic studies describe the extent and nature of alcohol use in the older population by reporting percentages of abstainers, daily drinkers, and heavy drinkers: abstainers, 31% to 58%; daily drinkers, 10% to 22%. Heavy drinking, defined as a minimum of 12 to 21 drinks per week, is present in 3% to 9% of the older population.

Longitudinally designed community studies provide valuable insight regarding the natural course of drinking patterns among older adults. Most of the literature on drinking indicates that although older adults are likely to decrease the quantity of alcohol consumed on a given day, the frequency of use or pattern of use changes very little over time.

About two-thirds of elderly alcoholic patients started drinking at a young age; late-onset drinking accounts for the remaining one-third of older adults who abuse alcohol. Late-onset drinkers tend to have a higher level of education and income than those who started drinking at a younger age. Stressful life events, such as bereavement or retirement, may trigger late-onset drinking in some, but not all, persons.

Cultural and Demographic Factors

Numerous studies indicate that the prevalence of alcohol use and alcohol-related problems is much higher for older men than for older women. Among younger adults, however, the ratio of male to female drinkers has changed since the 1980s: more women than men present for alcoholism treatment. These changes are likely to be reflected in the next generation of older women. Similar patterns by gender are seen with illicit drug use, except that benzodiazepines are much more commonly used by older women than by older men.

Conclusions from the few studies addressing differences among various ethnic groups are less clear. Varying with the study, older Black and Hispanic Americans consume amounts of alcohol similar to or lower than the amounts consumed by older White Americans. More relevant risk factors for alcohol consumption among older adults, rather than race or ethnicity, are increased leisure time and higher disposable income.

Clinical Settings

The prevalence rate for alcohol problems among hospitalized older adults and those living in retirement communities is substantially higher than for community-dwellers. A survey among residents of a Veterans Affairs nursing home found that 35% of those interviewed had a lifetime diagnosis of alcohol abuse.

RISKS AND BENEFITS OF SUBSTANCE USE

Benefits of Alcohol Consumption

Moderate alcohol consumption among otherwise healthy older adults has been promoted in the clinical and lay press as having significant beneficial effects, especially with regard to cardiovascular disease and mortality. Alcohol in moderate amounts may promote relaxation and reduce social anxiety. However, although there are benefits from moderate drinking, the practice is not recommended for older adults who currently do not drink. There is no evidence to support a therapeutic effect of alcohol for heart disease or any other condition in persons who previously did not drink. Many older adults do not drink because of past problems with drinking (personal, family), the cost of drinking, and the adverse effects of intoxication.

Excess Physical Disability

Substance abuse has clear and profound effects on the health and well-being of older adults. They are prone to the toxic effects of substances on many different organ systems because of both age-related changes and in association with other illnesses common in late life. The social and economic impact is also tremendous. Substance abuse has adverse effects on self-esteem, coping skills, and interpersonal relationships, which may be compounded by losses that are common in the late stages of life.

Levels of alcohol consumption above seven drinks per week, so called at-risk drinking, are associated with a number of health problems, including increased risk of stroke caused by bleeding, impaired driving skills, and increased rate of injuries (e.g., falls and fractures). The risk of breast cancer in women who consume three to nine drinks per week increases by approximately 50% over that of women who have fewer than three drinks per week. Alcohol is also known to interfere with the metabolism of many medications, including OTCs as well as prescribed medications (e.g., digoxin, warfarin), and potentiates harmful interactions with psychoactive medications (e.g., benzodiazepines and antidepressants).

Older adults who consume more than an average of four drinks per day or whose drinking has led to a diagnosis of alcohol dependence are at greatest risk for excess physical disability and physical illness related to the drinking. The most common problems associated with alcohol dependence are alcoholic liver disease, chronic obstructive pulmonary disease, peptic ulcer disease, and psoriasis. Unexplained multisystem disease is justification to probe more closely for alcohol misuse. With smoking, the risks are much clearer, including increased rates of pulmonary disease, especially cancer. Research is beginning to demonstrate that the disability associated with substance abuse is reversible.

Mental Health Problems

Substance abuse can be a significant factor in the course and prognosis of nearly all mental health problems of late life. Alcohol, benzodiazepine, opioid, and cigarette use are all associated with mood disturbances. Persons with both alcoholism and depression tend to be at increased risk of suicide and more socially dysfunctional behavior than nondepressed persons with alcoholism.

The complex role of alcoholism in the development of Alzheimer's disease is not fully understood, but alcoholism is believed to be associated with dementia. The criteria for alcohol-related dementia are:

- Clinically evident dementia at least 60 days after last alcohol exposure;
- A history of significant use of alcohol for at least 5 years, that is, at least 35 drinks per week for men and 28 per week for women; and
- Significant use of alcohol within 3 years of the onset of cognitive deficits.

Clinical features supporting the diagnosis of alcohol-related dementia include end-organ damage (e.g., liver disease), cognitive stabilization or improvement after abstinence, and evidence of cerebellar atrophy (i.e.,

shrinking in the size of the brain) in brain imaging. More research is needed to understand the potential benefits of long-term abstinence from alcohol in terms of the effect this will have on mood and memory.

IDENTIFICATION AND ASSESSMENT OF SUBSTANCE ABUSE

Older adults suspected of being substance misusers may present with nontraditional signs of substance abuse. Some older adults may be unable to tolerate even normal amounts of alcohol; some may have negative effects even with limited use; and others, especially late-onset alcoholics, may never develop physiological dependency. Almost 40% of older adults at risk for substance abuse do not self-identify. Nontraditional approaches are needed, for example, educating friends and families about substance abuse to sensitize them to clues that are not seen by clinicians and health care providers. The assisted living nurse can say something like, "I am concerned about you; I am wondering if alcohol (your daily martini) might be why your diabetes is not responding to diet and medications." Clinical examination is the most valuable tool for identifying substance-use problems: observing for conjunctival injection (i.e., bloodshot eyes), hand tremor, and abnormal skin vascularization (i.e., increased visibility of veins on the face, nose particularly), among other signs. Screening questionnaires for alcohol abuse can also be used. There are two commonly used self-administered questionnaires to screen for alcohol misuse: the Michigan Alcoholism Screening Test (MAST) and the CAGE (see Chapter 19, "Prevention"). The CAGE identifies a lifetime problem (i.e., of alcohol abuse), not a current one. It can be modified to use as a screen for other substances although it is less effective in screening female older adults than male older adults. The MAST is very sensitive for identifying individuals with alcohol problems

Another tool, the Alcohol Use Disorders Identification Test (AUDIT) is reportedly useful in identifying alcohol misuse among ethnic minority older adults. The American Geriatrics Society (n.d.) guideline, *Substance Abuse Among Older Adults*, addresses screening recommendations for older adults and age-related physiologic changes that may occur with late-life alcoholism. Medications that may interact adversely with alcohol are outlined, and chronic conditions that may be triggered or worsened by alcohol use are noted. To assist the clinician in early detection, the risk factors for alcoholism in late life are summarized; guidelines for inquiring about alcoholism and specific laboratory values that may be abnormal are also provided. Different risk levels are outlined, as are definitions for abuse and dependence and various interpersonal and pharmacologic intervention strategies.

Biologic markers, specifically blood tests, of substance use can be useful in managing patients with known substance-use disorders but are less valuable in detecting illness. These markers include γ-glutamyl transferase, mean corpuscular volume, and transferrin. Blood work results that show macrocytic anemia (large red blood cells), thrombocytopenia (low platelets), and elevated γ-glutamyl transferase (liver function tests) should raise concerns about the possibility of substance abuse. Urine drug screens are an effective method for screening for or identifying illicit drug use as well as prescription drug use.

TREATMENT

Older adults with a substance-use problem often present with a variety of treatment needs. It is important to have an array of services that can be tailored to individual needs and that have the flexibility to adapt to changing needs over time. Older adults can successfully be treated for substance misuse and abuse. The spectrum of interventions can range from prevention and education, for those who are abstinent or low-risk drinkers, to minimal advice or brief structured interventions, for at-risk or problem drinkers, to formalized alcoholism treatment, for those who meet criteria for abuse or dependence. The array of formal treatment options includes psychotherapy, education, rehabilitative and residential care, and psychopharmacologic agents. An example of the necessity to tailor care is the contrast between the at-risk drinker or benzodiazepine user and the severely dependent patient. It is unlikely that the at-risk user will need the intensity of services required for the severely dependent patient. Indeed, requiring the at-risk drinker to accept a set of rigorous services may be more detrimental than helpful.

Dependency on medications such as benzodiazepines is managed by tapering the dosage until the drug can be stopped and at the same time providing supportive counseling via groups, psychosocial support, and 12-step programs. The physical symptoms of withdrawal from narcotics can be controlled when necessary with oral clonidine. Assuring that the patient enters a long-term treatment program increases the likelihood of long-term success. For smoking cessation, it is important to prepare the person for quitting by dis-

cussing management strategies before quitting, setting a quit date, and implementing a monitoring plan to maintain success.

Detoxification and Stabilization

The initial assessment of any substance abuser should include an assessment of the person's potential to suffer acute withdrawal. Patients with severe symptoms of dependency or withdrawal potential and those with significant medical or psychiatric comorbidity may require inpatient hospitalization for acute stabilization prior to implementing an outpatient management strategy; for example, severe withdrawal from alcohol use can be life threatening. *Detoxification* is achieved by placing the patient on the minimum amount of drug that suppresses withdrawal symptoms and then decreasing the dosage.

It is not unusual for older adults who are substance abusers to go through withdrawal. Alcohol withdrawal, for example, can occur when an older person goes to the hospital following an acute event or accident. Early symptoms include tachycardia (i.e., increased heart rate), sweating, tremulousness, and hypertension and this may progress to delirium, psychosis, and seizures. It is helpful to give benzodiazepines such as lorazepam[OL] to help prevent or manage these symptoms.

Traditionally, outpatient substance abuse treatment has been reserved for clinics that specialize in substance abuse. This model is inadequate for addressing the broader public health demand; a variety of clinicians and clinical settings need to be involved. This is particularly important for older adults who frequently seek medical services but rarely seek specialized addiction services. The traditional addiction clinic is focused on supportive group psychotherapy and encouragement to attend regular self-help group meetings such as Alcoholics Anonymous, Alcoholics Victorious, Rational Recovery, or Narcotics Anonymous.

For older adults, peer-specific group activities are more effective than mixed-age group activities. Outpatient rehabilitation, in addition to focusing on active addiction issues, needs to address time management because abstinence reduces the time spent in maintaining the substance-use disorder. Management of this time—often the greater part of the person's day—is critical for treatment success. However, abstinence is not the only positive outcome of treatment; patients should be praised for making progress in cutting down on use as well as stopping use. This may be particularly relevant for medication misuse such as benzodiazepines, as it may be more difficult to eliminate their use. The Consensus Panel of the Mental Health Technical Assistance Center Substance Abuse and Mental Health Services Administration recommended that male older adults with drinking problems should be limited to one alcoholic drink per day (two, for a special occasion). The amount of daily alcohol for a woman is lower.

The risks of adverse events (e.g., falls) with benzodiazepines are greater with higher doses and medications with a longer half-life such as diazepam or clonazepam. The Consensus Panel recommended that insomnia treatment with benzodiazepines should be limited to 4 months and that medications that last for shorter periods of time be used. A stepped approach should be used so that individuals are weaned to shorter-acting benzodiazepines if they are on longer-acting medications. Continued attempts should be made to wean the individual of the benzodiazepine; social services and financial support are helpful to stabilize the resident in early recovery.

Brief Interventions

Low-intensity, brief interventions can be cost-effective as an initial approach for at-risk and problem drinkers in primary care settings. Brief alcohol intervention to reduce hazardous drinking by older adults that used advice protocols demonstrated that protocols are acceptable to and effective for this population.

Pharmacotherapy

The use of medications to support abstinence may be of benefit, but it is not well studied. Small-scale studies demonstrate that naltrexone is well tolerated and efficacious in older adults. Studies are ongoing with using various antidepressants, including the selective serotonin reuptake inhibitors. Some of the general principles used in treating younger patients should be applied to older drinkers as well. For example, benzodiazepines are important in the treatment of alcohol detoxification, but they have no clinical place in maintaining long-term abstinence because of their abuse potential and the potential for fostering further alcohol or benzodiazepine abuse. Disulfiram may benefit some well-motivated patients, but cardiac and hepatic disease limits the use of this agent by the older adult who abuses alcohol. The use of methadone maintenance has proven efficacy in

opioid dependence. Older patients can be initiated and maintained on methadone, following the same principles of use as for younger patients. Comorbid medical and psychiatric disorders must be identified and properly treated, and may necessitate the need for referral to, or consultation with, a psychiatrist with expertise in these areas. Buprenorphine and buprenorphine with naloxone are approved for outpatient treatment of opioid dependence. However, given the complexity of treatment of this condition, systematic training, practice, monitoring, regulation, and evaluation are necessary in a multidisciplinary treatment setting to optimize outcomes. Guidelines for developing treatment programs using buprenorphine are available on the Web site of the Substance Abuse and Mental Health Services Administration (U.S. Department of Health and Human Services, 2004).

Establishing abstinence from nicotine follows the same principles as that from other addicting substances. Initially, pharmacologic substitution with either nicotine gum or patch is followed by a gradual decrease in dosage. Several trials demonstrate that antidepressant medications improve rates of continued abstinence, but only bupropion has been approved for this purpose by the U.S. Food and Drug Administration. As with other abstinence regimens, psychotherapy plus pharmacotherapy is better than pharmacotherapy alone (see also Chapter 40, "Respiratory Diseases and Disorders").

RESOURCES

American Geriatrics Society. (n.d.). *Substance abuse among older adults.* Retrieved December 1, 2008, from http://www.healthinaging.org/agingintheknow/chapters/ch_36.asp

Blow, F.C., Brower, K.J., Schulenberg, J.E., Demo-Dananberg, L.M., Young, J.P., & Beresford, T.P. (1992). The Michigan Alcoholism Screening Test—Geriatric Version (MAST-G). *Alcoholism: Clinical and Experimental Research, 16,* 372.

Moore, A.A., & the American Geriatrics Society Clinical Practice Committee. (2003). *Clinical guidelines for alcohol use disorders in older adults.* Retrieved August 2005 http://www.americangeriatrics.org./products/positionpapers/alcohol.shtml

Oslin, D.W., Pettinati, H.P., & Volpicelli, J.R. (2002). Alcoholism treatment adherence: Older age predicts better adherence and drinking outcomes. *American Journal of Geriatric Psychiatry, 10*(6), 740–747.

U.S. Department of Health and Human Services. (2004). *Clinical guidelines for the use of buprenorphine in the treatment of opioid addiction. Treatment improvement protocol (TIP) series 40.* Retrieved April 22, 2009, from http://buprenorphine.samhsa.gov/Bup_Guidelines.pdf

Diseases

and

Disorders

Unfortunately, the risk of acquiring just about any medical problem increases with age, and the majority of older adults in assisted living communities have multiple comorbid conditions (e.g., cancer, hypertension, arthritis). Chronic diseases can result in a diminished quality of life and greatly increased personal and public health care costs. Much of the acute exacerbations of chronic illnesses, the associated disability, and death can be avoided through good care and aggressive monitoring. In addition to general healthy lifestyle behaviors, such as regular physical activity, smoking cessation,

moderate alcohol use, and a low fat, low sodium diet, specific interventions are helpful for each medical problem. This section, which covers each body system (cardiac, musculoskeletal, etc.) reviews the most common medical problems and how to evaluate the resident for evidence of these problems and manage them. The information provided will help the nurse working with the resident to know when a problem requires immediate medical attention and when the sign or symptom is a chronic problem associated with the underlying diagnosis.

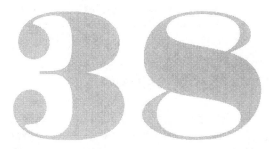

Dermatologic Diseases and Disorders

Sumaira Z. Aasi and Barbara Resnick

Skin disease increases with aging and sun exposure. Dermatologic (skin) care of the older adult requires awareness of the normal age-related changes that occur in the skin as well as the cumulative impact of ultraviolet (UV) radiation exposure. In addition, it is important to be familiar with the common skin diseases such as cancers, inflammatory diseases, and infections often seen in older adults.

AGING AND PHOTOAGING

Skin is composed of the epidermis, dermis, basement membrane zone (the area between the epidermis and dermis that serves to hold the two together), and the subcutaneous fat. In normal young skin the epidermis is close to the dermis. Over time, there is a decrease in the contact or closeness between the epidermis and dermis, thus making it more difficult to transfer nutrients to all the layers of the skin. There is also a change with age in the barrier function of the skin because fewer lipids (i.e., fats) are present in the top layer of the skin, leading to dryness and roughness. One small open area in the skin from this dryness puts the older adult at risk for infection. With age it takes longer for new epidermal cells to regenerate; thus, wound healing is slower. Collagen and elastin are proteins that constitute most of the skin and keep it strong and stretchable. Although not visible, the dermis has less collagen and elastin with age. The decrease in these proteins contributes to the sagging and wrinkling of the skin that is visible.

Changes in hair in the older adult include graying due to changes in follicular melanocytes (cells responsible for the color of skin and hair) and thinning due to changes in how hair grows over time.

Photoaging refers to the effects of UV exposure on skin. The depth of penetration of UV light depends on the wavelength; shorter wavelengths are more damaging to the skin. Ultraviolet B (UVB; 290 to 320 nm) radiation causes most of the acute and chronic damage. Ultraviolet A (UVA; 320 to 400 nm) also plays an important role because it makes up more of the sunlight that reaches the earth's surface and has greater depth of penetration into the skin.

Photodamaged skin, or skin damaged from the sun, appears wrinkled, coarse, or rough, and has mottled pigmentation (i.e., blotches of darkened areas). Also commonly found due to photodamage are seborrheic keratoses, which are noncancerous growths of the outer layer of skin that vary in color from light tan to black, size range, and have a pasted-on or stuck-on appearance). In addition, freckles, hypopigmentation (areas where the color has faded), and telangiectasias (dilated or easily visible blood vessels on the skin) can all occur from photodamage as can skin cancers. Prevention of photodamage involves the use of broad-spectrum sunscreens that protect against both UVB and UVA radiation as well as avoidance of direct sunlight and use of protective clothing, hats, and sunglasses (see Figure 38.1).

SEBORRHEIC DERMATITIS

Seborrheic dermatitis is a common chronic dermatitis (i.e., inflammation of the skin) characterized by redness and greasy-looking scales in areas rich in sebaceous glands (i.e., small glands in the skin that secrete an oily matter called sebum to lubricate the skin) such as at the hairline (i.e., scalp), on the forehead, and around the nose. Seborrheic dermatitis is frequently seen in those individuals with neurological problems such as Parkinson's disease and more commonly in males than females.

Although the cause of seborrheic dermatitis is unclear, it is thought that the normal yeast that lives on the skin (*Malassezia furfur*) may cause this inflammation of the skin. It is impossible to cure; symptoms are controlled with treatment: medicated shampoos that act against yeast, including selenium sulfide, ketoconazole, and various tar shampoos. In cases of significant inflammation, mild topical corticosteroids such as hydro-

cortisone 1% to 2% can be applied to the skin. Once the dermatitis is under control, the medicated shampoos are used for maintenance.

ROSACEA

Rosacea is a chronic inflammatory skin disease that results in a tendency to blush or flush easily, develop bumps or pus-filled pimples on the face, have dry skin, burning and itching of the eyes, and cause small visible blood vessels to become prominent, eventually causing rhinophyma or bumps on the nose. This is a common condition in fair-skinned persons and affects young to middle-aged as well as older adults. The flushing that occurs can be brought on by sunlight exposure, alcohol, hot beverages, and drugs that cause vasodilatation or widening of the veins. Medications such as oral niacin (for hyperlipidemia) and topical steroids can often induce or worsen rosacea.

Like seborrheic dermatitis, there is no cure for rosacea; treatment is chronic. Individuals with rosacea should avoid skin irritants or strong soaps and cleansers, should reduce sun exposure, and regularly apply sunscreens. Oral antibiotics such as tetracylines (doxy-

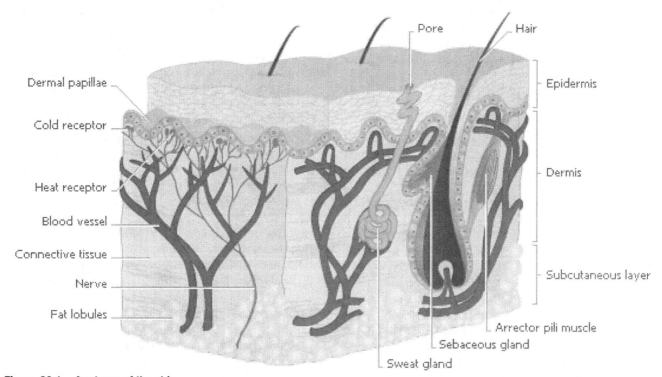

Figure 38.1   Anatomy of the skin.

cycline, minocycline) and erythromycin are used to treat the moderate to severe papular-pustular rosacea. Topical agents such as azelaic acid cream, erythromycin, clindamycin, and metronidazole can be used for mild rosacea or as maintenance once the oral antibiotics are discontinued. Severe rosacea can be treated with oral isotretinoin and in some cases surgical intervention may be needed to scrape off the areas of rosacea.

XEROSIS

Xerosis, or dryness of the skin, occurs commonly in older adults because of the reduced water content and barrier function of the aging epidermis. It is worsened by environmental factors, such as decreased humidity from cold weather or central heating, irritation by hot water, and too frequent washing with harsh soaps and cleansers. Skin findings are often more pronounced on the legs. Varying with the severity of the dryness, xerosis can present as rough, itchy skin or as scales that give the skin a dry, cracked appearance. Therefore, it is helpful to encourage the older adult to use tepid water when bathing and to apply skin lubricants immediately after bathing. Moisturizing agents containing lactic acid or α-hydroxy acids can reduce the roughness and scaliness. When irritation or inflammation is a prominent finding, short-term use of mild topical corticosteroids provides relief.

NEURODERMATITIS

Neurodermatitis is a nonspecific term used to refer to chronic, itchy conditions of unclear cause. It is most common in adults over the age of 60. The skin generally has signs of chronic scratching, such as hyperpigmentation or darkening and lichenification (i.e., leathery thickness) along with redness and scaling. Treatment consists of topical corticosteroids, as well as behavior modification to try and reduce the scratching.

STASIS DERMATITIS

Stasis dermatitis is skin irritation on the lower extremities, generally related to circulatory problems such as chronic venous insufficiency (i.e., changes in the valves of the vein that result in blood pooling in the lower legs and not returning to the heart to be recircu-

lated). It is often accompanied by intense itching and swelling around the ankles. Venous ulcers, especially on the shins or above the ankles, can develop spontaneously just because of the poor circulation in the lower extremities. Support stockings and exercise of the calf muscles to improve venous return are recommended. Walking and pumping (flexing the ankle as if pushing on a gas pedal) the feet are helpful. Topical treatment to relieve the itching should include corticosteroids and emollients. Eucerin, for example, is recommended as a good emollient; it moisturizes with petroleum and mineral oil. The cream version can be rather greasy; the lotion is less so. Petroleum jelly is a low cost alternative.

Sensitization to ingredients in topical medications and emollients, including topical antibiotics, is common. A new lotion or treatment should be tested before the resident uses it liberally. Testing can be done by placing the lotion or treatment on a small area of the skin over a 24-hour period to give the skin some time to react.

VENOUS AND ARTERIAL ULCERS

An ulcer is a wound with loss of epidermal and dermal layers, in contrast to an erosion, which is loss of the epidermal layer only. Chronic leg wounds are defined as open wounds that fail to heal within a period of 6 weeks. Venous disease causes 72% of leg ulcers, 22% have a mixed arterial and venous etiology, and only 6% are due to pure arterial disease. Table 38.1 differentiates between venous and arterial ulcers with regard to common location, drainage differences, and shape.

In addition to direct treatment of the ulcers, the older adult should be encouraged to make some lifestyle changes to prevent worsening of the ulcer or underlying condition and to promote wound healing. For arterial ulcers, exercise, diet low in cholesterol, smoking cessation, weight loss, and better diabetic control should be encouraged. These activities will likewise help vascular ulcers in addition to the use of knee or thigh-high support hose, elevation of the legs when possible, and avoidance of foods and medications that can cause fluid retention (e.g., salt and medication that cause sodium retention or swelling such as nonsteroidal anti-inflammatory medications, anti-epileptic agents, or calcium channel blockers). Wounds that persist and do not heal for months may benefit from further evaluation by wound experts or surgeons. (For information on pressure ulcers, see Chapter 33.)

38.1 | Differentiation Between Venous and Arterial Ulcers

	VENOUS ULCERS	ARTERIAL ULCERS
Comorbid conditions	Varicose veins Venous insufficiency	Peripheral artery disease with poor circulation. Intermittent claudication (i.e., pain in the calf when walking or at rest)
Location	Generally over the shin or above the ankle	Over the toes, foot, heel, or ankle
Shape	Irregular in shape	Punched out circular shape
Wound appearance	Often covered with slough (yellow tissue)	Often covered with slough but also may be necrotic (black, hard tissue)
Pain	Usually without pain	Painful
Swelling	Usually swelling up to the ankle or above	No swelling
Treatment	Compression to decrease the swelling. Occlusive dressings with absorbent properties to manage the drainage and debride slough	Dressings or ointments to debride slough or necrotic tissue

INTERTRIGO

Intertrigo is an inflammation (i.e., rash) of the body folds (adjacent areas of skin). An intertrigo usually develops from the chafing of warm, moist skin in the areas of the inner thighs and genitalia, the armpits, under the breasts, the underside of the belly, behind the ears, and the web spaces between the toes and fingers. It usually appears red and raw-looking, and may also itch, ooze, and be painful. Intertrigos occur more often among overweight individuals, those with diabetes, those restricted to bed rest or diaper use, and those who use medical devices, like artificial limbs, that trap moisture against the skin. Once the irritation occurs, it is not unusual for the individual to develop a secondary candidal or mixed bacterial colonization. Frequent airing of the area, attempts to keep the area dry and clean, and use of topical antifungal powders and creams, such as 2% miconazole powder or nystatin cream or Goldbond Powder constitute the treatment. Occasionally, a very mild topical corticos-

teroid such as 1% to 2% hydrocortisone is needed for a short period to reduce inflammation and irritation (see also the section "Candidiasis" later in this chapter).

BULLOUS PEMPHIGOID

This is a chronic autoimmune blistering disorder characterized by large tense blisters on normal or erythematous skin. They are usually filled with clear fluid but on occasion may be bloody. These blisters can be found anywhere on the body. Though it may last for months to years, bullous pemphigoid is often a self-limited disease. The blisters heal without scar formation. Treatment depends on severity. When the lesions are together in one place such as just on the leg, they may be treated with topical corticosteroids. More extensive disease can be treated with oral corticosteroids, especially for control of acute flare-ups. Because of the adverse effects of corticosteroids, particularly in older adults, local treatment is usually tried first.

PRURITUS

Pruritus, or itching, is a very common skin complaint. Among older adults, pruritus can be very severe at times, compromising quality of life. Although xerosis is the most common cause of pruritus in the older adult, systemic diseases such as kidney disease, chronic liver disease, thyroid disease, anemia, cancers, or drug side effects must also be considered. Generalized pruritus can also be associated with pervasive anxiety disorder, depression, and even psychosis.

Treatment depends on the underlying cause; symptomatic relief can often be achieved with topical corticosteroids, emollients, or menthol in calamine preparations. Oral antihistamines such as Benadryl should be used with caution in older adults as they may cause confusion, dry mouth, and urinary and bowel problems.

PSORIASIS

Psoriasis affects 2% of the population and generally is first noted in individuals in their mid-20s and then again when they are 50 to 60 years of age. There is a genetic predisposition. Psoriasis is a chronic skin disease characterized by scaling and inflammation that results in patches of thick, red skin covered with silvery scales. These patches, sometimes referred to as plaques, usually itch and/or burn. Psoriasis most often occurs on the elbows, knees, scalp, lower back, face, palms, and soles of the feet, but it can affect any skin site. The disease may also affect the fingernails, toenails, and the soft tissues inside the mouth and genitalia. About 15% of people with psoriasis have joint inflammation that produces arthritis symptoms, a condition called psoriatic arthritis.

Treatment generally involves topical ointments such as corticosteroids, vitamin D derivatives (calcipotriene), topical retinoids (tazarotene), salicylic acid, or tar compounds. Some of these treatments may be irritating or messy to apply. Older adults who do not improve with topical treatments may be candidates for options such as phototherapy (i.e., light therapy) or immunosuppressive agents.

HERPES ZOSTER (SHINGLES)

More than two-thirds of reported cases of herpes zoster occur in persons aged 50 years and older. Individuals with herpes zoster are contagious (mostly by direct contact with the blisters) to those who lack immunity but are less contagious to those individuals who had varicella (i.e., chicken pox) virus earlier in their lives. Symptoms can include pain, burning, paresthesia (i.e., numbness), tenderness, pruritus, or hyperesthesia (i.e., increased sensation or sensitivity of the skin) for several days before the rash appears. This pain will be around the affected dermatone (i.e., the area of the skin supplied by nerve fibers originating from a single dorsal nerve root. Shingles will affect just one side of the body.

Ten percent to 15% of cases of herpes zoster occur around the eye; these individuals should be referred to an ophthalmologist to evaluate the resident for potential damage to the eye and altered vision. Pain is the chief complaint; it can precede, occur with the rash, and/or persist after the rash. Pain that persists or appears after the rash has healed or at 30 days after onset of rash is called *post-herpetic neuralgia*. Age is the most significant risk factor; post-herpetic neuralgia occurs in 70% of zoster patients age 70 and older and can be difficult to treat.

Classically, shingles start as small blisters on a red base, with new blisters continuing to form over a period of three to five days. The blisters follow the path of individual nerves that comes out of the spinal cord (called a dermatomal pattern). They will only be present on one side of the body (e.g., the right side of the face). The entire path of the nerve may be involved or there may be areas with blisters and areas without blisters. The vesicles, or blisters, initially start with clear fluid and then over 24 hours become pus filled, then burst, and eventually crust over in 7 to 10 days. The entire course, however, may take three to four weeks from start to finish. Treatment in all residents should be initiated early, within 72 hours of the onset of rash. Antiviral medications such as acyclovir or famciclovir are often prescribed for 7 to 10 days. Early treatment halts progression of disease, increases the rate of clearance of virus from the blisters, decreases the incidence of spread in the individual to other skin areas, and may decrease pain and the incidence of post-herpetic neuralgia. Other treatments are for comfort and include the use of pain medication if needed, dressing changes to the open blisters, wet compresses, and topical antibiotics such as bacitracin to treat secondary bacterial infections in the blisters if this occurs. Long-term pain management may be needed as indicated for those with post-herpetic neuralgia (see Chapter 21, "Chronic Pain and Persistent Pain").

CANDIDIASIS

Factors that contribute to intertrigo also predispose a person to candidiasis or fungal infection. Candidiasis is similar to intertrigo except that there generally are small pustules along the edges of the area of redness and irritation. Candida pustules can also occur on the back of bedridden residents and on other areas prone to moisture. Oral candidiasis or *thrush* may also develop in older adults who use corticosteroid inhalers for pulmonary problems, are on antibiotics or immunosuppressive medications (e.g., prednisone) or among those with diabetes mellitus. Treatment resembles that for intertrigo: keep the moist areas dry, improve hygiene, and treat with topical or oral anticandidal agents such as nystatin or ketoconazole.

SCABIES

Scabies is an infestation with the human mite *Sarcoptes scabiei* that spreads by person-to-person contact and thus can occur in residents in assisted living settings. An adult female mite becomes fertilized on the skin and burrows into the top superficial layer, where she lays eggs. The clinical manifestations occur days to weeks later when the person develops a hypersensitivity reaction to the mite saliva and excretions. Infested people complain of severe pruritus, especially of the hands, armpits, genitalia, and peri-umbilical region. Clinically, erythematous papules (i.e., circumscribed, solid elevation with no visible fluid) and linear burrows (i.e., crooked, raised lines) are observed. Itchiness and scratching can be severe to the point of causing bleeding. Diagnosis is confirmed by a dermatologist by scraping a suspected lesion and finding mite excreta, eggs, or, rarely, the mite itself, under the microscope

An outbreak of scabies should be reported when a facility experiences two or more concurrent cases of scabies affecting residents and/or staff members. Two or more consecutive cases of scabies occurring within 4 to 6 weeks of each other should also be considered to be an outbreak. A person is considered to be no longer able to spread the scabies 24 hours after start of effective therapy. The time between contact with the mite and the appearance of the symptoms of the pruritic rash varies. Symptoms can occur 1 to 4 days following mite infestation. The infested individual may be asymptomatic yet able to transmit the mite to others. After infestation occurs, the mite deposits eggs under the skin of the human host. After larvae hatch from the eggs, they travel to the surface of the skin. Transmission can occur as early as 2 weeks after the original infestation of the individual. While scabies is readily transmissible with skin to skin contact, the mite can only survive in the environment for 48 hours without a human host. The bedding and clothing of an infested individual may contain viable mites, but exposure to a human host must occur within a short period of time for transmission to occur.

In general, vacuuming and general cleanliness should provide adequate environmental control. Fumigation is not necessary; furniture should not be discarded. Clothing or bedding that were used by an infested individual during the 7 days before effective treatment should be laundered and dried with the hot cycle or dry cleaned. Items that cannot be laundered or dry cleaned should be placed in a plastic bag and sealed for 7 days to allow time for mites and eggs to die. During an identified scabies outbreak, staff members who have been providing care to an identified case should not be rotated to other resident care units until 24 hours after completion of the staff member's scabicidal treatment. The resident should also be isolated from other residents for 24 hours.

Treatment, often initiated when there is strong clinical suspicion of infestation, involves eradicating the mite, decreasing the pruritus, and treating any contacts. Topical permethrin 5% is most commonly used. It is applied from the neck to the toes and rinsed off after 8 to 12 hours. This treatment should be repeated in 1 week to prevent development of resistance. Persons who may have been exposed should also be treated. Topical corticosteroids may help to reduce pruritus, but it is important to reassure residents that the itching may persist for weeks or months after the mite infestation is removed.

LOUSE INFESTATIONS

Lice can infest the body (pediculosis corporis), scalp (pediculosis capitis), or pubic hair (pediculosis pubis). With pediculosis corporis or capitis, lice are spread from person to person through physical contact or fomites. Pediculosis pubis is usually spread by sexual contact. In all cases, the complaint is of pruritus of the involved areas, and there can be secondary infection. In cases of pediculosis corporis, the lice feed on the body but live on clothing, where they lay eggs, often near the seams. In cases of pediculosis capitis, the lice lay eggs on the hair, close to the scalp. The eggs (or nits) are visible as white specks stuck on the hair. Treatment involves killing the lice and larvae, treating close contacts, and treating the secondary infection. Pyrethrin or its derivatives (permethrin) can be used as single 10-minute topical treatment for the infected person as well as those who have been exposed. Ideally a second treatment should be done 7 to 10 days after the first treatment to kill newly hatched lice. Combs, brushes, hats, clothing, bedding, and towels (bath, linen) must be washed with hot water. Combing the lice out of the hair regularly is useful. Treatment is ongoing until no further lice are visible in the hair.

BENIGN GROWTHS

Seborrheic Keratoses

Seborrheic keratoses, as described previously, are very common benign growths that present as tan to gray or black waxy or warty papules and plaques. They commonly occur on the trunk and extremities but can be found anywhere on the body. There is no need to remove these growths although they may bother the resident and thus he or she may request surgical removal.

Cherry Angiomas

Cherry angiomas are round to oval, bright red, dome-shaped papules ranging in size from less than 1 mm to several millimeters. They are benign but can bleed when picked at or irritated. There is no need to remove these lesions.

Actinic Keratoses

Actinic keratoses (also known as *solar keratoses*) are lesions caused by chronic UV radiation. They are considered premalignant growths, precursors of squamous cell cancer. The lesion is generally irregular in shape, occasionally scaly, red and either raised (papules) or not raised (macules) on sun exposed areas such as the face, ears, hands and arms. Actinic keratoses are often treated to prevent progression to squamous cell carcinoma. They respond to a variety of treatments, such as cryotherapy with liquid nitrogen (freezing), topical agents such as chemical acids like 5-fluorouracil, or surgical removal. Although cryotherapy treatment for 10 to 15 seconds is very effective, it can be somewhat uncomfortable and can cause pigmentary changes. When several lesions are present in an area, treatment that the older adult can perform independently may be recommended using topical 5-fluorouracil. Treated lesions can appear red and some discomfort might occur.

BASAL CELL CARCINOMA

Basal cell cancer is the most common cancer in the United States. As with other skin cancers, fair-skinned persons with chronic sun exposure are at risk. Most commonly a basal cell cancer appears as waxy papules with overlying telangiectasias. Some basal cell carcinomas have an open area in the middle and what is best described as rolled edges. These growths may or may not be dark in color. Treatment of basal cell carcinoma is surgical excision. Some basal cell carcinomas, particularly those located in cosmetically important areas, those that are nodular or morpheaform, and those that are recurrent should be excised by use of Mohs micrographic surgery to ensure adequate excision and tissue sparing. Like squamous cell carcinomas, basal cell carcinomas occurring in poor surgical candidates can also be treated with ablative methods, such as cryosurgery, radiation, and curettage with electrodessication.

SQUAMOUS CELL CARCINOMA

Squamous cell carcinoma is the second most common form of skin cancer. It affects people in mid- to late-life and occurs most commonly on sun-exposed areas. This carcinoma causes local tissue destruction if not treated. They have a low risk (but greater risk than basal cell carcinomas) to spread, known as metastasis. These growths present as chronic red papules with scaling, crusting, or ulceration. The person may tell you that the area simply won't heal. Treatment consists of surgical excision.

MELANOMA

The incidence of melanoma continues to increase; it affects all adult age groups. Risk factors for melanoma include very fair skin type, family history, and sunlight exposure, particularly intermittent blistering sunburns in childhood. Melanomas are usually asymptomatic; thus, regular skin examinations and early recognition are key for favorable prognosis. A new pigmented skin lesion or a change in the color, size, surface, or borders of a preexisting mole should be suspected for melanoma and biopsied. A useful mnemonic is ABCD: Asymmetry, Borders, Color, Diameter. Treatment consists of surgical excision and, depending on depth, may also involve sentinel node mapping and biopsy, lymph node dissection, or adjuvant therapy. Sentinel lymph node mapping is a method of determining whether the cancer has metastasized (spread) beyond the primary tumor and into the lymph system.

RESOURCES

Davies, A. (2008). Management of dry skin conditions in older people. *British Journal of Community Nursing, 13*(6), 250, 252, 254–257.

Lawton, S. (2007). Addressing the skin-care needs of the older person. *British Journal of Community Nursing, 12*(5), 203–204, 206,

Martin, E. S., & Elewski, B. E. (2002). Cutaneous fungal infections in the elderly. *Clinical Geriatric Medicine, 18*(1), 59–75.

Weinberg, J. M. (2007). Herpes zoster: Epidemiology, natural history, and common complications. *Journal of American Academy of Dermatology, 57*(6 Suppl.), S130–S105.

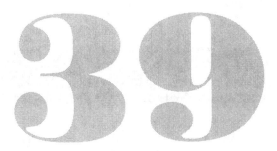

Oral Diseases and Disorders

Kenneth Shay, Bradford L. Picot, and Sandra J. Fulton Picot

The oral structures are used to initiate food intake, produce speech, and protect the digestive tract. Dysfunction and disease in the mouth can profoundly affect an older adult's overall health and social functioning. Evidence suggests a link between periodontal disease, diabetes, heart disease, and other systemic diseases in older individuals. Findings prevalent in older adults (e.g., decay, missing teeth, periodontal disease, and salivary hypofunction) are not normal; professional dental care should be provided.

AGING OF THE TEETH

Most age-related changes in teeth are subtle (see Table 39.1) but become significant in the presence of environmental factors or disease.

Moreover, older adults seem to be less sensitive to sensations in their mouth that might drive them to see a dentist. More likely, older adults come to the dentist complaining of food caught in carious lesions (i.e., cavities) or soft-tissue lacerations caused by fractured teeth rather than by pain from the dental disease itself. This might be explained by the diminished *pulp space* commonly seen among older adults.

The nerves and blood vessels of the tooth are located in the pulp; these nerves are responsible for the sensations that are felt in the tooth. The *dentin layer* of the tooth covers the pulp; it consists of tubules that communicate with the outside of the tooth as they pass through the enamel or outermost layer. Over time, odontoblastic cells within the pulp continue to generate dentin, thereby reducing the number and diameter of dentinal tubules. These processes decrease the communication between the nerves and the outside of the tooth as a result of which the older adult is less sensitive to stimuli in the oral cavity or abutting the teeth, such as temperature. Other changes in the teeth are staining, chipping, and cracking.

DENTAL DECAY

Dental *caries*, or tooth decay, occurs when oral bacteria break down enamel and dentin, the outer layers of the tooth. This can occur throughout life. Recurrent caries is decay that occurs in areas that were previously treated (i.e., a previous filling or crown).

Older adults usually have more restored teeth (that are usually older and more extensive) and thus are more likely to have recurrent caries than younger adults. In addition, older adults tend to have more caries of the root surfaces because gingival, or gum, recession decreases the amount of gum tissue over the tooth, thereby leaving a larger area of tooth exposed to breakdown from bacteria. Caries generally do not result

| Summary of Common Oral Health Changes Associated with Aging and Nursing Interventions |

ORAL CAVITY COMPONENT	COMMON CHANGES	NURSING INTERVENTIONS
Teeth	Plaque and calculus (hard yellowish deposit on teeth that is composed of mineral salts, food, and other debris that has hardened over time).	On admission, ask resident when he or she last saw a dentist; urge dental visits every 6 months.
		Older adults with decreased vision, use of their hands, or flexibility of the upper extremity may need help with care of the teeth and mouth.
		Routine brushing with toothpaste or rinses containing fluoride and plaque removal properties; flossing; gently brush tongue and roof of mouth after breakfast and before bedtime.
		Limit sticky foods (e.g., cakes).
	Teeth darken with aging, appearing yellow gray.	Use over-the-counter whiteners as stain removers. If ineffective, urge dental visits at least every 6 months for stain removal.
	Diminished tooth sensitivity; diminished susceptibility to effects of bacterial metabolites; increased tooth fragility leading to brittle, cracked, or chipped teeth.	Teach independent older adults or nurses of dependent older adults to check their mouths for asymptomatic dental problems during regular mouth care (after breakfast and before bedtime). Urge dental visits every 6 months.
	Normal age changes that result in increasing risk of asymptomatic dental problems including dental caries (cavities).	As above.
Edentulism (total tooth loss)	Total tooth loss related to poor socioeconomic status, poor oral hygiene, dental caries, periodontal diseases, oral cancer.	Routine brushing and flossing of teeth and/ or brushing tongue and roof of mouth (in cases in which there are not teeth); conduct regular inspections of mouth; urge regular dental visits every 6 months.
		Dentures improve speech and shape of face but may not improve chewing and eating. Clean dentures after each meal and soak in disinfectant several times per week; remove dentures for several hours each day, usually during sleep.
		Inspect mouth for poorly fitting dentures. Refer to dentist for adjustment or replacement.
		Implants may be helpful as they can be used to attach dentures.

(continued)

39.1 | Summary of Common Oral Health Changes Associated with Aging and Nursing Interventions *(continued)*

ORAL CAVITY COMPONENT	COMMON CHANGES	NURSING INTERVENTIONS
Gingiva (gum) and part of the periodontium	Gingival recession (receding gum) exposes the roots and results in exposed nerves thus increasing sensitivity to extreme food and liquid temperatures; increased susceptibility to dental caries. Gingival recession is caused by too much pressure on the handle of the tooth brush, pushing the gum backward from the teeth. Some medications can cause this as well.	When brushing their teeth, teach older adults to lighten their grip on the handle of their tooth brushes and use soft bristle tooth brushes.

Refer to dentist for periodontal disease screening. |
| Oral mucosa | Thinner, less hydrated; less elastic; slower healing and subject to more injuries; increased risk of infection. | Oral screenings for open areas and any other abnormalities by older adults or care provider after breakfast and bedtime tooth brushing. |
| Periodontium (consists of the tissues that surround and support the teeth, including the gum) | Buildup of plaque and tartar may lead to bleeding gums, less support surrounding teeth, malposition, loosening of teeth with eventual loss of teeth; bone and gum recession resulting in loose teeth and increased susceptibility to dental caries. Smoking and poor oral hygiene increase the risk. | Assess if older adult is a smoker and inspect mouth at admission and periodically.

Attention to oral hygiene. More frequent dental recalls. |
| Orofacial musculature | Atrophy or wasting of the muscles of the face and mouth result in slower chewing and increase risk of choking. | Urge older adults to cut their foods into smaller pieces and take extra time to chew completely before swallowing. |
| Xerostomia | Subjective feeling of dry mouth (not a normal part of aging) related mostly to medications (see text examples). Also, blocked salivary ducts, systemic disorders are causes.

With a dry mouth, there is an increased risk of dry and irritated soft tissues in the mouth, sores on the tongue, decreased antimicrobial activity, diminished moistures, caries, periodontal disease, fungal infection, burning pain, and difficulty with chewing and swallowing, taste changes, dental caries, and difficulty in wearing dentures. | Suggest to prescriber that medications that contribute to feeling of dry mouth be decreased, discontinued, or substituted, if possible.

Increase attention to oral hygiene and limited sugar in the diet; drink extra fluids (if not contraindicated); recommend saliva substitutes, oral lubricants, xylitol gum, and sugarless candy.

Screened and treated by dentist; daily application of fluoride in the form of PrevDent, 1% to 2% acidulated fluoride gel or .5% neutral sodium fluoride gel. |

(continued)

39.1

Summary of Common Oral Health Changes Associated
with Aging and Nursing Interventions *(continued)*

ORAL CAVITY COMPONENT	COMMON CHANGES	NURSING INTERVENTIONS
Oral lesions: Cancer	Early stage, often asymptomatic, but varies; appears as painless red, white (leukoplakia represents malignant or premalignant < 10% of the time), or mixed red and white (erythroplakia) areas of the oral mucosa that may be ulcerated or indurated; advanced stage symptomatic; increased risk with age, tobacco, and alcohol use; peaks around 65–74, but 10 years earlier among African Americans.	Early diagnosis is critical to survival. Teach older adult the risk of oral cancer especially with smoking and alcohol use. Look underneath the tongue, back and floor of the mouth, and lips. If the lesions do not disappear in 14 days or increase in size, refer to dentists who specialize in oral pathology. Oral cancer screening annually by dentist.
Oral lesions: HIV infection related	Oral lesions occur along the gum line. Oral (mucosal) ulcers are usually the earliest sign of HIV infection. Hairy leukoplakia and oral candidiasis correlate with low CD4 counts; hairy leukoplakia starts out as corrugated white lesions along the lateral border of the tongue and buccal mucosa. Kaposi sarcoma starts early as asymptomatic small purple/red macule (i.e., a flat lesion). It later increases in size, becomes more raised, painful, and prone to ulceration.	Refer resident to dentist or oral pathologist.

in pain in older adults and therefore may become advanced before discovery, often resulting in destruction of the tooth (i.e., inability to preserve it).

Advanced caries commonly results in necrosis (dead tissue) of the remaining pulp, which usually leads to an acute or chronic dental abscess. Even if these infections do not cause pain, they should not be ignored because the bacteria can spread to other parts of the body, causing infections in joint replacements or in the fluid around the heart.

The risk factors for dental caries are the same at any age. Older adults, however, tend to be at greater risk for developing caries because they tend to have poor oral hygiene related to decreased visual acuity, impaired manual dexterity, decreased upper-extremity flexibility, decreased saliva, diets with high levels of concentrated sweets (cake, cookies, candy), limited lifelong exposure to fluoride, and fewer dental visits, overall. Less than one-third of older adults have annual dental visits, and half have not seen a dentist in 5 years.

Prevention of caries requires daily oral hygiene with a fluoride toothpaste, flossing, mouth rinse, limited sugar intake, and regular dental examinations. Treatment of dental caries includes topical high-potency fluoride for remineralization (i.e., strengthening of the tooth), removal of the caries and replacement of removed tooth structure with fillings or crowns. A useful preventive strategy includes regular use of the topical antiseptic agent chlorhexidine gluconate, which is available as a .12% mint flavored oral rinse. Twice daily rinses reduce gingivitis (i.e., inflammation of the gums) and activation of bacteria that cause caries. When caries involves the dental pulp (i.e., the nerves of the tooth), root canal treatment becomes necessary, which in turn usually requires reinforcement of the remaining tooth structure with a crown.

DISEASES OF THE PERIODONTIUM

The most common form of periodontal disease is *gingivitis*: an inflammatory reaction of the gums to plaque (i.e., bacteria buildup) in the mouth, presenting as swelling of the gums and light bleeding on brushing. Gingivitis develops more rapidly in older adults than in younger adults. Fortunately, the changes that occur with gingivitis are rapidly reversible following removal of the plaque deposited on the teeth. If the inflammatory process is not treated it will progress to *periodontitis*: destruction of the hard and soft tissues around the teeth (periodontium) that can ultimately result in loss of teeth. In addition to age and poor oral health, smoking increases the risk of periodontitis.

The prevention and control of periodontal disease revolves around daily oral care: tooth brushing and flossing to remove bacterial plaque on the teeth, brushing of the tongue, and regular dental evaluations (every 6 to 12 months). Once periodontal disease has been discovered and is being treated, it is important to see the dentist every 3–4 months for regular cleanings. Topical antibiotics (chlorhexidine, tetracycline) and systemic antibiotics (minocycline, metronidazole) are increasingly used to treat periodontal disease.

EDENTULISM (ABSENCE OF TEETH)

Advanced age was once considered synonymous with the need for false teeth; this stereotype is fading. Nevertheless, removal of one or more teeth in an older adult is common. It may be easier and less costly for the older adult to have a loose, painful tooth removed than to undergo expensive and lengthy restorative dental treatment.

There are unique problems, however, associated with being edentulous. Functionally, the teeth aid in mastication (chewing) and enunciation (speaking). Aesthetically, the teeth support the lips and cheeks and keep the nose and chin at a fixed distance apart from each other. Facial appearance is dramatically changed when all teeth are gone because of the lack of tissue support and diminished vertical height in the lower half of the face. Chewing ability is severely compromised, yet the impact on nutritional intake is difficult to characterize. A longitudinal study using diet diaries demonstrated a relationship between loss of teeth and increased carbohydrate intake, decreased protein intake, and diminished intake of selected micronutrients.

Removable dentures to replace all or some lost teeth can aid in speech and restore the shape of the face. It is less certain that dentures restore the ability to chew. The data indicate that dentures restore, on average, only about 15% of the chewing ability associated with natural dentition. The range of foods regularly eaten by denture wearers is significantly restricted in comparison with the dietary range of persons with natural teeth. Denture wearers also have to chew more times before they swallow food, and they swallow their food in larger particles (i.e., boluses). Older adults who hope that dentures will restore oral intake in cases of malnutrition or unexplained weight loss are usually disappointed. Those who hope for a more socially acceptable appearance, clearer speech, and modest improvement in chewing comfort and range of dietary choices are more likely to be satisfied with dentures, however.

Dentures often are a considerable source of discomfort, dysfunction, and embarrassment for older people. They should be kept clean by removing and cleaning them after meals, and soaking them in a commercial disinfectant several times each week; they should be out of the mouth several hours each day. The best time is during sleep, when there is less salivation. Saliva helps to keep bacteria from growing. Therefore, during the night, with less saliva, there is a risk of greater bacterial growth than would occur during the day. Fractured or broken dentures, as well as denture looseness or soreness, should be brought to a dentist's attention without delay. However, since neither dental services nor dentures are currently covered by Medicare and fewer than 10% of older Americans have private dental insurance, many older adults continue to use inadequate or even damaging dentures. (Some states' Medicaid programs cover dentures, including replacement dentures if lost or damaged.)

Another more recent treatment for edentulism is *dental implants*. Dental implants are a titanium fixture that is surgically placed in the bone of the jaw (alveolar bone). It usually takes 4–6 months for the implant to grow into the bone and become stable. Dental implant treatment is a long, protracted process, is expensive, not Medicare covered, and variably covered by dental insurance plans. Implants have been used to restore single missing teeth or as attachments on which to snap dentures. As opposed to the 15% masticatory function restored with dentures, implants used with dentures (overdentures) restore 60% to 80% chewing function. Implants, unlike dentures, are only removable by a dentist.

SALIVARY FUNCTION IN AGING

Saliva is critical for protecting the tissues of the oral cavity and maintaining tissue function in speech, mastication, swallowing, and taste perception. It helps to control the environment of the mouth (the acidity) and contains a wide spectrum of antimicrobial factors, lubricates the oral surfaces, and keeps the taste pores open and working. Saliva also has remineralization properties helpful in preventing decay. Complaints of *xerostomia* (i.e., a subjective feeling of a dry mouth) are very common among older adults. Leading causes are commonly prescribed drugs that happen to have this adverse effect (i.e., anticholinergic drugs such as tricyclic antidepressants, opioids, antihistamines, and anti-arrhythmic agents, sedatives, tranquilizers, antihypertensives, and antiparkinsonian drugs).

Untreated xerostomia predisposes the individual to dry tissue of the mouth that can crack and bleed, fissures on the tongue, decreased antimicrobial activity, diminished lubrication, caries, periodontal disease, fungal infections, burning pain, and difficulty with mastication and swallowing. Treatment may include saliva substitutes, oral lubricants, and/or xylitol gum and candy (sugar free gum and candy), which provide symptom relief but do not have the protective properties of saliva. Daily application of fluoride in the form of PrevDent, 1% to 2% acidulated fluoride gel, or .5% neutral sodium fluoride gel can also help with xerostomia. Residents should be told that they are at increased risk for oral disease and should particularly try to limit sugar in their diet and optimize their daily oral hygiene practices.

MEDICATIONS

In addition to the medications predisposing the older adult to xerostomia, older adults take other meds that compromise dental health (see Table 39.2).

Residents with a history of stroke might be taking blood thinners such as Coumadin, warfarin, and Plavix. These meds require special titration if residents are in need of dental surgery such as extractions, periodontal surgery, or implants. A side effect of bisphosphonates, often taken by residents with osteoporosis or with weakened bone structure, includes osteonecrosis (i.e., death of the bone) of the jaw—often precipitated by surgery or severe infection in the oral cavity. While this can occur in other parts of the body, the jaw has a high rate of bone breakdown, providing a greater opportunity for osteonecrosis to occur. It is *very* important to send a list of the resident's medications with him or her when going to the dentist.

ORAL MUCOSAL PROBLEMS

Squamous cell cancer accounts for 96% of oral and oropharyngeal malignancies (see Table 39.1). Oral cancer is strongly linked with the use of tobacco, particularly cigarettes. Lip cancer has a strong correlation with pipe and cigar smoking. Alcohol enhances the effects of tobacco and thus increases the risk of cancer when both drugs are used regularly.

Early oral malignancies appear as painless red, white, or mixed red and white areas in the mouth that may be ulcerated. Red and mixed lesions (termed *erythroplakia*) should be biopsied immediately. White lesions (*leukoplakia*) are malignant or premalignant less than 10% of the time and generally can just be monitored to see if they disappear in approximately 14 days.

Other warning signs of oral cancers include soreness or lump in the throat, difficulty chewing, difficulty swallowing or moving the jaw or tongue, hoarseness, swelling of the jaw, numbness of the tongue or mouth, or ear pain. The treatment of localized oral squamous cell carcinoma is generally surgical, although large but localized tumors can be managed with radioactive implants.

Oral candidiasis, a fungal infection of the mouth, presents as diffuse erythema (i.e., redness), cracking at the corners of the mouth, curdlike white patches, or erythema in denture areas. It can cause taste dysfunction, burning, itching, and pain. Older adults are particularly susceptible to candidiasis because of denture use, salivary hypofunction, the prevalence of diabetes mellitus, and the use of antibiotics for pulmonary and urologic diseases. Residents who use inhaled corticosteroids (e.g., Spiriva) also are at higher risk and should be instructed to rinse out their mouths after using the inhaler. Management involves, first, excluding the cause of the disease (if possible), followed by administration of topical or systemic antifungal agents and optimal oral and denture hygiene.

Burning mouth syndrome is a chronic oral-facial pain disorder usually without other clinical signs. It typically affects women age 50 or over, with a particularly high attack rate among Asian Americans and Native Americans. The pain most commonly affects the

39.2 | Drugs That Cause Problems With Gustation (Taste), Olfaction (Smell), and Xerostomia (Dry Mouth)

GUSTATION

Acyclovir	Enalapril	Pentoxifylline
Allopurinol	Ethacrynic acid	Phenytoin
Amiloride	Ethambutol	Procainamide
Amitriptyline	Fenoprofen	Prochlorperazine
Amphotericin B	Gemfibrozil	Promethazine
Ampicillin	Hydrochlorothiazide	Propafenone
Baclofen	Imipramine	Propranolol
Buspirone	Labetalol	Ritonavir
Captopril	Levamisole	Saquinavir
Chlorpheniramine	Lomefloxacin	Sulfamethoxazole
Desipramine	Mexiletine	Sulindac
Doxepin	Nabumetone	Terfenadine
Dexamethasone	Nelfinavir	Tetracyclines
Diclofenac	Ofloxacin	Trifluoperazine
Dicyclomine	Nifedipine	Zidovudine
Diltiazem	Pentamidine	

OLFACTION

Amitriptyline	Enalapril	Pentamidine
Amphetamine	Flunisolide	Pirbuterol
Beclomethasone dipropionate	Flurbiprofen	Propafenone
Cocaine	Hydromorphone	Tocainide
Codeine	Levamisole	Zalcitabine
Dexamethasone	Morphine	

(continued)

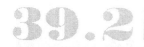

Drugs That Cause Problems With Gustation (Taste), Olfaction (Smell), and Xerostomia (Dry Mouth) *(continued)*

XEROSTOMIA (DRY MOUTH)

Anti-arrhythmic	Anticholinergics	Antidepressants
Antihistamines	Antihypertensives	Antiparkinsonian
Multiple drug interactions	Opioids	Sedatives

Nonpharmacologic Causes of Taste and Smell Problems in Older Adults

GUSTATORY DYSFUNCTION

Oral causes

   Burning mouth syndrome

   Candidiasis

   Laceration

   Malignancy

   Salivary hypofunction

   Therapeutic irradiation of head

   Thermal or chemical burn

Other causes

   Alzheimer's disease, other neurodegenerative disorders

   Central nervous system tumor

   Endocrinopathies (e.g., diabetes mellitus, Cushing's syndrome, adrenocortical insufficiency, hypothyroidism)

   Head trauma

   Nutritional deficiencies (vitamin B_{12}, zinc)

   Psychiatric disorder

   Stroke

(continued)

39.3 | Nonpharmacologic Causes of Taste and Smell Problems in Older Adults *(continued)*

OLFACTORY DYSFUNCTION

Upper aerodigestive and respiratory causes

    Dental infection

    Periodontal disease

    Poor oral hygiene, including poor denture hygiene

    Sinusitis

    Tobacco smoking or use of nasal snuff

    Tumor of airway or sinus

    Upper respiratory infection (bacterial or viral)

Other causes

    Alzheimer's disease, other neurodegenerative disorders

    Central nervous system tumor

    Exposure to volatile or particulate toxins

    Head trauma

    Nutritional deficiencies (niacin, zinc)

    Psychiatric disorder

    Stroke

lips, tongue, and palate (i.e., roof of the mouth). Multiple causes have been suggested, including xerostomia, denture use, candidiasis, nutritional deficiencies, and psychiatric disorders. Treatment is generally based on identifying the underlying cause and implementing a specific treatment to relieve the symptoms. For example, if candidiasis seems to be the cause, this is treated with antifungal medications.

TASTE PERCEPTION

The sense of taste might be more accurately termed *flavor*—that is, the full range of sensations that accompany eating, including temperature, texture, sound, and smell in addition to the perception of sweet, salt, sour, and bitter. Flavor perception is prone to impairment in the older adult because of changes in smell, sensations in the mouth, saliva production, and the presence of dentures, which present physical and temperature barriers to the food the individual is trying to taste. Flavor-enhancement strategies have positive effects on both food preference and caloric intake among frail older adults. The subjective perception of saltiness and sweetness decreases with age and may result in the increasing use of salt or eating particularly salty or sweet foods. There are many causes for the loss of taste (see Table 39.3). Some drugs have no primary effect on taste but cause diminished saliva flow that causes impaired taste perception.

RESOURCES

Angular chelitis in adults: Condition, treatment, and pictures—an overview. (2008). Retrieved October 30, 2008, from http://www.visualdxhealth.com/adult/angularCheilitisPerleche.htm

Detecting oral cancer: A guide for health care professionals. (2009). Retrieved October 31, 2008, from http://www.nidcr.nih.gov/OralHealth/Topics/OralCancer/DetectingOralCancer.htm

Helgeson, M.J., Smith, B.J., Johnsen, M., & Ebert, C. (2002). Dental considerations for the frail elderly. *Special Care in Dentistry, 22,* 40S–55S.

Little, J.W., Miller, C., Rhodus, N., & Falace, D. (2002). Dental management of older adults. In *Dental management of the medically compromised patient* (6th ed.). St. Louis, MO: Mosby.

McCorkle, W. (2006). Scientific sleuths: The art of the oral pathologist. *North Carolina Dental Review, 23,* 7–11.

Schiffman, S.S., & Zervakis, J. (2002). Taste and smell perception in the elderly: Effect of medications and disease. *Advances in Food and Nutrition Research, 44,* 247–346.

Shay, K. (2002). Infectious complications of dental and periodontal diseases in the elderly population. *Clinical Infectious Diseases, 34,* 1215–1223.

Respiratory Diseases and Disorders

E. Wesley Ely and Barbara Resnick

Normal changes that occur with aging in pulmonary function are a decrease in the size of the airways and decrease in the older adult's ability to expand his or her lungs because of kyphoscoliosis (i.e., curvature of the spine and other bony changes). Pulmonary function tests reveal a decline of forced vital capacity (i.e., total amount of air forced out of the lungs) and forced expiratory volume (i.e., total amount of air forced out of the lungs in a 1-second period). Table 40.1 describes various pulmonary function tests and anticipated results in older adults without pulmonary disease.

COMMON RESPIRATORY SYMPTOMS AND COMPLAINTS

Older adults may not report feeling short of breath because they think this is a normal symptom associated with aging. It is also commonly associated with being deconditioned, or in poor physical condition, because of lack of exercise and physical activity. These individuals adjust their activity level to compensate for the changes in their pulmonary function. Evaluation may indicate abnormalities such as asthma, emphysema, or pulmonary fibrosis, or a combination of these disorders.

Dyspnea

Dyspnea, a subjective sensation of feeling short of breath, becomes prominent in lung diseases such as chronic obstructive pulmonary disease (COPD) and pulmonary fibrosis. Importantly, the level of dyspnea is the best predictor of quality of life, yet it does not correlate with either oxygenation or pulmonary function tests. A resident who complains of dyspnea needs evaluation, especially if this is new in onset or worse than the resident's baseline. If possible, *pulse oximetry* should be done to determine if the individual has sufficient oxygen; levels of 90 or above are considered normal. In addition, counting respirations at rest—and with activity—will further help determine if the symptom of dyspnea is indicative of an acute medical problem. Respirations greater than 20 (per minute) when sitting should be reported to the resident's primary health care provider. However, respirations in the 35 to 45 range during physical activity can be considered a normal response to exertion. Common causes of dyspnea in older adults include COPD, cardiac disease, asthma, interstitial lung disease, and deconditioning.

Chronic Cough

Fortunately, most people can be reassured that chronic cough, though particularly annoying, usually has a

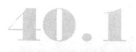

40.1 | Description of Pulmonary Function Tests and Results

ABBREVIATION	NAME	DESCRIPTION
FVC	Forced vital capacity	The total amount of air that can be forcibly blown out after full inspiration; measured in liters.
FEV_1	Forced expiratory volume in 1 second	The amount of air that can be forcibly blown out in one second; measured in liters. Along with FVC, this test is considered one of the primary indicators of lung function.
FEV_1/FVC	FEV1%	The ratio of FEV_1 to FVC. In healthy adults it should be approximately 75%–80%.
PEF	Peak expiratory flow	The speed of the air moving out of the lungs at the beginning of the expiration; measured in liters per second.
FET	Forced expiratory time	A measurement, in seconds, of the duration of the expiration.
TV	Tidal volume	The specific volume of air that is drawn into and then expelled out of the lungs.
MVV	Maximum voluntary ventilation	The maximum amount of air that can be inhaled and exhaled in one minute; measured in liters/minute.

benign cause. By far, the most common causes of chronic cough are postnasal drip, asthma, and gastroesophageal reflux. These three diagnoses account for over 90% of the causes identified in most series. As such, a reasonable approach to the treatment of chronic cough is empiric treatment for these conditions. Not infrequently, a combination of these conditions may be causative and require treatment for multiple causes when single therapies are ineffective. Less common yet important diagnostic considerations of cough in older adults include drug effects (e.g., angiotensin-converting enzyme inhibitors), heart failure, chronic cough after viral upper respiratory tract infection or secondary bacterial infections, recurrent aspiration, or cancer.

Wheezing

Wheezing is generally believed to be due to asthma when noted in younger individuals. In older adults, however, there can be many other causes of wheezing: postnasal drip, heart failure, pulmonary edema, or airway hyperresponsiveness as a result of chronic bronchitis.

MAJOR PULMONARY DISEASES IN OLDER PERSONS

Asthma

After childhood, there is a second peak in the prevalence of asthma after age of 65: 5% to 10% of older adults are diagnosed with adult-onset asthma. The rate of death from asthma among older adults has increased and now accounts for up to 45% of all asthma deaths. Treatment of asthma in older adults may be challenging because of their difficulty with peak expiratory flow monitoring and correct activation of the metered-dose inhaler. Neurologic, muscular, and arthritic diseases in older adults can also lead to suboptimal timing and are a barrier to the coordination needed for correct use of inhalers.

Inhaled corticosteroids (or other controller drugs such as leukotriene receptor antagonists) represent the mainstay of therapy in older adults. Prescribing the lowest effective dose and regular rinsing of the mouth after use of the inhaler can help prevent fungal infections. Inhaled short-acting beta (β)-agonists are used to relieve symptoms of shortness of breath on an as-needed basis.

Chronic Obstructive Pulmonary Disease

Approximately 15 million people in the United States have COPD; it is the fourth most common cause of death after heart disease, cancer, and stroke. Prevalence and mortality rate from COPD is increasing, especially among older adults. Wheezing is commonly associated with COPD, as is a barrel-shaped chest. Pulmonary function test results indicate a forced expiratory time of greater than 9 seconds.

Daily drug therapy for COPD consists of a β-agonist, ipratropium bromide or tiotropium, or both drugs in combination. For more severe disease, long-acting β-agonists are added. For example, salmeterol, used with a combined albuterol and ipratropium bromide metered-dose inhaler, can achieve improved adherence and long-term control by reducing the number of inhalers by one (i.e., the resident will use only the long-acting inhaler and the combination short-acting inhaler rather than three inhalers).

It is not generally recommended that treatment includes oral steroids. They may, however, be used during acute events such as when the resident has an upper respiratory infection superimposed on the COPD. There is generally no benefit to keeping the person on steroids for longer than 14 days. It is estimated, however, that possibly 5% to 10% of individuals benefit from long-term use of corticosteroids. There are significant risks, however, with prolonged use, including peptic ulcer disease, hypertension, cataracts, diabetes mellitus, osteoporosis, psychosis, seizures, poor wound healing, and infections.

Most individuals with COPD have a history of smoking; many may still be smoking. Smoking cessation at any age slows the decline in lung disease. Encouraging either a decrease or complete cessation of smoking is useful even for the oldest-old person (see Chapter 19,

"Prevention"). Residents with COPD should be encouraged to engage in physical activity to build their lung capacity and the efficiency of their cardiovascular system.

Pulmonary Fibrosis

Pulmonary fibrosis involves scarring of the lung, caused by environmental factors such as smoking, genetic factors, autoimmune disease (e.g., rheumatoid arthritis), and/or certain medications (e.g., amiodorone). The air sacs (i.e., alveoli) of the lungs gradually become replaced by fibrotic tissue. When the scarring occurs, the tissue becomes thicker, causing an irreversible loss of the tissue's ability to transfer oxygen into the bloodstream. Incidence of pulmonary fibrosis is increasing in older adults. Residents with pulmonary fibrosis may complain of dyspnea (often unrecognized because of a decrease in the activity level on the part of the resident) and cough. *Clubbing*, a thickening of the flesh under the toenails and fingernails, is often present. The nail curves downward, similar to the shape of the round part of an upside-down spoon. Treatment, which may include oral steroids, is generally based on the resident's symptoms.

Pulmonary Thromboembolism

The incidence of pulmonary thromboembolism increases in older adults. Age-specific risk factors include hypercoagulability (i.e., increased ability to develop a blood clot due to increases in clotting factors in the blood), a diagnosis of cancer, decreased mobility (due to stroke, heart failure, or arthritis), blood vessel injury (due to trauma such as a needle stick), or varicosities. Symptoms include low-grade fever, evidence or complaint of dyspnea, chest pain particularly when breathing in, confusion, slight elevation in white blood cell count, anxiety, and a sense of impending death. When a clot is identified, treatment focuses around anticoagulation; this can be done in the assisted living community if there are professional health care staff available to facilitate management and oversight of treatment. Anticoagulation therapy (warfarin) should continue for at least 6 months. (For information on pneumonia, see Chapter 41, "Infectious Diseases"; for information on lung cancer, see Chapter 51, "Oncology.")

RESOURCES

Alexander, J. L., Phillips, W. T., & Wagner, C. L. (2008). The effect
    of strength training on functional fitness in older patients with

chronic lung disease enrolled in pulmonary rehabilitation. *Rehabilitation Nursing, 33*(3), 91–97.

Centers for Disease Control and Prevention. (2008). Deaths from chronic obstructive pulmonary disease—United States, 2000–2005. *Morbidity Mortality Weekly Report, 57*(45), 1229–1232.

Knight, J., & Nigam, Y. (2008). Exploring the anatomy and physiology of ageing. Part 2—the respiratory system. *Nursing Times, 104*(32), 24–25.

Masotti, L. (2008). Diagnosis and treatment of acute pulmonary thromboembolism in the elderly: Clinical practice and implications for nurses. *Journal of Emergency Nursing, 34*(4), 330–339.

Schofield, I., Kerr, S., & Tolson, D. (2008). An exploration of the smoking-related health beliefs of older people with chronic obstructive pulmonary disease. *Journal of Clinical Nursing, 16*(9), 1726–1735.

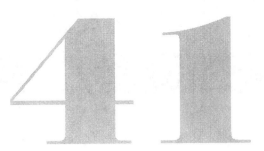

Infectious Diseases

Kevin Paul High and Barbara Resnick

Infection is the major cause of mortality in 40% of those age 65 years and older. It is also a significant cause of morbidity in older adults, often exacerbating underlying illness or leading to hospitalization. Further, because of their increased susceptibility to infection, older adults are likely to succumb to resistant infections. This chapter explores the biological, cultural, and societal factors that influence susceptibility to infection, the presentation of disease, and the management of infections in older adults.

PREDISPOSITION TO INFECTION

Fundamental alterations in the immune response occur with aging in large measure because of comorbidities but also because of age-related declines in immunity, a phenomenon known as *immune senescence* (Table 41.1). The main features of immune senescence are depressed T-cell responses and T-cell–macrophage interactions. Clinically, this results in a delayed hypersensitivity response and a decreased response to infectious organisms.

Although age itself influences immune function, comorbidities have the greatest impact on immune function. For example, reduced skin integrity and diminished cough or gag reflexes are normal age-related changes and decrease older adults' ability to fight infection. If the older individual also has chronic obstructive pulmonary disease, in which there is decreased ability to clear infectious particles and to destroy them at the alveolar areas (i.e., air sacs in the lungs), the risk of getting a lower respiratory tract infection will be even greater in comparison to older adults with age changes

alone. Comorbid diseases also indirectly complicate infections in elderly persons. For example, community-acquired pneumonia in otherwise healthy people under age 50 is typically treated on an outpatient basis and rarely causes mortality. In an older adult, however, community-acquired pneumonia in addition to multiple comorbid conditions, such as stroke or Parkinson's disease and congestive heart failure, increase the morbidity and mortality associated with the pneumonia.

A major influence on immune function in the older person is nutritional status. Global (protein and calorie) undernutrition is present in approximately 11% of older adults. Even mildly undernourished older adults (i.e., those with a serum albumin of 3.0 to 3.5 g/dL) have evidence of immune compromise. Nutritional interventions may boost immune function in some older adults, but this remains controversial.

Institutional/residential settings (e.g., assisted living communities) or group housing settings place older adults at increased risk for disease such as influenza. Widespread antibiotic use also increases the risk for acquiring diseases caused by resistant organisms such as methicillin-resistant *Staphylococcus aureus* (MSRA), vancomycin-resistant enterococci, and multiple resistant gram-negative rods.

RECOGNITION OF INFECTIONS IN OLDER ADULTS

Presentation

Older adults commonly present without the typical signs and symptoms of an acute infection. Fever, the most

41.1   Changes That Cause a Decrease in Immune Function With Aging (Immune Senescence)

AREA OF CHANGE	COMMENT
Skin, mucous membranes	Skin thins and dries with aging
Function of neutrophils	Decreased adherence to foreign particles and decreased destruction of these particles
Thymic hormones	Decrease in ability to fight infection
T cells	A decrease in their ability to fight infection with a shift from naive to memory subtypes
Natural killer cells	Number increases, but function declines
Proliferative responses	
IL-2, IL-2 receptor	Decrease in number, thus decreasing ability to fight infection
IL-4, IL-6, IL-10	Increase in these inflammatory markers and decreased ability to fight infection
IFN-γ	Increase in these inflammatory markers and decreased ability to fight infection
PGE$_2$	Increase in these inflammatory markers and decreased ability to fight infection
Autoimmunity	Increase in autoimmunity occurs with autoantibodies common, but of unclear significance

readily recognized feature of infection, may be absent in 30% to 50% of older adults with serious infections. The cause of impaired febrile responses in older adults is not well understood, although it is believed to be due to the body's reduced ability to regulate temperature at an older age.

Because of the altered febrile response to infection, fever in older adults can be redefined as a temperature > 2°F (1.1°C) over baseline (if a baseline is available) or, perhaps more practically, an oral temperature > 99°F (37.2°C) or a rectal temperature > 99.5°F (37.5°C) on repeated measures.

In addition to the absence of fever, other common atypical presentations of infection in older adults include decline in baseline functional status (i.e., bathing, dressing, or walking), confusion, falling, or exhibiting behavior change (e.g., less engaged in daily activities). There may be a subsequent decline in appetite and decreased food and fluid intake, as well as exacerbation of underlying illness (e.g., atrial fibrillation).

Antibiotic Management

Drug distribution, metabolism, excretion, and interactions may be altered with age. Aging in the absence of any comorbid disease is associated with reduction in renal function. As such, reduction in antibiotic dose may be required. It bears noting that antibiotic interactions can occur with many medications commonly prescribed for older adults. Digoxin, warfarin, oral hypoglycemic agents, theophylline, antacids, lipid-lowering agents, and antihypertensive medications can have significant interactions with commonly prescribed antibiotics. Drug concentrations can increase (e.g., as occurs with an increase in digoxin concentrations when digoxin is taken with macrolides, tetracyclines, and trimethoprim) or decrease (e.g., such as occurs when some fluoroquinolones are taken with antacids) with concomitant drug administration. Atrophic gastritis (i.e., chronic inflammation in the stomach lining that decreases acid production and other enzymes needed for digestion), a common problem in older adults, and use of H_2 blockers (e.g., Zantac) or proton-pump inhibitors (e.g., Prevacid) can reduce the absorption of some antibiotics, such as ketoconazole or itraconazole. Adherence to prescribed regimens may be limited as a consequence of poor cognitive function, impaired hearing or vision, multiple medications, and financial constraints. Minimum criteria for the appropriate initiation of antimicrobial therapy is shown in Table 41.2.

INFECTIOUS SYNDROMES

Bacteremia and Sepsis

Bacteremia is the presence of bacteria in the blood, normally a sterile environment. Detection of bacteria in the blood (most commonly with blood cultures) is always abnormal. Bacteria can enter the bloodstream and cause bacteremia associated with infections (e.g., pneumonia), during surgery, or when the individual has a catheter or intravenous line. Older adults with bacteremia are less likely than their younger counterparts to have chills or sweating, and fever is commonly absent. Management of bacteremia requires intravenous administration of appropriate antibiotics.

Pneumonia

Older adults account for more than 50% of all pneumonia cases; pneumonia mortality is more than three to five times that of young adults. Comorbidity, being 85 years of age and older, a decline in function (e.g., inability to independently perform activities of daily living), body temperature of < 36.1°C, hypotension (< 90 mm Hg systolic), or tachycardia (i.e., heart rate of > 110 beats per minute) are all predictors of mortality in community-acquired pneumonia of older adults.

Aspiration, defined as the inhalation of either oropharyngeal or gastric contents into the lower airway, is a common cause of pneumonia among older adults. Inhalation of these contents can lead to aspiration

41.2 | Suggested Minimum Criteria for Initiation of Antibiotic Therapy

CONDITION	MINIMUM CRITERIA
Urinary tract infection, without catheter	Fever *and* one of the following: new or worsening urgency, frequency, suprapubic pain, blood in the urine, incontinence
Urinary tract infection, with catheter	Fever *or* one of the following: new-onset delirium or shaking chills
Skin and soft-tissue infection	Fever *or* one of the following: redness, tenderness, warmth, new or increasing swelling of affected site
Respiratory infection	■ Fever > 102°F (38.9°C) *and* one of the following: respiratory rate > 25, productive cough ■ Fever > 100°F and < 102°F; *and* one of the following: respiratory rate > 25, pulse > 100, rigors, new-onset delirium ■ Afebrile with COPD; *and* new or increased cough with purulent sputum ■ Afebrile without COPD *and* new or increased cough *and* either respiratory rate > 25 or new-onset delirium
Fever without source of infection	■ At least one of the following: new-onset delirium, shaking chills ■ Antibiotics might be started as a diagnostic test and then discontinued in 3–5 days if no improvement

Note: COPD = chronic obstructive pulmonary disease.

pneumonia and might be seen or reported with the following signs and symptoms:

- Cough
- Fever or chills
- Malaise, myalgias (muscle achiness)
- Shortness of breath, dyspnea on exertion
- Pleuritic chest pain (sharp pain usually on one side of the chest)
- Putrid expectoration
- Nonspecific symptoms including headache, nausea/vomiting, anorexia, weight loss

Treatment requires the use of antibiotics.

Prevention of pneumonia in older adults is challenging and requires a multipronged approach. Immunization with a pneumonia vaccine (see Chapter 19, "Prevention"), smoking cessation, swallowing evaluation, and management of all other chronic medical problems are important preventive interventions.

Influenza

Influenza causes approximately 40,000 deaths annually in the United States, nearly all of them among the older adult population. Primary symptoms of influenza are: fever, chills, headache, muscle aches, dizziness, loss of appetite, and tiredness. Symptoms may also include sweating, sore throat, dry cough, runny nose, burning eyes, nausea, and weakness. Symptoms usually appear 1 to 4 days after exposure to the virus through droplets in the air or direct contact of bodily fluids (saliva, mucous) from an infected individual. Overall, symptoms are similar to those of the common cold. However, they tend to develop quickly and are often more severe than the typical sneezing and congestion of the common cold. Fever rises quickly and can reach 104 degrees Fahrenheit. Although the fever may subside after 2 or 3 days, the resident may be exhausted for days. Influenza almost never causes symptoms in the stomach and intestines. The illness that some call stomach flu is not influenza, but a different virus. Influenza vaccine is 60% to 80% efficacious in older adults for preventing severe disease, hospitalization, and death.

For those who do get influenza, several drugs are available for treatment or prophylaxis following exposure to influenza. M2 inhibitors (e.g., amantadine and rimantadine) are effective in treatment and prevention but can cause many side effects in older adults; they are not generally used. Neuraminidase inhibitors (e.g., zanamivir and oseltamivir) are safer treatment options for older adults. Treatment of influenza is most effective if initiated within 24 hours of symptom onset.

Urinary Tract Infection

Urinary tract infection (UTI) is among the most common infections in older adults and is particularly prevalent among older adults with indwelling catheters.

Asymptomatic Bacteruria

Many older adults have asymptomatic bacteruria (i.e., bacteria in the urine), and numerous studies suggest that there is no clinical benefit for treatment of this condition. Rather, treatment is associated with significant adverse effects, expense, and the potential for development of resistant organisms. Thus, no treatment is recommended. Unfortunately, it is sometimes difficult to determine what is symptomatic. The presentation of infection can be quite subtle in older adults. Change in functional (or mental) status often prompts the collection of a urine specimen even in the absence of fever, dysuria, or other typical clinical features. It may be helpful to simply observe these individuals for a few days rather than expose them to a course of (unnecessary) antibiotic therapy.

Symptomatic Urinary Tract Infection

Symptomatic bacteruria involving infection in the lower urinary tract (i.e., every part of the urinary system except the kidneys) is characterized by dysuria, frequency, and urgency. These infections require therapy the length and type of treatment of which may vary, based on the type of bacteria noted in the urine and allergies or intolerable side effects to antibiotics on the part of the resident. A 3-day course of antibiotics is sufficient for symptomatic bacteruria of the lower urinary tract.

Upper UTIs (i.e., those that include the kidney) are generally characterized by fever, chills, nausea, and flank pain. These infections typically require more prolonged therapy lasting 7 to 21 days. Urine cultures and sensitivities are done to guide antimicrobial therapy. Prophylactic antibiotics to prevent recurrent UTIs in older women are not recommended because of the high incidence of the development of resistant organisms. Intravaginal or systemic estrogen replacement and/or the daily intake of at least 300 mL of cranberry juice may be helpful in prevention of infections in older women.

Urinary Tract Infection in Men

UTIs are generally less common in men. When they do occur, it is usually because of a backup of urine in the bladder (i.e., urinary retention) due to an enlarged prostate, or impaired emptying due to autonomic neuropathy. Autonomic neuropathy is a type of peripheral neuropathy that affects involuntary body functions (e.g., bladder function, heart rate, blood pressure) by interrupting signals from the brain. Treatment involves antibiotics and monitoring to be sure the individual is emptying his bladder adequately (see Chapter 26, "Urinary Incontinence").

Tuberculosis

Worldwide, approximately 1.7 billion persons are infected with *Mycobacterium tuberculosis* (MTB); the number is 16 million in the United States. Adults age 65 and older account for one-fourth of all active tuberculosis cases in the United States. The current incidence of MTB in older adults is due to exposure in the early 1900s, when it was estimated that 80% of all persons were infected with MTB by the age of 30. Most active cases of tuberculosis in older adults are due to reactivation of the disease.

As with most other infections in older adults, tuberculosis may not present in classic fashion (i.e., cough, sputum, fever, night sweats, weight loss). Rather, the person may complain of fatigue and anorexia, or show a decline in function, or have a low-grade fever. It is possible for the older adult to have extrapulmonary disease, which is evidence of MTB in another organ of the body (e.g., the brain, bones, or bladder). Diagnosis of active disease usually requires isolation of the organism from sputum, urine, or some other clinical specimen.

The most confusing aspect of MTB is interpretation of the purified protein derivative (PPD) skin test results. In all populations, *induration* (i.e., a hard, red, raised area) of ≥ 15 mm 48 to 72 hours after placement of a 5-tuberculin-unit PPD indicates a positive test. Induration ≥ 10 mm is considered *a positive test in assisted living residents*, recent converters (previous PPD < 5 mm), immigrants from countries with a high number of cases of MTB, underserved populations in the United States (e.g., homeless persons, Black Americans, Hispanic Americans, and Native Americans), and persons with specific risk factors (e.g., gastrectomy; > 10% below ideal body weight; chronic kidney failure; diabetes mellitus; or immune suppression, including that caused by corticosteroids or malignancy). In residents infected with human immunodeficiency virus (HIV), those with a history of close contact with persons with active MTB, and those with chest radiographs consistent with MTB, ≥ 5 mm induration is considered a positive PPD test.

In assisted living settings, it is important to use a *two-step procedure* for PPD testing. Two-step testing requires retesting of residents within 2 weeks of initial testing. If the second skin test results in ≥ 10 mm of induration or the increase in the size of the induration from the first to the second skin test is ≥ 6 mm, the resident is considered PPD positive. Treatment of MTB typically involves four-drug therapy (isoniazid, rifampin, pyrazinamide, and ethambutol or streptomycin).

Infective Endocarditis

Infective endocarditis is an inflammation of the inner layer of the heart, the endocardium (i.e., the tissue that lines the chambers of the heart), and the heart valves. Diagnosis is often difficult in the older adult as fever and leukocytosis (i.e., elevated white count) are less common in older adults than in younger individuals. The practice of giving antibiotics prior to a dental procedure is no longer recommended *except* for individuals with cardiac conditions associated with the highest risk of adverse outcomes resulting from bacterial endocarditis, including prosthetic cardiac valve, previous endocarditis, or congenital heart disease. Antibiotic prophylaxis is *not* recommended for the following dental procedures or events: routine anesthetic injections (i.e., injections of novocaine) through noninfected tissue, taking dental radiographs, placement of removable prosthodontic or orthodontic appliances, adjustment of orthodontic appliances, or routine cleaning. Antibiotic prophylaxis is not recommended for individuals undergoing gastrointestinal or genitourinary procedures.

Prosthetic Device Infections

Permanent implantable prosthetic devices are common in older adults. Prosthetic joints, cardiac pacemakers, artificial heart valves, intraocular lens implants, vascular grafts, penile prostheses, and a variety of other devices are more often placed in older than in younger adults. Prosthetic device infections are usually separated into early versus late infection because the causative agents differ significantly. Early prosthetic device infection (PDI), most commonly defined as occurring less than 60 days after device implantation, is primarily due to contamination at the time of implantation or events associated with the acute hospitalization (such as occult bacteremias due to intravenous catheters). Late PDI is usually caused by bacteria from the skin, respiratory, gastrointestinal, or genitourinary tracks. Treatment includes antibiotics and in some situations removal of the hardware.

Bone and Joint Infections

Bone and joint infections, in the absence of prostheses, can also occur in older adults. Infection in the joint occurs most commonly when individuals have rheumatoid or osteoarthritis, or gout. Treatment usually involves antibiotics, although in some situations surgery is needed. Infection of the bone (i.e., osteomyelitis) can occur from a pressure ulcer or following a surgical intervention. Treatment often involves intravenous antibiotics to reach the site of the infection.

HIV Infection and AIDS

HIV infection in older adults was initially limited to those who had received blood transfusions for surgical procedures. However, increasing numbers of older Americans with HIV have acquired their infection via sexual activity. Older adults constitute approximately 10% of all new diagnoses of acquired immunodeficiency syndrome (AIDS) in the United States. Nonspecific symptoms such as forgetfulness, anorexia, weight loss, and recurrent pneumonia are often dismissed as age-related, and HIV testing can be delayed. Untreated HIV infection in older adults tends to pursue a more rapid downhill course, perhaps because of impaired T-cell replacement mechanisms with advanced age and the impact of additional comorbidities. Older adults are treated in the same way as younger individuals: with highly active antiretroviral therapy (HAART). HIV prevention should be discussed with residents, specifically focusing on safe sexual practices and increasing awareness of the benefits of testing and effective HIV therapy.

Gastrointestinal Infections

Gastrointestinal infections are common among older adults. Diverticulitis (i.e., inflammation or infection of a diverticula or pouch of the bowel), appendicitis (i.e., infection of the appendix), and cholecystitis (i.e., infection of the gallbladder) can all occur and present with fever, elevated white blood cell counts, or any significant symptoms other than a mild change in appetite, constipation, or fatigue in older adults. It is important to be aware of the possibility of these infections among older adults presenting with these vague symptoms.

Infectious diarrhea, specifically, *Clostridium difficile* (i.e., C. Diff) commonly occurs in older adults. C. difficile is a bacterium that causes frequent, watery, foul-smelling stools. Recent treatment with an antibiotic increases the risk for C. difficile, although this infection can occur simply by passing it from one person to the next via the hands of a health care provider. Standard treatment for C. difficile is metronidazole (Flagyl); oral vancomycin (Vancocin) is used when the symptoms and evidence of infection persist following a course of treatment. *Probiotics* are organisms, such as bacteria and yeast, that help restore a healthy balance to the intestinal tract. They are found in yogurt or in a pill form and should be encouraged for all those who have C. difficile or are at risk for acquiring this infection (also see Chapter 45, "Gastrointestinal Diseases and Disorders").

Methicillin-Resistant Staph Aureus

Methicillin-resistant *Staphylococcus aureus* (MRSA) is a strain of staphylococcus resistant to the broad-spectrum antibiotics commonly used to treat it. Older adults and people with weakened immune systems are at most risk for MRSA that can be contracted either in the hospital or in the community. Staph skin infections, including MRSA, generally start as small red bumps that resemble pimples or boils. These can quickly turn into deep, painful abscesses that may even require surgical draining. Sometimes, the bacteria remain confined to the skin. But they can also penetrate into the body, causing potentially life-threatening infections in bones, joints, surgical wounds, the bloodstream, heart valves, and lungs. These infections are generally treated with a course of antibiotics.

Individuals can either be carriers of MRSA or have active disease. A *carrier* is someone who does not have symptoms of MRSA (i.e., evidence of an affected area with drainage) but has the bacteria living on his or her skin, in his or her nose, bladder, or other areas within the body. This is referred to as an infection that is *colonized*. In many cases it is possible for a carrier to be declared clear of the MRSA virus. A resident may become free of bacteria by washing daily with chlorhexidin (over-the-counter products include Betasept, Calgon Vesta, Dyna-Hex, Hibiclens, Hibistat, Spectrum-4) and applying bacitracin ointment into the nostrils with a q-tip for a period of 6 to 8 weeks or longer.

Prevention of the spread of MRSA is particularly important in assisted living communities. At present, there is no clear guideline whether or not to use contact isolation (i.e., resident is isolated in a room; staff wear gloves, gowns, and masks as per universal precautions). The Centers for Disease Control (CDC) recommend the use of standard precautions to prevent the spread of infections in health care settings. *Standard precautions* combine the major features of universal precautions (UP) and body substance isolation (BSI) and are based on the principle that all blood, body fluids, secretions, and excretions except sweat, nonintact skin, and mucous membranes may contain transmissible infectious agents. Standard precautions include a group of infection prevention practices that apply to all persons, regardless of suspected or confirmed infection status, in any setting in which health care is delivered. These include: hand hygiene; use of gloves, gown, mask, eye protection, or face shield, depending on the anticipated exposure; and safe injection practices. Also, equipment or items in the resident's environment likely to have been contaminated with infectious body fluids must be handled in a manner to prevent transmission of infectious agents (e.g., wear gloves for direct contact, contain heavily soiled equipment, properly clean and disinfect or sterilize reusable equipment before use on another resident). The application of standard precautions during resident care is determined by the nature of the interaction and the extent of anticipated blood, body fluid, or pathogen exposure.

RESOURCES

Martin, C. P., Fain, M. J., & Klotz, S. A. (2008). The older HIV-positive adult: A critical review of the medical literature. *American Journal of Medicine, 121*(12), 1032–1037.

Onur, O. E., Guneysel, O., Akoglu, H., Aydin, Y. D., & Denizbasi, A. (2008). Oral, axillary, and tympanic temperature measurements in older and younger adults with or without fever. *European Journal of Emergency Medicine, 15*(6), 334–337.

Richards, C. L., Jr. (2006). Preventing antimicrobial-resistant bacterial infections among older adults in long-term care facilities. *Journal of the American Medical Directors Association, 7*(3 Suppl.), S88, S89–S96.

Trick, W. E., Weinstein, R. A., DeMarais, P. L., Tomaska, W., Nathan, C., McAllister, S. K., et al. (2004). Comparison of routine glove use and contact-isolation precautions to prevent transmission of multidrug-resistant bacteria in a long-term care facility. *Journal of the American Geriatrics Society, 52*(12), 2003–2009.

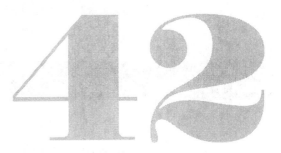

Cardiovascular Diseases and Disorders

Wilbert S. Aronow and Yael Sollins

The incidence of coronary vascular disease (CVD) is approximately 40% per 1,000 person-years in men and 22% in women, with the incidence being particularly high among racial and ethnic minorities. The consequences of CVD in these individuals are significant and include hypertension, stroke, myocardial infarction (MI), peripheral vascular disease, atrial fibrillation, and congestive heart failure. The estimated cost of CVD was $393.5 billion in 2005, nearly $175 billion more than cancer or HIV infections. Control of CVD risk factors is fundamental in reducing the incidence of CVD and in preventing adverse clinical outcomes such as stroke, long-term morbidity, and premature cardiovascular death. Prevention strategies include engaging in regular exercise, achieving and maintaining a desirable weight, eating a heart-healthy diet, smoking cessation, and adhering to medication management recommendations for hypertension, hyperlipidemia, diabetes, atrial fibrillation, and valvular heart disease.

AGE-RELATED CARDIOVASCULAR CHANGES

No changes should be noted in the older adult's ejection fraction (i.e., the portion of blood that is pumped out of a filled ventricle as a result of a heartbeat), stroke volume (i.e., the amount of blood pumped out with a contraction of the ventricle), or the cardiac output (i.e., the amount of blood pumped out of the heart in 1 minute) (see Table 42.1).

Epidemiology

Coronary artery disease (CAD) is the most common cause of death in persons age 65 years and older. Autopsy findings indicate that 70% of persons older than 70 years have CAD with ≥ 50% atherosclerotic obstruction or blockage of one or more coronary arteries. More than 30% of older adults have clinical manifestations of CAD such as a prior stroke, poor circulation of the lower extremities, or heart damage from an MI. The prevalence of CAD among 1,802 community-dwelling persons (mean age = 80 years) was approximately the same for Whites, African Americans, Hispanics/Latinos, and Asian Americans: 60% of persons hospitalized with acute MI are age 65 years and older. The prevalence of CAD and the incidence of new coronary events are similar among men and women aged 75 years and older, but it is higher among men younger than 75. Eighty-three percent of MIs in women occur after menopause. Women are less likely than men to survive the initial MI.

Risk Factors

Modifiable risk factors for CAD in older adults include cessation of cigarette smoking, treatment of hyperlipi-

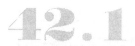

Changes That Occur in the Cardiovascular System With Age	
AREA OF CHANGE	**CHANGES**
Structural heart changes	Myocardial cells decrease in size Decreased distensibility of the aortic artery Decreased tone of the arteries Increased weight/size of the heart Increased size of the myocardial cells Increased thickness of the left ventricle wall and size of the left atrium Increased stiffness of the arteries Increased elastin levels, making it more difficult for the vessels to expand
Functional changes	Decreased diastolic pressure during the initial filling of the ventricles when the heart contracts Decreased filling of the heart chambers Decreased response to stimulation, so the heart is not as quick to have an increase in heart rate when working hard (e.g., exercising)

demia, treatment of hypertension, ingestion of a diet low in saturated fat and cholesterol, maintenance of ideal body weight, and regular physical activity. These personal and medically guided actions will reduce CAD and new coronary events. If hypertension is present, the goal is to lower the blood pressure to < 140/90 mm Hg. If CAD is present and the serum low-density lipoprotein cholesterol (LDL-C) is > 125 mg/dL, even if following the American Heart Association (AHA) step II diet, then lipid-lowering drug therapy (preferably statins) is recommended.

Treatment recommendations for the management of hyperlipidemia by the Adult Treatment Panel III (ATP-III) of the National Cholesterol Education Program (NCEP) include the following:

- Cholesterol: < 200
- High density lipoprotein (HDL): > 60
- LDL-C: < 100
- Triglycerides: < 150

In high-risk persons, treatment should be aggressive: recommended LDL-C treatment goal should be < 100 mg/dL and ideally drop to < 70 mg/dL. For moderately high-risk persons (2 + risk factors and 10-year risk of 10% to 20%), the recommended LDL-C goal should at least be < 130 mg/dL.

Signs and Symptoms of CAD

In older persons, *myocardial ischemia* (defined as impaired oxygen return to the heart due to poor blood flow from blocked arteries) caused by CAD is more commonly manifested by *dyspnea on exertion* than by chest pain typical of *angina pectoris*. In older persons, angina pectoris can present as back or shoulder pain or as burning epigastric pain. Substernal (below the sternum) anginal pain is less common in older adults. Angina pectoris pain in older adults can be less severe and of shorter duration than presentation in a younger individual. Myocardial ischemia can cause clinical heart failure (HF) and acute pulmonary edema. HF generally is associated with increased shortness of breath due to fluid accumulation throughout the body (legs, lungs, abdomen, face).

Symptoms of an acute MI in older adults may vary and range from 19% to 66% of individuals presenting with chest pain, 20% to 59% with dyspnea, 15% to 33% with neurologic symptoms, and 0% to 19% with gastrointestinal symptoms. Other symptoms associated with acute MI in older adults include peripheral gangrene, increased claudication (cramping in the calves with activity), palpitations, kidney failure, weakness, pulmonary embolism, restlessness, sweating, and sudden death. Older adults with acute MI are more likely than younger persons to die from the MI and to have pulmonary edema, HF, left ventricular (LV) systolic dysfunction (impaired pumping of the LV), cardiogenic shock, conduction disturbances requiring insertion of a pacemaker, atrial fibrillation (AF), or atrial flutter.

Diagnostic Testing

Coronary angiography is the gold standard for detecting CAD and determining its severity. Resting electrocardiography (ECG) may be used to diagnose MI or ischemia, whether silent or symptomatic, in older adults. Exercise stress testing can also be useful in the diagnosis as well as prognosis of CAD. An older adult who is unable to perform exercise stress testing because of musculoskeletal disorders or pulmonary disease can have a stress test using intravenous dipyridamole-thallium imaging. Echocardiography can be useful for identification of changes in the function of the heart muscle, acute myocardial ischemia, complications due to acute MI, blood clots, heart enlargement, and associated valvular heart disease.

Management

Clinical management decisions are based on research and clinician experience/expertise. Residents need to understand the logic or rationale of the clinical decisions, to the extent possible, to help them adhere to the treatment regimen.

Stable Angina Pectoris

The first step is management of reversible factors that can aggravate angina pectoris and myocardial ischemia: anemia, infection, obesity, hyperthyroidism, uncontrolled hypertension, arrhythmias such as AF with a rapid ventricular rate, and severe valvular aortic stenosis. Smoking should be stopped. Treatment of hypertension and hyperlipidemia can be initiated. An exercise program will improve exercise tolerance. Aspirin 160 to 325 mg daily decreases the incidence of MI, stroke, and vascular death.

■ Blockers are effective anti-anginal agents and are the drug of choice to prevent myocardial ischemia. They reduce MI, sudden coronary death, and mortality, and should be given to all persons with CAD for whom β-blockers are not contraindicated, for example, those with HF (except for β-blockers specifically indicated for HF) or bradycardia (heart rate of less than 60).

Nitrates relieve and prevent angina pectoris. Nitroglycerin administered as a 0.3 to 0.6 mg sublingual tablet or as a 0.4 mg sublingual spray is the drug most commonly used to relieve an acute anginal attack. Long-acting nitrates help prevent recurrent episodes of angina. A 12- to 14-hour nitrate-free interval every 24 hours is necessary to avoid nitrate tolerance, as individuals build up a tolerance to nitrates and they thus become less effective when used for long periods of time. Persistent angina that is interfering with quality of life, despite treatment with multiple medications (nitrates, β-blockers, and calcium channel blockers), might require coronary artery bypass graft (CABG) surgery or percutaneous transluminal coronary angioplasty (PTCA).

Acute Myocardial Infarction

As soon as acute MI is suspected, aspirin should be administered (160 mg to 325 mg daily) and continued indefinitely. The first dose of aspirin should be chewed. Clopidogrel 75 mg daily may be used for persons unable to tolerate aspirin. Treatment (in the hospital) is then initiated with a β-blocker and additional medications depending on the person's symptoms and comorbid medical problems. In some situations, such as if the ischemia lasts for at least 30 minutes and is repetitive, reperfusion therapy with either thrombolytic therapy or PTCA may be recommended.

Treatment After Myocardial Infarction

Every attempt to control coronary risk factors must be made after the MI. Aspirin 160 to 325 mg daily should be administered indefinitely as should β-blockers if not contraindicated. Angiotensin-converting enzyme (ACE) inhibitors are recommended during and after acute MI. ACE inhibitors reduce MI size and permanent damage to the ventricles, both of which have a beneficial effect on morbidity and mortality. ACE inhibitors are also recommended for use indefinitely in older adults after an MI unless there are specific contraindications to their use, such as angioedema, which is swelling in the deep layers of the skin, renal artery stenosis, and previous allergy to ACE inhibitors. Calcium channel blockers (e.g., verapamil) should not be used after MI unless other medications do not resolve the persistent angina pectoris.

Coronary Revascularization After Myocardial Infarction

The benefits of revascularization, specifically CABG surgery, which involves using blood vessels from another part of the body to bypass clogged heart arteries, focus on improving length and quality of life. For example, the individual will have less chest pain and shortness of breath associated with activity.

DYSLIPIDEMIA

Double-blind, randomized controlled studies conclusively demonstrate an absolute reduction in cardiovascular mortality and morbidity in older adults with dyslipidemia treated with statins compared to persons younger than 65 years of age. In older adults with prior MI and a serum LDL-C of ≥ 125 mg/dL, statins reduce new coronary events in persons age 60 to 100 years and new stroke in persons age 60 to 90 years. Older adults in whom the serum LDL-C was reduced to < 90 mg/dL had the greatest reduction in new coronary events and in stroke. See Table 42.2 and Table 42.3 for treatment indications and drug regimens regarding dyslipidemia.

HEART FAILURE: EPIDEMIOLOGY AND ETIOLOGY

HF is the most common cause of hospitalization and rehospitalization in older adults. The prevalence and incidence of HF increase with age. CAD, hypertension, valvular heart disease, and cardiomyopathies are the most common causes of HF in older adults.

Not only do older adults experience an age-related decrease in heart function, they are more likely to have LV diastolic dysfunction because of hypertension, myocardial ischemia due to CAD, valvular aortic stenosis, hypertrophic cardiomyopathy, and other cardiac disorders. The prevalence of an abnormal LV ejection fraction associated with HF increases with age and is higher in older women than in older men. The LV ejection fraction is measured by echocardiography and helps determine the most appropriate therapy for HF. An ejection fraction of ≥ 50% is considered normal.

Signs and Symptoms of Heart Failure

Dyspnea is the most common symptom of HF and may progress from exertional dyspnea to dyspnea at rest, and to the development of acute pulmonary edema. Pulmonary congestion from fluid in the lungs may cause coughing and wheezing. Decreased cardiac output can

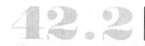 | Treatment Indications for Dyslipidemia

RISK CATEGORY	CONDITIONS	LDL-CHOLESTEROL GOAL	INITIATE NONPHAR-MACOLOGIC MANAGEMENT	CONSIDER DRUG THERAPY
Low	0–1 risk factor[a]	< 160 mg/dL	≥ 160 mg/dL	≥ 190 mg/dL; optional: 160–189 mg/dL
Moderate	2 + risk factors; 10-year CAD risk < 10%	< 130 mg/dL	≥ 130 mg/dL	≥ 160 mg/dL
Moderately high	2 + risk factors; 10-year CAD risk 10%–20%	< 130 mg/dL	≥ 130 mg/dL	≥ 130 mg/dL; optional: 100–129 mg/dL
High	CVD, DM, or 10-year CAD risk > 20%	< 100 mg/dL	≥ 100 mg/dL	≥ 100 mg/dL
Very high	DM + CVD; acute coronary syndrome; multiple severe or poorly controlled risk factors	< 70 mg/dL; optional: < 70 mg/dL	≥ 100 mg/dL	≥ 100 mg/dL; optional: 70–99 mg/dL

Note: CAD = coronary artery disease; CVD = cardiovascular disease; DM = diabetes mellitus; HDL = high-density lipoprotein; LDL = low-density lipoprotein. CVD is signified by CAD, angina, peripheral artery disease, transient ischemic attack, stroke, abdominal aortic aneurysm, or 10-year CAD risk > 20%.
[a]Risk factors are cigarette smoking, hypertension, HDL < 40 mg/dL, family history of premature CAD, male age ≥ 45 year, female age ≥ 55 year.

42.3 | Drug Regimens for Dyslipidemia

CONDITION	DRUG	DOSAGE	FORMULATIONS
Elevated LDL, normal TG	Statin (HMG-CoA reductase inhibitor):		
	Atorvastatin	10–80 mg qd	T: 10, 20, 40, 80
	Fluvastatin	20–80 mg qd in P.M., max 80 mg	C: 20, 40; T: ER 80
	Lovastatin	10–40 mg qd in P.M. or bid	T: 10, 20, 40
	Pravastatin	10–40 mg qd	T: 10, 20, 40, 80
	Rosuvastatin	10–40 mg qd	T: 5, 10, 20, 40
	Simvastatin	5–80 mg qd in P.M.	T: 5, 10, 20, 40, 80
Elevated TG (> 500 mg/dL)	Fenofibrate	54–160 mg qd	T: 54, 160
	Gemfibrozil	300–600 mg po bid	T: 600
Combined elevated LDL, low HDL, elevated TG	Fenofibrate, gemfibrozil, or HMG-CoA if TG < 300 mg/dL	As above	As above
Alternative for any of above	Niacin	100 mg tid to start; increase to 500–1000 mg tid; ER 150 mg qhs to start, increase to 2,000 mg qhs as needed	T: 25, 50, 100, 250, 500, ER 150, 250, 500, 750, 1,000; C: TR 125, 250, 400, 500
Elevated LDL or combined with inadequate response to one agent	Lovastatin/niacin combination	20 mg/500 mg qhs to start; increase to 40 mg/ 2,000 mg as needed	T: 20/500, 20/750, 20/ 1,000
	Colesevelam	Monotherapy: 1,850 mg po bid; combination therapy: 2,500–3,750 mg/ d in single or divided doses	T: 625
	Ezetimibe	10 mg qd	T: 10
	Ezetimibe/simvastatin[a] combination	1 tab qd	T: 10/10, 10/20, 10/40, 10/80

Note: bid = twice a day; C = capsule; d = day; ER = extended release; HDL = high-density lipoprotein; HMG-CoA = 3-hydroxy-3-methyl-glutaryl-CoA; LDL = low-density lipoprotein; max = maximum; po = by mouth; qd = once a day; qhs = each bedtime; T = tablet; TG = triglycerides; tid = three times a day; TR = trace.

[a]Safety guidelines: Measure liver function tests at baseline and at 3 months, then periodically. Watch for statin-induced myopathy (muscle pain).

cause weakness, a feeling of heaviness in the limbs, nocturia, oliguria, confusion, insomnia, headache, anxiety, memory impairment, bad dreams or nightmares, and, rarely, psychotic manifestations. Increased fluid in the liver can occur and may cause epigastric or right upper quadrant heaviness or a dull ache, a sense of fullness after eating, anorexia, nausea, and vomiting. Right ventricular failure causes edema that first occurs in the dependent parts of the body. Chest x-ray for residents with suspected HF will show pulmonary vascular congestion in those with LV failure.

Management

Precipitating causes of HF, such as excess sodium ingestion (e.g., pickles, potato chips), myocardial ischemia, infection, anemia, fever, hypoxia, tachyarrhythmias, bradyarrhythmias, hyperthyroidism, hypothyroidism, and obesity must be identified and treated. Sodium intake should be decreased to between 1,500 and 2,400 mg/day, equal to about 1 teaspoon of salt. The Dietary Approaches to Stop Hypertension (DASH) eating plan is commonly recommended as the ideal approach to manage cardiovascular risk. This diet consists of fruits, vegetables, whole grains, low-fat dairy products, poultry, and fish. Drugs known to precipitate or aggravate HF, such as nonsteroidal anti-inflammatory drugs (NSAID), calcium channel blockers, and most antiarrhythmic drugs, should be stopped. It is critical, therefore, to check with residents to be sure they are not taking over-the-counter pain medications (e.g., NSAIDS).

Persons with HF who are dyspneic at rest or at a low activity/exertion level may benefit from a formal cardiac rehabilitation program. Disease management strategies, either self- or nurse-directed, are effective at reducing rehospitalization rates among older adults with HF. Frequent weighing, careful attention to symptoms, and adjustment of diuretic dosing are components of HF disease management. A weight gain of more than 2 pounds in a single day should be reported to the resident's primary health care provider. ACE inhibitors improve symptoms, quality of life, and exercise tolerance. They decrease mortality and hospitalization for HF associated with abnormal LV ejection fraction and should be administered unless there are specific contraindications to their use.

Residents on an ACE inhibitor should be monitored for orthostatic hypotension (Exhibit 42.1), although it is only necessary to inform the primary health care provider if there are complaints of dizziness. It is important, also, to monitor the estimated glomerular filtration rate (GFR) because ACE inhibitors can impair kidney function. Contraindications to use of ACE inhibitors are symptomatic hypotension, progressive azotemia (i.e., a higher than normal blood level of urea or other nitrogen-containing compounds in the blood), facial swelling, hyperkalemia (i.e., elevated potassium levels), intolerable dry cough, and rash. For those who cannot tolerate an ACE inhibitor, a drug from the group referred to as angiotensin II type 1 receptor antagonists can be tried.

As previously noted, continuous administration of β-blockers after MI reduces mortality, sudden cardiac death, and recurrent MI, especially in older adults. These benefits are even more marked in persons with a history of HF. β-blockers are beneficial in the treatment of HF associated with normal LV ejection fraction by:

- Reducing the heart rate to < 90 beats per minute, thereby increasing the time the LV has to fill and increasing the volume of blood that is pumped throughout the body
- Decreasing myocardial ischemia
- Reducing elevated blood pressure
- Preventing further enlargement of the heart

42.1   Evaluating Residents for Orthostatic Hypotension

Step I. Have the patient lie supine for 5 minutes.

Step II. Take the resting blood pressure and heart rate.

Step III. Have the person come to stand and obtain a blood pressure and heart rate after standing for 1 minute and then again at 3 minutes after coming to stand.

Patients unable to stand may be assessed while sitting upright.

The increase in heart rate, and thus stress on the heart muscle, that occurs with exercise can also be prevented with modest doses of β-blockers, especially in older adults.

Diuretics are also used in the treatment of HF. Mild HF can be treated with a thiazide diuretic. However, a thiazide diuretic is ineffective if the estimated GFR is < 30 mL per minute (estimated GFR is calculated based on the individual's blood urea nitrogen and creatinine level and provided on the lab printout). Older adults with moderate or severe HF should be treated with a loop diuretic (e.g., furosemide), so named because of where it works in the kidney. Those with severe HF or concomitant renal insufficiency may need metolazone in addition to the loop diuretic. Aldosterone antagonist diuretics can be used in older adults who have a normal estimated GFR and a normal serum potassium. The minimum effective dose of diuretic should be given. Digoxin may also be used in the treatment of older adults with HF, particularly if they have a supraventricular tachyarrhythmias such as AF. Conversely, calcium channel blockers such as nifedipine, diltiazem, and verapamil exacerbate HF in older adults with HF and abnormal LV ejection fraction and should be avoided.

Prevention of Acute Heart Failure

The number-one cause of acute HF is fluid retention, usually associated with increased sodium intake or retention. Residents should be encouraged to adhere to a low-sodium diet of no more than 2,400 mg/day. Daily weights are advisable; the primary care clinician should be notified immediately if there is a gain of more than 2 pounds in 1 day. Over-the-counter drugs to avoid that can exacerbate sodium and fluid retention include sodium-based antacids, high-dose aspirin, NSAIDs, ginseng (germanium), ginkgo, echinacea, and decongestants. Black licorice candy has the same negative effect.

VALVULAR HEART DISEASE

Valvular Aortic Stenosis

Valvular aortic stenosis (AS) in older adults is usually due to stiffening, scarring, and calcification of the valve leaflets. Angina pectoris, syncope or near syncope, and HF are the three classic manifestations of severe AS. Echocardiography is used to diagnose AS and determine severity. Surgical intervention is an option for individuals with symptoms such as exertional syncope. Balloon aortic valvuloplasty is an alternative for those who are not candidates for aortic valve surgery.

Aortic Regurgitation

Acute aortic regurgitation (AR) in older adults results in the heart being unable to keep up with the demand for blood; fluids can back up in the body and cause shortness of breath. Aortic regurgitation may be due to infective endocarditis, rheumatic fever, aortic dissection, trauma following prosthetic valve surgery, or rupture of the sinus of Valsalva. It causes sudden severe HF. Prophylactic antibiotics should be used to prevent bacterial endocarditis in older adults with chronic AR, according to American Heart Association guidelines (available at http://www.amhrt.org).

Mitral Regurgitation

Causes of mitral regurgitation (MR) include CAD, mitral valve prolapse, and rheumatic heart disease. Symptoms associated with severe MR are primarily those of HF, especially dyspnea. Echocardiography is used to diagnose the presence and monitor the severity of MR.

Mitral Stenosis

The most common causes of mitral stenosis (MS) are rheumatic fever and endocarditis. Generally, early in the disease process, there are no symptoms and the older individual may only know he has MS because he has a diastolic murmur. In later stages of the disease, there may be shortness of breath, dizziness, or chest pain. Echocardiography is used to diagnose the presence and severity of MS. Long-term oral warfarin therapy is used to reduce the risk of thromboembolic events (blood clots). Treatment options also include balloon valvuloplasty or surgery.

ARRHYTHMIAS

Ventricular Arrhythmias

The presence of three or more consecutive premature ventricular complexes (PVCs) on an ECG constitutes ventricular tachycardia (VT), which is considered sustained if it lasts ≥ 30 seconds and nonsustained if it lasts < 30 seconds. Nonsustained VT and simple ventricular arrhythmias (VAs), defined as those that are not frequent, are generally not treated with antiarrhythmic drugs but with β-blockers if there are no contraindications. Alternatively, automatic implantable cardioverter-defibrillators (AICDs) are used in older adults who are willing to undergo this type of intervention. In helping a resident make a decision about whether or not to have an AICD inserted, consider the pros and cons, benefits, burdens, and/or risks. While the AICD may be life-prolonging, it can result in some discomfort when triggered.

Atrial Fibrillation

AF is the most common type of arrhythmia in adults; it is more common as people age. Cardiac conditions associated with the development of AF are hypertension, rheumatic mitral valve disease, CAD, and HF. Noncardiac causes include hyperthyroidism, hypoxic pulmonary conditions, surgery, and alcohol intoxication. People with AF may have an irregular heart rate (i.e., the heart may beat quickly, slow down, and then speed up again), palpitations and lightheadedness, or more vague symptoms, such as malaise; they are also at increased risk for thromboembolic disease/events. Treatment of AF in older adults with HF requires evaluation of their heart rate and rhythm and prevention of a clot. Medications, such as β-blockers, are commonly used to slow the heart rate, and anticoagulation (warfarin) is initiated if not contraindicated or refused by the resident/family. Some residents may undergo electrical cardioversion to restore their heart rhythm to normal. Generally, AF can be easily managed by slowing the heart rate with medications such as calcium channel blockers or β-blockers; this does not require hospitalization. For the majority of older adults, the AF will change back to normal sinus rhythm on its own. These individuals are treated with medications, however, to help prevent the AF from frequently recurring.

Bradyarrhythmias

Numerous drugs can cause bradyarrhythmias (i.e., a slow heart rate of less than 60 beats per minute) and conduction disturbances. Individuals who are in good physical condition (e.g., runners) may have normally slow heart rates even as low as 40. It is important, therefore, to get a good history and baseline heart rate on residents at the time of move-in. Hyperkalemia, hypokalemia, hypothyroidism, and hypoxia can cause abnormalities in conduction. Bradyarrhythmias can cause dyspnea, weakness, fatigue, falls, angina pectoris, HF, episodic pulmonary edema, dizziness, faintness, slurred speech, personality changes, paresis, and convulsions

in older adults. For disorders that cannot be reversed, such as sick sinus syndrome (i.e., when the heart fluctuates between going too fast and too slow), or a blockage in the conduction system, a permanent pacemaker can be implanted.

PERIPHERAL ARTERIAL DISEASE

Aneurysms and Dissections

Aneurysms (i.e., a localized widening of an artery or vein) and dissections (i.e., a tear in the aorta) are primarily disorders of older adults. Aneurysms most commonly occur in the abdominal aorta, thoracic aorta, popliteal arteries, and iliac arteries, and they are usually atherosclerotic. Symptomatic aneurysms are medical emergencies that require immediate surgery. Symptoms may include the following:

- Sudden and severe pain, or an unusual pulsing sensation over the involved blood vessel can indicate an aneurysm.
- Pain in the abdomen or lower back extending into the groin and legs can indicate an abdominal aneurysm.
- Chest pain, hoarseness, persistent coughing, and difficulty swallowing can indicate a thoracic aneurysm.
- Throbbing sensation or lump directly behind the knee can indicate an aneurysm in this area.
- Severe headache may indicate a dissecting (rupturing) aneurysm in the head.

Occlusive Peripheral Vascular Disease

The prevalence of occlusive peripheral vascular disease (PVD) increases with age. Significant independent risk factors for symptomatic PVD in older men and women are age, cigarette smoking, hypertension, diabetes mellitus, and a high serum LDL-C and low serum HDL cholesterol. Persons with diabetes mellitus commonly have more distal and diffuse atherosclerosis. Atherosclerotic vascular disease affecting the lower extremities may cause asymptomatic arterial insufficiency or symptomatic disease including intermittent claudication (i.e., cramping or pain in the calves when walking) or pain at rest, ulceration, and gangrene. Only one-half of older adults with documented PVD are symptomatic (unable to walk far or fast enough). However, ischemic muscle symptoms might not occur because of comorbidities such as arthritis or pulmonary disease. Atypical symptoms might not be recognized as intermittent claudication, or there may be sufficient collateral arterial channels to tolerate arterial obstruction. Hence, there are no symptoms.

The diagnosis of PVD is usually made by a thorough history and physical examination. Asymptomatic arterial insufficiency can be identified by a low ankle-brachial index (ABI), determined by dividing the systolic blood pressure measured at the ankle by that obtained in the brachial artery of the arm on the same side of the body. Lower extremity arterial disease is defined as an ABI < 0.9. Medical therapy for PVD includes cessation of cigarette smoking and treatment of other risk factors, such as high cholesterol. Exercise therapy is the most effective medical treatment for intermittent claudication. Aspirin therapy or the use of clopidogrel is often recommended, as this can delay the progression of PVD and will reduce the incidence of stroke, MI, or vascular death. Surgical interventions may be an option for very severe disease. Properly fitted shoes, daily foot washing, and keeping the skin moist with topical emollients to prevent cracks and fissures (places for bacterial infection) may prevent the infections. Careless nail clipping or injury from walking barefoot must be avoided. Fungal infection of the feet must be treated. Socks should be wool or other thick fabrics. Padding or shoe inserts may be used to prevent pressure ulcers. When a foot wound develops, specialized foot gear, including casts, boots, and ankle foot orthoses, are helpful in relieving pressure on the wound.

VENOUS DISORDERS

Chronic deep venous insufficiency is common in older adults and presents with the following: edema of the lower extremities, pigmentation changes (spotty) or darkening in the color of the leg, or irregular shaped ulcers on the lower extremities (particularly above the ankle) that drain serosanguinous fluid. Treatment consists of limb elevation, any type of supportive stockings, and exercise to increase muscle tone.

RESOURCES

American Health Association. (n.d.). *Guidelines for blood lipids.* Retrieved July 15, 2008, from http://wwwamericanheartorg/presenterjhtml?identifier = 183#total

Aronow, W.S. (2003a). Epidemiology, pathophysiology, prognosis, and treatment of systolic and diastolic heart failure in elderly patients. *Heart Disease, 5*(4), 279–294.

Aronow, W.S. (2003b). Hypercholesterolemia: The evidence supports use of statins. *Geriatrics, 58*(8), 18–20, 26–28, 31–32.

Aronow, W.S. (2004). Management of peripheral arterial disease of the lower extremities in elderly patients. *Journals of Gerontology Series A: Biological Sciences and Medical Sciences, 59*(2), M172–M177.

Chobanian, A.V., Bakris, G.L., Black, H.R., Cushman, W.C., Green, L.A., Izzo, J.L., Jr., et al. (2003). The seventh report of the Joint National Committee on Prevention, Detection, Evaluation, and Treatment of High Blood Pressure: The JNC 7 report. *Journal of the American Medical Association, 289*(19), 2560–2572.

Goldstein, L.B., Adams, R., Alberts, M.J., Appel, L.J., Brass, L.M., Bushnell, C.D., et al. (2006). Primary prevention of ischemic stroke: A guideline from the American Heart Association/American Stroke Association Stroke Council: Cosponsored by the Atherosclerotic Peripheral Vascular Disease Interdisciplinary Working Group; Cardiovascular Nursing Council; Clinical Cardiology Council; Nutrition, Physical Activity, and Metabolism Council; and the Quality of Care and Outcomes Research Interdisciplinary Working Group: The American Academy of Neurology affirms the value of this guideline. *Stroke, 37*(6), 1583–1633.

Grundy, S.M., Cleeman, J.I., Merz, C.N., Brewer, B., Jr., Clark, L.T., Hunninghake, D.B., et al. (2004). Implications of recent clinical trials for the National Cholesterol Education Program Adult Treatment Panel III Guidelines. *Circulation, 110*(2), 227–239.

43

Hypertension

Mark Andrew Supiano and Jennifer Hauf

Hypertension affects approximately 50 million individuals in the United States and approximately 1 billion individuals worldwide. As the population ages, the prevalence of hypertension will increase even further unless broad and effective preventive measures are implemented. Recent data from the Framingham Heart Study suggest that individuals who are normotensive at 55 years of age have a 90% lifetime risk for developing hypertension, and less than 40% of older adults are adequately controlled. The relationship between blood pressure (BP) and risk of cardiovascular disease events is continuous, consistent, and independent of other risk factors. The higher the individual's BP, the greater the risk of myocardial infarction, heart failure, stroke, and/or kidney disease. For individuals aged 40 to 70 years, each increment of 20 mm Hg in systolic BP or 10 mm Hg in diastolic BP doubles the risk of cardiovascular disease across a BP range from 115/75 to 185/115 mm Hg. Fortunately, there are many effective interventions, behavioral and pharmacologic, that can manage BP. Appreciating these treatments and helping residents weigh the pros and the cons of treatments is an important component to nursing care in assisted living communities.

EPIDEMIOLOGY AND PHYSIOLOGY

BP, particularly systolic pressure, increases with increasing age. The risk associated with hypertension does not decline with age, and the criteria that define hypertension, outlined in the Seventh Report of the Joint National Committee on Prevention, Detection, Evaluation, and Treatment of High Blood Pressure (JNC 7; see Table 43.1), are not age adjusted. Epidemiologic studies, including the National Health and Nutrition Examination surveys, suggest that the prevalence of hypertension in persons age 65 years and older is between 50% and 70%; it is highest among older Black Americans. Among the older hypertensive population, the prevalence rate is higher for women, particularly for those above the age of 75 years. Since the early 1900s, the use of antihypertensive medications has increased, as a result of which the prevalence rates of elevated BP, left ventricular hypertrophy (i.e., enlarged ventricle or chamber of the heart), and cardiovascular and stroke mortality have all declined. However, these trends have not occurred among the older population; BP remains poorly controlled in many older adults despite treatment for hypertension.

Many of the physiologic changes that occur with aging contribute to the increase in BP, but lifestyle factors such as obesity and physical inactivity, and the presence of comorbid diseases, are also important contributors. Several physiologic changes combine to increase peripheral vascular resistance—resistance to the flow of blood in the arterial vessels—which is the physiological cause of what is referred to as hypertension. Arterial stiffness provides the best explanation for the relatively greater increase in systolic pressure and the increase in pulse pressure (i.e., the difference between systolic and diastolic pressure) observed with aging. Several mechanisms contribute to arterial stiffness. Reduced sensitivity of the baroreflex, the mechanism

43.1 | Classification of Blood-Pressure Levels From the Joint National Committee on Prevention, Detection, Evaluation, and Treatment of High Blood Pressure

CATEGORY	SYSTOLIC (MM HG)		DIASTOLIC (MM HG)
Normal	< 120	and	< 80
Prehypertension	120–139	or	80–89
Hypertension			
Stage 1	140–159	or	90–99
Stage 2	> 160	or	> 100

that controls the ability of the body to adjust the BP to changes in position such as lying to standing, might be related to decreased arterial distensibility. Alterations in kidney function as well as sodium balance further contribute to the increased incidence of hypertension with age. Approximately two-thirds of older hypertensive persons have sodium-sensitive hypertension, that is, high BP that improves with low sodium intake (see Figure 43.1).

CLINICAL EVALUATION

Accurate measurement of BP is the most critical aspect of the diagnosis of hypertension in the older adult. Because variability in BP increases with age, the diagnosis should be made by using the average of several BP readings taken on each of three visits. Ambulatory BP monitoring (i.e., BP monitoring done over a 24-hour period) may be necessary for residents with extreme BP variability or possible white-coat hypertension.

Once an elevated BP is noted, it is helpful to explore any factors that might be contributing to the high reading. Medication side effects, poor adherence to hypertensive treatment, high salt intake, pain, anxiety, or stress are some examples of immediate causes of elevated BP. The residents should also be monitored for evidence of target organ damage, disease noted secondary to the high BP such as damage to the heart, brain, eyes, and kidney. Although most older adults have essential hypertension (i.e., hypertension that occurs without any specific medical problem), secondary hypertension is also possible. Secondary hypertension is present when the high BP is a result of (i.e., secondary to) another condition, such as kidney disease or tumors (e.g., pheochromocytoma and paraganglioma). Regardless of age,

it is useful to explore with the resident's lifestyle factors that could be adjusted to improve the resident's BP, such as smoking history, dietary intake of sodium and fat, alcohol intake, and level of usual physical activity (see also Chapter 18, "Physical Activity," and Chapter 19, "Prevention").

TREATMENT

Based on results of several randomized placebo-controlled clinical trials, and meta-analyses of more than 40 randomized clinical trials of antihypertensive therapy, the overwhelming consensus among clinical experts is that treatment of hypertension in older adults is safe and effective in reducing cardiovascular (e.g., chronic heart failure) and cerebrovascular (e.g., stroke) morbidity and mortality. The treatment effect was largest in men, in those age 70 and over, and in those who had pulse pressures of greater than 40 mm Hg when at rest. *Pulse pressure* is the change in BP seen during a contraction of the heart. This is calculated by subtracting the diastolic pressure (the bottom number when obtaining a BP reading) from the systolic pressure (the top number). The resting pulse pressure in healthy adults is about 40 mm Hg.

It is important to balance the beneficial effects of antihypertensive therapy with the potential impact on the person's functional status and quality of life. A treatment approach that is not likely to produce adverse effects and targets a reduction in systolic BP to 135 to 140 mm Hg and diastolic BP to 85 to 90 mm Hg should be developed. For individuals with type 2 diabetes, a systolic BP goal of less than 130 mm Hg is recommended. For persons with markedly elevated systolic BP, an intermediate target, such as 160 mm Hg, may be an appropriate initial goal.

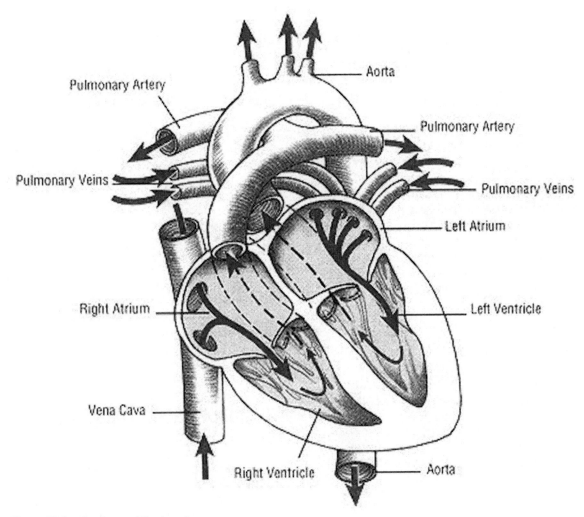

Figure 43.1 Anatomy of the heart.

Lifestyle Modification

Nonpharmacologic therapy may be effective for older adults with stage 1 hypertension (140 to 159 mm Hg systolic or 90 to 99 mm Hg diastolic BP) and is particularly important as it may help to decrease the amount of medication needed. Lifestyle modifications that target the typical characteristics of the older hypertensive person—overweight, sedentary, and salt-sensitive—are likely to be effective (see also Chapter 18, "Physical Activity," and Chapter 19, "Prevention").

Pharmacologic Treatment

The approach to pharmacologic management of the older hypertensive person is generally based on the JNC 7 guideline. The prescribed drug might be selected based on other comorbid conditions (e.g., diabetes mellitus, coronary artery disease or history of myocardial infarction, heart failure, prostatism), racial and ethnic background, and, of course, the person's tolerance to treatment.

Guidelines suggest that for simple, uncomplicated hypertension, the initial antihypertensive drug of choice is a low-dose thiazide-type diuretic. Most residents will not reach their systolic BP goal on a single medication; JNC 7 recommends considering starting individuals on two drugs if the initial BP is more than 20 mm Hg above the target level. The second drug added is generally an angiotensin-converting enzyme (ACE) inhibitor. Beyond these general recommendations for initial therapy, there is no universally accepted approach to choosing alternative agents or combination therapies; these decisions should be made on an individual basis that considers the advantages and disadvantages of the drug together with the resident's comorbidities. Given the many choices of antihypertensive medications available, it is best to avoid the centrally acting agents (e.g., clonidine, methyldopa), as these agents are more likely to cause orthostatic hypotension.

Diuretics

Therapy with low-dose thiazide-type diuretics (e.g., hydrochlorothiazide ≤ 25 mg daily, or the equivalent) improves BP safely and with few adverse effects. Importantly, these medications are low cost and only need to be taken once a day. Although there is a risk of hypokalemia (i.e., low potassium), hyperuricemia (i.e., elevation in uric acid, which can cause gout), hyponatremia (i.e., low sodium), and glucose intolerance (i.e., increased blood sugar), these problems are less likely to occur if the medication is used in low dosages.

Angiotensin-Converting Enzyme Inhibitors

ACE inhibitors are effective in lowering BP in older hypertensive adults. Drugs in this class are generally well-tolerated (with the exception of cough during ACE inhibitor therapy), and they do not adversely affect the central nervous system (e.g., cause changes in memory or wakefulness) or metabolic profile (e.g., alter electrolytes such as potassium or sodium). In addition, this type of medication is particularly beneficial for older adults who have diabetes mellitus or evidence of heart disease.

Angiotensin-Receptor Blockers (ARBs)

There is no reason to start initial treatment for hypertension with an ARB unless the person is unable to tolerate ACE inhibitor therapy.

Calcium Channel Antagonists (CCAs)

Although CCAs are not recommended as first-line therapy, they may be considered as second-line drugs, generally in combination with a thiazide-type diuretic. These drugs reduce peripheral vascular resistance but can cause unpleasant side effects such as constipation and swelling of the feet.

β-Receptor Antagonists

β-receptor antagonists are recommended in the JNC 7 report as another option for second-line drug therapy.

These drugs are less effective alone than therapy with a low-dose thiazide diuretic in terms of reducing BP and preventing cardiovascular events, stroke, and death. In addition, β-blockers are more likely to be discontinued because of adverse effects such as symptoms of dizziness or swelling of the feet. Because of their effectiveness in the management of symptomatic coronary artery disease, in secondary prevention following myocardial infarction, and in certain heart failure conditions, β-receptor antagonists are often used to treat BP when the older individual has these comorbid conditions.

α-Receptor Antagonists

Although these medications are effective in reducing BP in older adults, they are more likely to cause side effects such as postural hypotension and increase the risk of acute heart failure. α-receptor antagonist therapy, usually in combination with another drug, might be considered for treating older hypertensive men with prostatism, because these drugs have been shown to be efficacious in improving obstructive urinary symptoms.

MONITORING OF BLOOD PRESSURE

Frequency of follow-up visits to the primary health care provider and frequency of BP measurement should reflect the resident's degree of BP elevation, with closer follow-up for those with more severe hypertension (i.e., systolic BP greater than 180 mm Hg). With the exception of hypertensive emergencies (see the following section), attempts to reduce the individual's BP too rapidly are unnecessary and likely deleterious. For most residents, an interval of 1 to 2 months is appropriate between visits to the health care provider to determine the need for dose adjustment. No more than weekly BP monitoring at the assisted living community is sufficient, unless there are concerns about adverse drug effects such as orthostatic hypotension.

The older adult's adherence to the antihypertensive medication regimen is particularly important for the primary health care provider to know, prior to changing any medication (dose or type). If possible, send the BP record with the resident and the list of *all* medications and any relevant information about lack of adherence (e.g., refusal to take the medication; timely refill by a resident who is self-administrating). It is also helpful to inform the primary health care provider about lifestyle activities, including smoking, drinking, exercise, use of any herbal products or over-the-counter medications. Increased alcohol intake or use of nonsteroidal anti-inflammatory drugs such as Aleve, for example, may worsen BP control.

SPECIAL CONSIDERATIONS

Hypertensive Emergencies and Urgencies

Elevated BP in the absence of signs or symptoms of target-organ damage (e.g., heart attack or stroke) does not constitute a hypertensive emergency or urgency. A rapid and overly aggressive reduction in BP in a resident with incidentally discovered elevated BP is potentially harmful and may produce complications, such as coronary or cerebral hypoperfusion syndromes (i.e., decreased blood flow to the brain or the heart).

Examples of true hypertensive *emergencies* in older adults include hypertensive encephalopathy (i.e., the occurrence of neurologic symptoms such as change in cognition or function due to neurological causes), acute heart failure with pulmonary edema, dissecting aortic aneurysm (i.e., a tear or burst in the aortic artery causing massive bleeding), and unstable angina (i.e., chest pain). These residents need to be sent to the acute care hospital. Even in these situations, BP should not be lowered more than 25% within the first 2 hours, with a goal of achieving 160/100 mm Hg gradually over the first 6 hours of therapy.

Hypertensive *urgencies*, situations in which BP should be lowered within 24 hours to prevent the risk of target-organ damage, are more common than true emergencies. Most can be managed with oral administration of antihypertensive medications to achieve a gradual BP reduction.

Special Considerations in Hypertension Measurement and Management

There are many challenges to obtaining an accurate sense of the individual's BP; it can change markedly throughout the course of the day. In general, BP appears to be highest in the morning before breakfast. Postprandial (i.e., after eating) hypotension is common among older adults and likely affects about one-third of these individuals. This occurs because blood is diverted to the stomach to digest food and thus blood flow to the rest of the body is decreased and overall BP goes down.

It is not well-known if there is a significant advantage to the treatment of hypertension with antihypertensive therapy in old-old individuals (i.e., those greater than 90 years of age), especially if the person has to endure drug side effects. Even a recommendation that is seemingly benign—to eat a low sodium diet—can cause a decrease in appetite and weight loss that can result in other clinical problems such as protein-energy malnutrition. In all situations it is critical to work with the resident, his or her primary health care provider, and family or proxy as appropriate to weigh the benefits and risks of treatment of hypertension.

RESOURCES

Aronow, W. S. (2008). Treatment of hypertension in the elderly. *Geriatrics, 63*(10), 21–25.

Beckett, N. S., Peters, R., Fletcher, A. E., Staessen, J. A., Liu, L., Dumitrascu, D., et al. (2008). Treatment of hypertension in patients 80 years of age or older. *New England Journal of Medicine, 358*(18), 1887–1898.

Fowler, M. B. (2008). Hypertension, heart failure, and beta-adrenergic blocking drugs. *Journal of the American College of Cardiology, 52* (13), 1073–1075.

Leibovitch, E. R. (2008). Hypertension, refining our treatment. *Geriatrics, 63*(10), 14–15, 17–20.

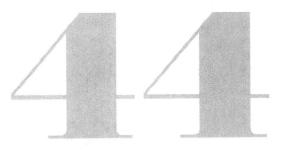

Endocrine and Metabolic Diseases and Disorders

David A. Gruenewald, Alvin M. Matsumoto, Caroline Blaum, and Krystal L. Thomas

Although there are some normal age-related changes in the endocrine system, the major endocrine changes occur during times of physical and emotional stress. For example, fasting blood glucose levels change very little with normal aging, increasing 1 to 2 mg per dL per decade of life. In contrast, infection or use of certain medications such as corticosteroids may result in a marked increase in the glucose level of an older adult. In some cases, a loss of function in one aspect of the endocrine system may be compensated for by another system in the body: reduction in testicular testosterone production in older men may be partially compensated for by an increase of pituitary luteinizing hormone secretion by the brain. This stimulates testosterone production in the testes and decreases breakdown and destruction of the testosterone that is available.

As with diseases in other organ systems, endocrine disorders in older adults often present with nonspecific or atypical symptoms and signs. Diabetes mellitus, for example, may present with increased thirst, hunger, and urinary frequency. Rather, the older adult with a high blood sugar may be confused, depressed, or apathetic. Diagnosis of the most common endocrinopathies (i.e., problems with the endocrine system) in older adults, such as hyperparathyroidism, diabetes mellitus, hypothyroidism, and hyperthyroidism, are generally discovered as a result of abnormalities found on routine laboratory screening.

THYROID DISORDERS

Thyroid function is based on a feedback system involving the pituitary gland, found in the brain, and the thyroid gland, found in the neck. The thyroid gland is under the control of the pituitary gland, a small gland the size of a peanut at the base of the brain. The function of the thyroid gland is to take iodine, found in many foods, and convert it into thyroid hormones: thyroxine (T4) and triiodothyronine (T3). Thyroid cells are the only cells in the body that can absorb iodine. These cells combine iodine and the amino acid tyrosine to make T3 and T4, which are then released into the bloodstream and transported throughout the body where they control metabolism (i.e., conversion of oxygen and calories to energy). Every cell in the body depends on thyroid hormones for regulation of their metabolism. The normal thyroid gland produces about 80% T4 and about 20% T3; however, T3 possesses about four times the hormone strength as T4. When the level of thyroid hormones (T3 and T4) drops too low, the pituitary gland produces thyrotropin or thyroid stimulating hormone (TSH), which stimulates the thyroid gland to produce more hormones. The pituitary senses the thyroid hormone production and responds by decreasing its TSH production.

One can imagine the thyroid gland as a heating system and the pituitary gland as the thermostat. Thyroid hormones are like heat. When the heat gets back to the thermostat, it turns the thermostat off. As the room cools (i.e., the thyroid hormone levels drop), the thermostat turns back on (TSH increases) and the furnace produces more heat (thyroid hormones). The hormone secreted by one gland is sensed and responded to by the other; a balance is maintained. Low levels (less than 5 units) of TSH are sufficient to keep the normal thyroid gland functioning properly. When the thyroid gland becomes inefficient, such as in early hypothyroidism, the TSH becomes elevated (greater than 5 units). The rise in TSH represents the pituitary gland's response to a drop in circulating thyroid hormone and is the first indication of thyroid gland failure.

Thyroid function is generally unchanged or minimally changed in healthy older adults. Certain medications, however, can cause thyroid disease. Amiodorone, used to treat cardiac arrhythmias, for example, can cause either hypo- or hyperthyroidism.

Nonspecific, atypical, or asymptomatic presentations of thyroid disease are common in older adults and can be detected by laboratory testing. Thyroid disease is so common in older adults it is generally routinely checked for on an annual basis by lab tests. However, treatment of thyroid disease may not affect any symptoms experienced by the older individual.

Hypothyroidism

Underactive thyroid gland is common in older adults, affecting 2% to 14% of the older population. Mild hypothyroidism causes underproduction of thyroid hormone and increases TSH secretion (remember, TSH increases to make the thyroid gland produce more thyroid hormone). As in younger people, most cases of hypothyroidism in older adults are due to autoimmune disease: the body's immune system functions abnormally and attacks the thyroid gland. Other causes include drugs that depress thyroid function and decreased activity of the pituitary gland. Hypothyroidism is more common in older women but can be seen in either gender.

Symptoms of hypothyroidism are often atypical in older adults (See Table 44.1). Some clinical features of hypothyroidism (e.g., dry skin, decreased skin turgor, slowed mentation, weakness, constipation, anemia, hyponatremia, arthritis, paresthesias, gait disturbances) may misleadingly suggest other diseases. Furthermore, these symptoms usually have a slow onset and a slow rate of progression. In addition, older patients with mild hypothyroidism who develop serious nonthyroidal illness may rapidly become severely hypothyroid. Cognitively impaired older adults with hypothyroidism

44.1 | Symptoms of Hypothyroidism

TYPICAL SYMPTOMS	OTHER OR TYPICAL SYMPTOMS
Fatigue	Decreased sweating
Weight gain or extreme thinness	Chest pain
Decreased tolerance for cold	Coarse or slow-growing hair
Coarse skin, dry, decreased skin turgor	Anemia
Deepened or hoarse voice	Fluid retention, especially around the eyes
Constipation	Dull facial expression and droopy eyelids
Mental impairment— slow mentation	Placidity or nervousness
Depressed mood	Sleepiness or insomnia
Slow, rapid or irregular heartbeat	Decreased tolerance for medication
Diffuse edema	Gait disturbance
	Numbness and tingling of hands and feet
	Muscle weakness
	Alternation in hearing, taste, and smell

rarely recover normal cognitive function with thyroid replacement. Those without underlying cognitive impairment may, however, show an improvement in cognition, functional status, and mood with treatment of the hypothyroidism.

Thyroid replacement usually starts at a low dosage (e.g., 25 µg per day) in older adults, increasing the dose every 4 to 6 weeks until TSH levels normalize. The goal is to reduce or eliminate symptoms of hypothyroidism. Giving too much thyroid replacement too quickly can cause cardiac symptoms, such as increased heart rate, angina or congestive heart failure. Over replacement of thyroid hormone should be avoided because it can alter bone turnover (i.e., breakdown of bone) and contribute to osteoporosis as well as worsen heart disease. With correction of the hypothyroid state, the body will once again work at optimal efficiency. The clearance rate of medications such as anticonvulsants, digoxin, and opiate analgesic agents may improve and might require a change in the dosage of those medications.

Hyperthyroidism (Thyrotoxicosis)

Hyperthyroidism develops in 0.5% to 2.3% of older people; 15% to 25% of all cases of thyrotoxicosis occur in adults age 60 and over. In the United States, most cases in older adults are due to Graves' disease, which occurs when the immune system mistakenly attacks the thyroid gland and causes it to overproduce the hormone thyroxine. Hyperthyroidism often presents with vague, atypical, or nonspecific symptoms in older adults (Table 44.2).

Older persons may present with apathetic thyrotoxicosis. This presentation of hyperthyroidism is quite different from the typical hyperactive presentation of thyroid disease seen in younger individuals (increased activity, inability to sleep, increased heart rate, anxiety). The older adult with apathetic thyrotoxicosis presents with depression, inactivity, lethargy, or withdrawn behavior, often in association with symptoms such as weight loss, muscle weakness, or cardiac symptoms (e.g., increased heart rate, fatigue, dizziness). Older individuals who experience an increased heart rate due to hyperthyroidism are at risk for developing atrial fibrillation (i.e., an irregular heart rhythm that generally is rapid with a pulse rate greater than 120 beats per minute). Hyperthyroidism can also contribute to osteoporosis as it increases bone turnover.

Nodular Thyroid Disease and Thyroid Cancer

The incidence of multinodular goiter increases with aging: approximately 90% of women age 70 and over, and 60% of men age 80 and over, have thyroid nodules. The highest incidence of goiter is seen in individuals with an iodine-deficient diet. Most goiters are nonpalpable.

Solitary thyroid nodules are more likely to be malignant in people over 60 years of age, especially men. Any new solitary nodule or an enlargement of an existing nodule needs to be evaluated.

44.2 | Symptoms of Hyperthyroidism

Feeling warm or hot all the time

Tremors

Sweating

Itching skin or urticaria

Pounding, rapid, irregular heartbeat

Atypical chest pain

Weight loss, despite overeating

Marked anxiety and restlessness

Sleeplessness

Fatigue and weakness

Protruding eyes and double vision

Diarrhea

Hair loss

Heart failure

Constipation

Muscle atrophy or weakness

Nausea and vomiting

Febrile illness

Note: Bold items more common in older adults.

DISORDERS OF PARATHYROID AND CALCIUM METABOLISM

Important changes occur with aging in several systems that regulate calcium levels in the body. This can have an impact on bone breakdown, cause a reduction in bone mass, and, in some cases, lead to osteoporosis.

Hyperparathyroidism

Hyperparathyroidism is overactivity of the parathyroid glands resulting in excess production of parathyroid hormone (PTH), which regulates and helps to maintain calcium and phosphate levels. Overactivity of one or more of the parathyroid glands causes high calcium levels (i.e., hypercalcemia) and low levels of phosphate in the blood. Most people with hyperparathyroidism have no symptoms. Of those who present with symptoms, they are commonly associated with the effects of an increased calcium level. Calcium is involved in nervous system function. Thus, most symptoms of parathyroid disease are neurological in origin, the most common symptoms being fatigue, tiredness, or lack of energy. Other very common symptoms include memory problems, depression, problems with concentration, and problems sleeping. Other manifestations usually involve the kidney (i.e., renal calculi or stones) and the skeletal system (bone pain due to the development of osteoporosis).

Vitamin D Deficiency

Calcium and vitamin D are needed to make bone. Dietary calcium intake is inadequate in older adults because of decreased absorption of calcium. In addition, vitamin D deficiency is common in older adults because of decreased sunlight exposure associated with lifestyle changes (e.g., advisement to stay out of the sun) and a decrease in the skin's ability to produce vitamin D. Low calcium and vitamin D levels result in weaker bones and risk of fractures. Furthermore, vitamin D deficiency is associated with muscle weakness and may contribute to fall risk in some older adults.

Adequate dietary calcium and vitamin D supplementation may reverse age-related hyperparathyroidism, increase bone mineral density, and reduce falls and osteoporotic fracture rates, although the effectiveness of vitamin D alone in preventing osteoporotic fractures is unclear. For many older people, an elemental calcium intake of at least 1,000 to 1,500 mg per day is desirable, together with at least 400 IU of vitamin D per day. Some older adults are unable to take daily oral supplements; they may benefit from 50,000 IU of oral vitamin D every month.

Hypercalcemia

Primary hyperparathyroidism and malignancy are the most common causes of hypercalcemia (i.e., increase in serum calcium level) in older adults. Generally, there are no symptoms of hypercalcemia, but some individuals may complain of fatigue, depression, increased thirst and urination, muscle weakness, anorexia (i.e., diminished appetite), nausea, vomiting, and abdominal pain. These individuals may have changes in memory and behavior, as well.

Paget's Disease of Bone

Paget's disease is characterized by localized areas of increased bone remodeling and growth of bone. This bone, however, is not good, strong bone; there is increased risk of fracture. Prevalence of Paget's disease increases with age and affects 2% to 5% of people age 50 years and over. The most commonly affected sites are the pelvis, spine, femur, tibia, and skull. Although Paget's disease is usually asymptomatic, when it is symptomatic, pain is the most common presenting symptom, either localized to the affected bones or resulting from secondary osteoarthritic changes, often in the hips, knees, and vertebrae. When bone deformities occur, the long bones of the lower extremities are usually affected, often with bowing (i.e., bending into the shape of a bow) of the involved extremity. Skull involvement may result in pressure on the eighth cranial nerve and sensorineural hearing loss. Treatment is not usually necessary for asymptomatic disease, unless there is concern for hearing loss from skull involvement, nerve root or spinal cord compression from vertebral involvement, or hip fracture from femoral neck involvement. Bisphosphonates (see Chapter 29, "Osteoporosis") suppress the accelerated bone turnover and bone remodeling that is characteristic of this disease. Therefore, this group of drugs is the best treatment option for individuals with Paget's disease.

HORMONAL REGULATION OF WATER AND ELECTROLYTE BALANCE

Unlike young adults, older adults are predisposed to having too much or too little water in the body, and/or low levels of sodium (i.e., *hyponatremia*). This is due to an increase in antidiuretic hormone (ADH), which is released from the pituitary gland and acts on the kidneys to increase their reabsorption of water into the blood and causes impaired kidney function, heart failure, hypothyroidism, and diuretic use. These conditions predispose the older adult to hyponatremia by impairing the body's ability to conserve or retain water. Some medications (e.g., chemotherapeutic agents, narcotics, antiseizure medication, antianxiety medications, antidepressants such as the selective serotonin reuptake inhibitors [SSRIs], sulfonylureas) cause the pituitary gland to release an excessive amount of ADH, resulting in a syndrome of inappropriate antidiuretic hormone (SIADH). Any of these problems, therefore, predispose older adults to insufficient amounts of water by reducing the ability of the kidneys to conserve sodium or to concentrate urine (and, therefore, retain the maximal amount of water in the body).

The signs and symptoms of insufficient amounts of fluid in the body (i.e., dehydration) can vary, with some individuals having no signs or symptoms and others having multiple observable problems and complaints. Specifically, symptoms can include postural hypotension (see Chapter 24, "Dizziness"), increased heart rate, weight loss of 3 to 5 pounds in only 1 to 2 days, decreased urine output or very dark urine, confusion, or change in behavior. For example, a resident may have low body fluid because of poor intake coupled with a period of diarrhea from a drug side effect or change in diet. Treatment in these situations would include increasing fluid intake.

Older adults are also at risk for *hyperkalemia* (i.e., elevated serum potassium), especially those with diabetes mellitus or kidney disease. Some medications, specifically angiotensin-converting enzyme inhibitors, nonsteroidal anti-inflammatory drugs, β-blocking agents, and diuretics with aldosterone-antagonist properties (e.g., aldactone) contribute to hyperkalemia. Symptoms are usually described as numbness and weakness of the extremities. This condition is usually picked up on routine lab chemistries. *Hypokalemia* also commonly occurs in older adults and is likely due to diuretics, which can cause an excessive loss of potassium, or to vomiting or excessive diarrhea.

DISORDERS OF THE ADRENAL CORTEX

The adrenal cortex produces three hormones: glucocorticoids (e.g., cortisol, which has anti-inflammatory properties), mineralocorticoids (e.g., aldosterone, which controls blood pressure), and androgens (e.g., testosterone). Over- or underproduction of these hormones can have an impact on the older adult.

Hypoadrenocorticism or Adrenal Failure or Addison's Disease

Basal serum cortisol levels, controlled by the adrenal cortex, do not change with aging. Chronic glucocorticoid therapy (i.e., treatment with steroids) is the most

common cause of adrenal failure in older adults, because the adrenal gland does not have to make cortisone when it is given via a pill. Other possible causes of adrenal failure include tuberculosis, cancer, or bleeding in the adrenal gland from anticoagulation. In addition, Addison's disease, a primary cause of adrenal failure, affects about 1 in 100,000 people. Most cases of Addison's Disease are caused by the gradual destruction of the adrenal cortex (i.e., the outer layer of the adrenal glands) by the body's own immune system. About 70% of these cases are caused by autoimmune disorders in which the immune system makes antibodies that attack the body's own tissues or organs and slowly destroy them. Adrenal insufficiency occurs when at least 90% of the adrenal cortex has been destroyed. Older adults with chronic adrenal insufficiency may present with nonspecific symptoms such as anorexia, weight loss, or impaired functional status; hyperkalemia may not be present initially.

Hyperadrenocorticism (Cushing's Syndrome) or Excessive Amounts of Glucocorticoids

The use of oral glucocorticoids for asthma or pain management associated with inflammation of the bones or muscles is the most common cause of Cushing's syndrome (i.e., excessive amounts of glucocorticoids) in older adults. Adverse effects can include psychiatric and cognitive symptoms, osteoporosis, myopathy (i.e., muscle weakness), and elevated blood glucose. It is important to closely monitor these individuals for weight gain, fluid retention, infections, diabetes, thinning of the skin, and weakening of the bone.

Diabetes

Diabetes mellitus is a metabolic disease characterized by *hyperglycemia* (i.e., high blood sugar) due to abnormalities in insulin secretion, insulin action, or both. Estimates of the prevalence of diabetes among individuals 65 years of age and older range between 15% and 20%. The prevalence of diabetes mellitus is higher among Black and Hispanic people in comparison to White persons.

PATHOPHYSIOLOGY OF DIABETES IN OLDER ADULTS

Diabetes is basically a disease of the pancreas. The American Diabetes Association classifies diabetes mellitus affecting older adults into three types: type 1, the result of an absolute deficiency in insulin secretion due to autoimmune destruction of the beta (β) cells of the pancreas (the body destroys the β cells); type 2, due to tissue resistance to insulin action and relative insulin deficiency (the most common among older adults); and a third category reserved for other specific types of diabetes such as those due to injury to the pancreas or diseases that cause the body to be unable to use insulin correctly. Beta cells are a type of cell in the pancreas that make and release insulin, a hormone that controls the level of glucose in the blood. There is a baseline level of insulin maintained by the pancreas, but it can respond quickly to spikes in blood glucose by releasing stored insulin while simultaneously producing more from the β cells. The response time is fairly quick, taking approximately 10 minutes.

Most older adults with type 2 diabetes have had years of high blood glucose, insulin resistance, and generally have the *metabolic syndrome,* a group of metabolic risk factors that include the following:

■ Abdominal obesity: excessive fat tissue in and around the abdomen;
■ Atherogenic dyslipidemia: blood fat disorders including high triglycerides, low high-density lipoprotein cholesterol and high low-density lipoprotein cholesterol, all of which result in blockages in the walls of the arteries;
■ Elevated blood pressure;
■ Insulin resistance or glucose intolerance: the body is unable to properly use insulin or blood sugar;
■ Prothrombotic state: an increased tendency to develop blood clots in major arteries or veins; and
■ A proinflammatory state: increased proteins in the blood that cause inflammation in various parts of the body and result in such things as weight loss and muscle wasting and weakening.

Reasons for the increased prevalence of type 2 diabetes among older adults are not fully known. There appears to be an interaction among several factors, including genetics, lifestyle, and aging influences. Obesity and decreased physical activity, common among older adults, contribute to impairment in insulin action. In addition, some medications commonly used by older adults (e.g., diuretics, estrogen, sympathomimetics, glucocorticoids, niacin, olanzapine) can alter carbohydrate metabolism and increase glucose levels. Illnesses, such as infections, myocardial infarction, and stroke, and stress on the body, such as undergoing a surgical procedure, can cause hyperglycemia.

The prolonged impact of hyperglycemia from diabetes leads to changes in the tissues and organs of the body including the kidneys, heart and vascular system, and the central nervous system.

DIABETES DIAGNOSIS AND EVALUATION

The current American Diabetes Association diagnostic criteria for diabetes mellitus do not include any adjustments that are based on age. There are three ways to establish the diagnosis of diabetes mellitus as shown in Table 44.3.

In clinical practice, the presence of two fasting glucose levels of ≥ 126 mg/dL is the most common method of diagnosis. Older adults with a fasting blood glucose from 110 to 125 mg/dL are defined as having *impaired fasting glucose* (IFG), a condition associated with increased risk for diabetes development. Some older adults have isolated postchallenge (i.e., after eating) hyperglycemia (IPH) but do not have high fasting blood glucoses. It has been demonstrated repeatedly that in people with glucose intolerance, progression to type 2 diabetes can be prevented by medications and lifestyle changes.

MANAGEMENT

General Principles of Diabetes Management

The resident's primary health care provider should work with him or her, and the caregivers, to develop

| 44.3 | Criteria for the Diagnosis of Diabetes Mellitus |

I. Symptoms of polyuria, polydipsia, and unexplained weight loss plus a casual plasma glucose concentration of ≥ 200 mg/dL (11.1 mmol/L). *Casual* is defined as any time of day without regard to time since last meal.

II. Plasma glucose concentration after an 8-hour fast of ≥ 126 mg/dL (7.0 mmol/L).

III. Plasma glucose concentration of ≥ 200 mg/dL (11.1 mmol/L) measured 2 hours after ingestion of 75 g of glucose in 300 mL of water administered after an overnight fast.

goals for diabetes management that ideally consist of the following:

■ Control of the hyperglycemia and its symptoms
■ Management of the associated risks for vascular disease (i.e., coronary disease or heart disease, cerebrovascular disease or stroke, and peripheral vascular disease including decreased sensation, burning, or pain in the feet), vision changes, and kidney disease
■ Evaluation and treatment of diabetes complications (e.g., foot ulcers, skin infections, bladder infections, hyper- and hypoglycemia)

Another consideration in treating older diabetic adults is life expectancy and the time needed for clinical benefit from a specific intervention. Clinical trials have demonstrated that approximately 8 years are needed before the benefits of glycemic control are reflected in a reduction in vascular complications such as diabetic retinopathy or kidney disease, but only 2 to 3 years are required to see benefits from better control of blood pressure and lipids. It is important to remember that the median remaining life expectancy for a 70-year-old woman is 14 years—plenty of time for the development of diabetes complications. Therefore, for a newly diagnosed person in her or his early 70s, diabetes management is no different from that of younger people. In all cases, resident preferences and quality of life must be considered.

Management of Hyperglycemia

There are many options for drug therapy in older adults with type 2 diabetes who have no preferred treatment plans. Treatment may include any of the classes of drugs shown in Tables 44.4 and 44.5, used alone or in combination. Oral treatment may be sufficient for some individuals, while others may be best controlled with insulin administration. The assisted living nurse may want to recommend the use of an insulin pen, for example, if this will optimize the resident's and/or nursing assistant's ability to administer insulin when needed. Ongoing management of blood sugars should certainly be considered and implemented, although there are no clear guidelines as to how often finger sticks should be checked. Individuals on insulin will need more regular testing, whereas those who are stable on oral treatments can be tested less frequently. It is important to establish a realistic plan with which the resident is comfortable, that the nursing staff can implement, and in which the level of oversight is such that episodes of hyper- or hypoglycemia can be prevented.

44.4 | Noninsulin Agents for Treating Diabetes Mellitus

DRUG	DOSAGE	HOW THE DRUG WORKS
Oral agents		
Second-generation sulfonylureas		
Glimepiride (Amaryl)	4–8 mg daily, begin 1–2 mg	Increases insulin production
Glipizide (generic or Glucotrol)	2.5–40 mg daily in a single or divided dose	Increases insulin production
(Glucotrol XL)	5–20 mg daily	Increases insulin production
Glyburide (generic or Diaβeta, Micronase)	1.25–20 mg daily in a single or divided dose	Increases insulin production
Micronized glyburide (Glynase)	1.5–12 mg daily	Increases insulin production

(continued)

44.4 | Noninsulin Agents for Treating Diabetes Mellitus *(continued)*

DRUG	DOSAGE	HOW THE DRUG WORKS
α-Glucosidase inhibitors		
Acarbose (Precose)	50–100 mg tid, just before meals; start with 25 mg	Delays glucose absorption
Miglitol (Glyset)	25–100 mg tid, with 1st bite of meal; start with 25 mg qd	Delays glucose absorption
Biguanides		
Metformin (Glucophage)	500–2550 mg divided	Decreases liver production of glucose
(Glucophage XR)	1500–2000 mg qd	Decreases liver production of glucose
Meglitinides		
Nateglinide (Starlix)	60–120 mg tid	Increases insulin secretion
Repaglinide (Prandin)	0.5 mg bid–qid if $HbA_{1c} < 8\%$ or previously untreated 1–2 mg bid–qid if $HbA_{1c} \geq 8\%$ or previously treated	Increases insulin secretion
Thiazolidinediones		
Pioglitazone (Actos)	15 or 30 mg qd; max 45 mg/d as monotherapy, 30 mg/d in combination therapy	Reduces the cells resistance to insulin so increases the use of insulin in the body
Rosiglitazone (Avandia)	4 mg qd–bid	Reduces the cells resistance to insulin so increases the use of insulin in the body
Combination drugs		
Glipizide and metformin (METAGLIP)	2.5/250 once; 20/2,000 in two divided doses	Increases insulin production and decreases liver production of glucose
Glyburide and metformin (Glucovance)	1.25/250 mg initially if previously untreated; 2.5/500 mg or 5/500 mg bid with meals; max 20/2,000/d	Increases insulin production and decreases liver production of glucose
Rosiglitazone and metformin (Avandamet)	4/1,000–8/2,000 in two divided doses	Reduces the cell's resistance to insulin so increases the use of insulin in the body and decreases liver production of glucose

(continued)

44.4 | Noninsulin Agents for Treating Diabetes Mellitus *(continued)*

DRUG	DOSAGE	HOW THE DRUG WORKS
Injectable Agents		
Exenatide (Byetta)	5–10 µg SC bid	Incretin mimetic, which means that when food is eaten and there is an increase in glucose, the drug causes an increase in the release of insulin. This has the advantage of very low risk of hypoglycemia since it only works when the blood sugar is elevated
Pramlintide (Symlin)	60 µg SC before meals	Amylin analogue that decreases the liver's release of glucagons and slows the emptying of the stomach, which decreases appetite

Note: qid = four times a day; qd = every day; SC = subcutaneous; tid = three times a day.

Management of Hypoglycemia

If the resident complains of being, or is observed to be, shaky, nervous, tired, sweaty, cold, hungry, confused, lightheaded, irritable, or impatient, he or she should be checked for hypoglycemia. If the blood sugar is greater than 70 mg/dl, it is unlikely that blood sugar level is the cause of the symptoms. There are some individuals, however, who become accustomed to having relatively high blood sugars (in the 200 range), and these individuals may feel symptomatic when their blood sugars drop into the low 100s.

If the resident is symptomatic and the blood sugar is less than 70 mg/dl, they should be directed to quickly eat or drink 15 grams of carbohydrate, such as 1/2 cup of fruit juice (e.g., orange, cranberry), 1–2 teaspoons of sugar or honey, 1/2 cup of regular soda, 5–6 pieces of hard candy, glucose gel or tablets (take the amount noted on the package to total 15 grams of carbohydrate), or 1 cup of milk. For individuals with some swallowing difficulty or who are unwilling or unable to eat or drink at the time, the nurse, nursing assistant, or other caregiver can be taught to squeeze decorative cake frosting between the gum and the cheek. This will dissolve and get absorbed into the bloodstream within minutes.

The resident's blood sugar should be checked again in 15 minutes. If it is still below 70 mg/dl, the resident should eat another 15 grams of carbohydrate. For emergency situations in which the resident is nonresponsive with a low blood sugar, a glucagon kit should be available in the facility and staff should be trained on the use of this kit. The kit includes a prefilled syringe of glucagon for easy oral administration.

DIABETES EDUCATION AND SELF-MANAGEMENT SUPPORT

Diabetes self-management and support must cover several areas. It is extremely important that the older adults, and all caregivers, be educated about hypo- and hyperglycemia, including precipitating factors, prevention, symptoms (Table 44.6), monitoring, treatment, and when to notify the primary health care provider. Diet and physical activity remain important components of the initial and ongoing management of residents with diabetes. Specific dietary recommendations must be tailored for each individual and include assessment of cholesterol intake and weight management. Physical activity programs should also be individualized.

44.5 | Insulin Preparations

PREPARATIONS	ONSET	PEAK	DURATION
Insulin lispro (Humalog)	15 min	0.5–1.5 h	6–8 h
Insulin (e.g., Humulin, Novolin)			
Regular	0.5–1 h	2–3 h	8–12 h
Neutral Protamine Hagedorn or NPH	1–1.5 h	4–12 h	24 h
Insulin aspart (NovoLog)	30 min	1–3 h	3–5 h
Long-acting (Ultralente)	4–8 h	16–18 h	> 36 h
Insulin Glargine (Lantus)	1–2 h	—	24 h
Insulin, zinc (Lente)	1–2.5 h	8–12 h	18–24 h
Isophane insulin and regular insulin inj. (Novolin 70/30)	30 min	2–12 h	24 h

44.6 | Signs and Symptoms of Hyper- and Hypoglycemia

HYPOGLYCEMIA	HYPERGLYCEMIA
Confusion	High levels of sugar in the urine
Abnormal behavior (functional changes)	Frequent urination
Both confusion and abnormal behavior	Increased thirst
Visual disturbances (double vision and blurred vision)	Confusion
Seizures	Dry mouth
Loss of consciousness	
Heart palpitations	
Tremor	
Anxiety	
Sweating	
Hunger	

The resident should be assessed regularly for level of physical activity and informed about the benefits of exercise and available resources for becoming more active (http://www.easyforyou.info).

Ongoing education is needed for older adults and their caregivers with regard to any changes in management, particularly if new medications are started. Finger sticks to monitor glucose levels are needed to prevent and manage episodes of hypo- or hyperglycemia. Education should also include risk factors and methods to prevent and manage infections (fungal and bladder infections, in particular), foot ulcers, foot numbness, visual changes, and the other associated complications of diabetes such as cognitive impairment, hyponatremia, or urinary frequency.

RESOURCES

Dale, D., Federman, D., & Antman, K. (2006). *ACP medicine* (vols. 1 and 2). New York: WebMD, Inc.

Holman, R. R., Paul, S. K., Bethel, M. A., Matthews, D. R., & Neil, H. A. (2008). 10-year follow-up of intensive glucose control in type 2 diabetes. *New England Journal of Medicine, 359*(15), 1577–1589.

Porsche, R., & Brenner, Z. R. (2006). Amiodarone-induced thyroid dysfunction. *Critical Care Nurse, 26*(3), 34–41.

Summaries for Patients. (2008). Comparison of two types of insulin added to diabetes pills in poorly controlled type 2 diabetes. *Annals of Internal Medicine, 149*(8), 1–46.

Zhang, X., Gregg, E. W., Cheng, Y. J., Thompson, T. J., Geiss, L. S., Duenas, M. R., et al. (2008). Diabetes mellitus and visual impairment: National health and nutrition examination survey, 1999–2004. *Archives of Ophthalmology, 126*(10), 1421–1427.

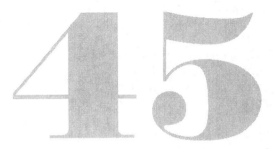

Gastrointestinal Diseases and Disorders

George Triadafilopoulos and Jennifer Hauf

The structure and function of the gastrointestinal tract are affected both by physiologic changes of aging and by the effects of accumulating disorders involving many body systems. In association with age, there are changes in connective tissue that limit the elasticity of the gut and additional alterations in the nerves and muscles of the gut that impair motility. Some disease states, like atherosclerosis and diabetes mellitus, can adversely influence gastrointestinal function and lead to symptoms and complications. Gastrointestinal problems may quickly compromise the older adult's ability to maintain adequate nutrition and hydration and can cause fatigue, weakness, weight loss, and decreased quality of life.

ESOPHAGUS

Gastroesophageal Reflux Disease (GERD)

GERD is a chronic symptom of mucosal damage produced by the abnormal reflux of gastric contents into the esophagus. Highly specific symptoms for GERD include heartburn, regurgitation, or both, that occur often after meals, are aggravated by lying down or bending forward at the waist, and are relieved by antacids. Among persons age 65 and over, symptoms of heartburn or acid regurgitation occur at least weekly in 20% of the population and at least monthly in 59% of the population.

In more than 80% of older adults, GERD is caused by transient inappropriate lower esophageal sphincter relaxation that leads to acid reflux into the esophagus. Some persons may have reduced lower esophageal sphincter tone that permits reflux when intra-abdominal pressure rises. Sliding hiatal hernia occurs in about 30% of older adults age 50 years or over and may contribute to acid reflux and regurgitation. Poor esophageal peristalsis (i.e., movement that allows passage of food, fluid, and gas) leads to delayed clearance of the refluxate and increased exposure of the esophagus to abdominal acid. Older adults who take medications with anticholinergic properties (e.g., Benadryl, oxybutinin) generally have reduced salivary secretions. Salivary secretions are important, as these secretions protect the lining of the esophagus from refluxed acid, which can damage the esophageal tissue.

Older adults with mild symptoms of regurgitation should be treated with acid-suppressing drugs to decrease the risk of damage to the esophageal tissue. If symptoms are not relieved by treatment, then further evaluation by the primary health care provider is recommended. The presence of anemia, dysphagia, gastrointestinal bleeding, recurrent vomiting, and weight loss suggests complicated GERD. Older adults with these signs and symptoms should be referred to their primary health care provider because the next step will generally be endoscopy to observe for tissue damage in the esophagus.

A group of drugs called proton-pump inhibitors are the treatment of choice for older adults with GERD. Some of these medications (e.g., omeprazole; Prilosec OTC) are currently available over-the-counter. These drugs heal esophagitis in 85% of cases and eradicate heartburn and regurgitation in 80% of cases. In comparison, H$_2$ antagonists (e.g., ranitidine) ameliorate symptoms and heal esophagitis in only 60% of cases. For the dysphagic older adult, various formulations of proton-pump inhibitors, such as orally disintegrating tablets, are available. Generally, therapy is continued for at least 8 weeks. After this period, the resident is given a trial period off medication to determine if symptoms reoccur. Recurrence is common after therapy is stopped, and lifelong therapy is usually needed. It should be recognized, however, that ongoing treatment with these medication is not without risk. Gastric acidity normally protects the individual against ingested pathogens that can cause pneumonia; therefore, suppression of the acid increases the risk of pneumonia.

Drug-Induced Esophageal Injury

Decreased esophageal peristaltic clearance, common among older adults, may be associated with pill retention, as a result of which esophageal injury can occur because of prolonged contact of the caustic contents of the medication with the esophageal mucosa. Given that salivation and swallowing are markedly reduced during sleep, pill intake immediately before going to sleep and without adequate fluid can increase risk of pill retention and injury. Taking medications with at least 8 fluid ounces of water helps dissolve tablets or capsules and may reduce the risk of injury or gastrointestinal complaints. Those with medication-induced esophageal injury complain of sudden painful swallowing (odynophagia) to a degree that even swallowing saliva is difficult.

Tetracyclines, particularly doxycycline, are the most common antibiotics that induce esophagitis. Aspirin and all of the nonsteroidal anti-inflammatory drugs (NSAIDs) can also damage the esophagus. Other offenders include potassium chloride, quinidine, iron, and alendronate (an agent increasingly used for treatment of osteoporosis in older adults). Alendronate should be used cautiously in residents with esophageal dysfunction. It must be taken on an empty stomach with at least 8 ounces of water that should be consumed with the medication to minimize the risk of the tablet getting stuck in the esophagus and causing damage. In addition, residents should stand or sit upright for at least 30 minutes after taking the alendronate to facilitate

drug absorption; the resident should not eat during this 30 minute interval.

Esophageal Cancer: Endoscopic Palliation

Esophageal cancer is commonly diagnosed at an advanced, incurable stage in older adults who are, therefore, not candidates for resection of the tumor. These residents are plagued by symptoms of esophageal obstruction or fistula formation, dysphagia, aspiration, and weight loss. In such instances, palliative treatments can sometimes be done such as laser therapy or a single stent placement into the esophagus to open the esophagus and facilitate swallowing.

STOMACH

Dyspepsia

Dyspepsia implies chronic or recurrent pain or discomfort in the upper abdomen. Major causes of dyspepsia are gastric or duodenal ulcers, gastroesophageal reflux, and gastric cancer. Endoscopy may or may not show evidence of reflux.

Because the incidence of gastric cancer increases with age, upper endoscopy should be considered in older adults presenting with new onset of dyspepsia. Treatment is targeted at the underlying diagnosis. For residents with evidence of an ulcer and documented *H. pylori* infection at the site of the ulcer, a trial of *H. pylori* therapy should heal the ulcer and decrease the likelihood that the ulcer will reoccur. For most older adults with functional (or nonulcer) dyspepsia, reassurance and a course of medication that decreases the secretion of acid (either H$_2$-receptor antagonists or proton-pump inhibitors) is usually recommended.

Medication-Induced Gastric Complications

The risk of ulcers and their complications is three times greater among NSAID users than in nonusers. For those age 60 or over, the relative risk increases even more, to fivefold. Older adults with NSAID-induced ulcers tend to present with anemia, bleeding, or perforation without the warning symptoms of dyspepsia or abdominal pain. When NSAIDs are used, even if these are COX-2 inhibitors, the individual should also take a proton-pump inhibitor.

Peptic Ulcer Disease

In the United States, *H. pylori* infection is responsible for about 80% of duodenal ulcers and approximately 60% of gastric ulcers. The majority of older adults with ulcers complain of dyspepsia, although bleeding, anemia, and acute abdominal pain may also occur. Typically, the diagnosis of peptic ulcer is made by upper gastrointestinal endoscopy.

Biliary Disease

Gallstones primarily form in the gallbladder and may obstruct the cystic or common bile duct, causing biliary pain, cholecystitis, and cholangitis. When stones obstruct the gallbladder, pancreatitis may occur. Biliary pain is characterized as acute, severe upper abdominal pain, usually in the epigastrium or right upper quadrant; it may last for more than 1 hour. Pain may radiate to the back or scapula and is often associated with restlessness, nausea, or vomiting. Episodes are typically separated by several weeks. Postprandial epigastric fullness (i.e., a sense of fullness in the mid-upper stomach after eating), fatty food intolerance, and regurgitation are nonspecific symptoms and may or may not be due to gallstones. In older adults who complain of biliary pain but have had a cholecystectomy, it is possible that they have a retained common bile duct and a stone could be embedded within this area.

COLON

Constipation

Chronic constipation, stool evacuation less than three times per week, affects about 30% of adults age 65 years or older and is more common among women. Some older adults may complain of straining at defecation or a sense of incomplete defecation despite a daily bowel evacuation. A more objective diagnosis of constipation is based on colonic transit times, which is the time it takes for the passage of stool through the colon. Normal transit time is about 6 hours in the small intestine and 36 to 72 hours in the large intestine.

Older adults are at risk for constipation because of normal age-related changes that result in decreased sensation of the need to defecate and a slowing of the motility of the gastrointestinal tract. Nerves in the rectum become less receptive and less able to distinguish between flatus, solid, or liquid matter exiting from the anus. Other factors contributing to constipation include comorbid conditions such as endocrine/metabolic diseases, myopathic conditions, neurologic disease, psychological conditions, and functional impairments. Medications commonly administered to older adults can also cause or contribute to constipation, such as analgesics, antacids, antidepressants, antihistamines, antihypertensives, anticholinergics, antiparkinsonism drugs, iron salts, NSAIDs, sedatives, and opiates. Lastly, poor mobility, low-fiber diets, and dehydration also increase the risk for constipation.

Most individuals with constipation have *colonic inertia*, defined as the delayed passage of radiopaque markers (or stool) through the colon. *Outlet delay*, when the stool passes normally through to the rectum but then remains there, is another cause of constipation. This is typically seen in older females with weak pelvic muscles.

Treatment of Constipation

In addition to the impact on quality of life, chronic constipation can lead to fecal impaction, and subsequent urinary and fecal incontinence. Treatment is a resident-sensitive mix of nonpharmacological and pharmacological measures.

Nonpharmacological Methods

Lifestyle interventions that specifically address diet, fluid intake, and activity may be helpful in preventing constipation in older adults. Increased dietary fiber, with a goal of consuming 24 grams of fiber per day, can improve *propulsion time*, increase the rate of passage of stool through the colon, and help produce stools that are softer and easier to expel. Adequate hydration and exercise to optimize bowel function may also be helpful. These interventions will not, however, be sufficient to treat constipation once it occurs (i.e., water and exercise will not provide the bowel stimulation needed to cause evacuation once constipation is present).

A comprehensive review of current prescribed medications can also be done to determine if there are medications that are likely to be contributing to constipation. If possible, it may be helpful to replace a constipating medication with one that is less-constipating, or at least reducing the dose. Lastly, encouraging the resident to recognize and respond to the urge to defecate rather than ignore it will help in preventing constipation.

Pharmacological Methods

Pharmacological treatment of constipation involves laxatives that are divided into the following classes: *bulk *laxatives, stool softeners, osmotic laxatives,* and *stimulant laxatives* (see Table 45.1). Bulk laxatives are organic polymers that absorb water from the intestinal lumen to improve stool bulk and soften stool consistency. These agents take several days to work. It is critical that the individual drink sufficient amounts of fluid to avoid mechanical obstruction. Laxatives will not be useful if the resident has a slow transit time that is causing the constipation or anorectal dysfunction thus making it difficult for him or her to eliminate stool once it is in the rectum.

Stool softeners lower intestinal surface tension that permits water to enter the bowel more readily. These agents may have some role in the prevention of constipa-

tion, but they are not effective as a treatment once constipation has occurred. *Saline/osmotic laxatives* contain poorly absorbed molecules that pull fluid into the colon from the blood stream (e.g., milk of magnesia). Newer saline/osmotic laxatives are the polyethylene glycols (PEGs) such as lactulose that appear to be safe and effective although they tend to cause significant gas production. *Stimulant laxatives* increase intestinal motility and secretion of water into the bowel, usually producing bowel movements within hours. These agents tend to be associated with abdominal discomfort, electrolyte imbalances, cramping, hepatotoxicity (liver damage), and allergic reactions.

45.1 | Descriptions of the Different Laxatives Used for Constipation

DRUG CLASS/DRUG	MECHANISM OF ACTION	ADVERSE EFFECTS	DOSAGE
Bulk-forming Psyllium	Increases water and water-absorbent properties of stool	Flatulence, abdominal cramps, rarely allergic reaction	10–20 g in evening with 1.4 dL of water
Osmotic laxatives Milk of Magnesia	Produces osmotic gradient and retains fluid in colonic lumen leading to improved propulsion	Flatulence, hypermagnesemia in residents with renal failure, hypokalemia	2.25–4.5 tbsp in the morning with 2 dL liquid
Lactulose	Produces osmotic gradient and colonic water retention	Flatulence, abdominal cramps, hypokalemia	10–30 mL daily to BID
Polyethylene glycol	Binds and retains water in the colonic lumen	Abdominal pain; rarely flatulence	10–3 g daily to BID
Chloride channel activator	Enhances intestinal fluid secretion and may restore mucosal barrier function	Nausea, abdominal discomfort, headache	24 mcg po BID
Stimulant laxatives Anthraquinones (senna, cascara)	Induces active secretion of water and electrolytes; myenteric plexus stimulation	Abdominal cramps, hypokalemia	12–30 mg daily
Bisacodyl	Direct stimulation of small intestine and colonic peristalsis	Abdominal cramps, flatulence, rectal burning	5–10 mg at night up to three times per week
Phosphate enema	Rectal distension stimulates evacuation	Anorectal irritation; hyperphosphatemia in chronic renal failure	When needed

Note: BID = twice a day; po = by mouth.

For older adults with normal colonic transit time, fluids, dietary fiber, and bulk laxatives, such as psyllium seed or calcium polycarbophil, are effective in maintaining bowel function so that constipation does not occur. Management of older adults with slow-transit constipation generally will require a daily osmotic laxative such as sorbitol, lactulose, or a polyethylene glycol solution. Individuals with anorectal dysfunction may need a stimulant laxative to evacuate the stool from the rectum. When fecal impaction occurs, the colon should be evacuated with enemas or polyethylene glycol electrolyte solution until cleansing is complete. Recurrence of fecal impaction should be avoided by establishing an appropriate diet, fluid, activity, and laxative plan.

Fecal Incontinence

Fecal incontinence, defined as recurrent uncontrolled passage of fecal material for at least 1 month, affects quality of life and can lead to social isolation. It may be minor, with inadvertent passage of flatus or soiling of underwear with liquid stool, or it may be major, with involuntary leakage of feces. Fecal incontinence affects 2% to 7% of adults, most of whom are older adults.

Fecal continence depends on many factors, such as physical and mental function, stool consistency, colonic transit, rectal strength, internal and external anal sphincter function, as well as anorectal sensation and reflexes. Normal defecation is a complex process that starts with entry of stool into the rectum that leads to reflex relaxation of the internal anal sphincter so that the stool can pass. Decreased anal sphincter tone can result from trauma (e.g., vaginal deliveries, anal surgery, radiation) or neurologic disorders (e.g., spinal cord injury or a secondary effect of diabetes mellitus) and result in being unable to tighten the sphincter and control the passage of stool.

Impaction is a common cause of fecal incontinence in older adults. The history and physical examination often provide clues to the cause of fecal incontinence. Asking about recent bowel activity, exploring symptoms of fullness, examination of the abdomen to see if it is hard, distended, and/or uncomfortable when palpated, and doing a rectal exam to see if there is stool in the rectum help identify evidence of impaction. In the event of impaction, or evidence of a large amount of stool in the rectum, enemata are likely needed (possibly given daily over a few days to fully evacuate the bowel). Following an impaction, work with the resident and his or her primary health care provider to establish a bowel regimen that will avoid future impactions.

Management of fecal incontinence should focus on trying to reduce how often the individual passes stool and making the stool consistency easier to manage. If the person tends to have frequent, loose stools, an antidiarrheal drug, such as loperamide, may be an effective way in which to decrease episodes of incontinence. A bulking agent, such as methylcellulose, can help firm the stool and make management easier for the resident and caregiver. Residents with incontinence related to cognitive impairment or physical debility may benefit from a regular defecation program. Such a program would include six to eight, 8-ounce glasses of fluid daily, regular physical activity as per resident ability, and, as needed, an appropriate laxative based on assessment of the resident's bowel patterns and stool consistency.

Diverticular Disease

Diverticular disease is very common in older adults and means that the individual has developed small pouches in the lining of the colon (i.e., large intestine) that bulge outward through weak spots. Each pouch is called a diverticulum; multiple pouches are called diverticula. The condition of having diverticula is called diverticulosis. When the pouches become inflamed, the condition is called diverticulitis. Most older adults with diverticular disease have no symptoms, although 20% will develop diverticulitis, and 10% may develop bleeding from the diverticula. The mere presence of diverticulosis does not require specific therapy. However, these individuals are encouraged to eat a diet high in fiber, as this may reduce the risk of developing diverticulitis or bleeding.

Some older adults with diverticulosis may complain of nonspecific abdominal cramping, bloating, flatulence, and irregular bowel habits. Diverticular bleeding is usually painless and self-limited; it rarely coexists with acute diverticulitis. Diverticulitis usually presents with left lower quadrant pain and a low-grade fever; nausea, vomiting, constipation, diarrhea, and dysuria or frequency may occur. If the resident has left lower abdomen tenderness or some distension, the primary health care provider should be contacted. Mild diverticulitis is usually treated with clear liquids and oral antibiotics.

Irritable Bowel Syndrome

Irritable bowel syndrome (IBS) is a functional gastrointestinal disorder characterized by abdominal pain, bloating, and either constipation or diarrhea, or both. Although psychosocial factors are commonly involved in IBS, they are not known to have a causative role. These signs and symptoms are *not* indicative of IBS: weight loss, first onset of symptoms after age 50, nocturnal diarrhea, rectal bleeding or obstruction, anemia, an elevated white blood count, abnormal blood chemistries, positive fecal cultures for infection. Treatment usually focuses on managing the symptoms and includes medications to prevent or decrease colon spasms, antidiarrheals, and/or fiber supplements.

Gastrointestinal Bleeding

Older adults commonly have a positive stool test for occult blood or are diagnosed with unexplained iron-deficiency anemia. Although colorectal cancer is a leading concern, many other causes, such as esophagitis, peptic ulcers, esophageal and gastric malignancies, intestinal or colonic angiodysplasia, benign colon polyps, inflammatory bowel disease, or hemorrhoids may be the cause. Unfortunately, the stool test can result in a false-positive: the test was positive but not really indicative of any serious finding. Given the high incidence of bowel cancer in older adults, however, the primary health care provider, resident, and family/proxy can then explore further testing to determine the cause of the bleeding and next steps.

Clostridium Difficile Infection and Pseudomembranous Colitis

C. difficile infection is generally precipitated by the use of antibiotics, such as cephalosporins, penicillins, or clindamycin, but it can also be passed from one resident to the next. Clinically it presents with watery, foul-smelling diarrhea, crampy abdominal pain, fever, abdominal tenderness and distention, and an elevated white blood cell count. The diagnosis is best made by sending a stool specimen for culture so that *C. difficile* cytotoxins can be identified. Antibiotic treatment is needed and usually is with metronidazole 250 mg orally every 6 hours for 10 days; it is effective in 85% of cases. If this does not eliminate the infection—based on the resident being pain free and without diarrhea—vancomycin (125 mg every 6 hours) is used. Relapses may occur in up to 20% of cases and require additional treatment. With multiple recurrences of *C. difficile*, vancomycin taper regimens are recommended. Prevention of transmission of *C. difficile* is critical and includes good hand washing between residents. It is critically important to educate all staff and families that alcohol-based cleaners will not kill *C. difficile*. Hand washing

with soap and water, however, is effective and should be stressed (also see Chapter 41, "Infectious Diseases").

Colonic Polyps and Colon Cancer

A colonic polyp is a small clump of cells that form on the colon lining. Although the great majority of colon polyps are harmless, some may become cancerous over time. The risk of developing colonic polyps is greater among those who are 50 years of age or older, male, overweight, a smoker, eat a high-fat, low-fiber diet, or have a personal or family history of colon polyps or colon cancer. Polyps are usually asymptomatic, but they may bleed or predispose the individual to cancer. Detection and removal of polyps decreases the risk of developing colorectal cancer.

Colorectal cancer is the third leading cancer in the United States and the second leading cause of cancer death. The risk of colorectal cancer increases dramatically with age, with more than 90% of cases occurring in people over age 50. Signs and symptoms indicative of colon cancer include a positive stool for occult blood, abdominal pain, altered bowel function, or pencil-thin stools. When any of these signs or symptoms are present, the primary health care provider will generally refer the individual for a colonoscopy. Residents may need help with the preparation for the colonoscopy. The goal of colonoscopy preparation is to eliminate all fecal matter from the colon so that the physician conducting the colonoscopy will have a clear view. There are several ways to achieve this: a clear liquid diet the day before the colonoscopy; a laxative such as Golytely (also called Colyte, or Nulytely), phospho-soda, or sodium phosphate tablets (Osmo-Prep and Visicol). On the day of the test, in addition to having nothing by mouth (i.e., NPO), a Dulcolax suppository or Fleets enema might also be administered.

RESOURCES

Calfee, D. P. (2008). Clostridium difficile: A reemerging pathogen. *Geriatrics, 63*(9), 10–21.

Holman, C., Roberts, S., & Nicol, M. (2008). Preventing and treating constipation in later life. *Nursing Older People, 20*(5), 22–24.

Miyamoto, M., Haruma, K., Kuwabara, M., Nagano, M., Okamoto, T., & Tanaka, M. (2007). Long-term gastroesophageal reflux disease therapy improves symptoms in elderly patients: Five-year prospective study in community medicine. *Journal of Gastroenterology and Hepatology, 22*(5), 639–644.

Morley, J. E. (2007). Constipation and irritable bowel syndrome in the elderly. *Clinics in Geriatric Medicine, 23*(4), 823–832, vi–vii.

Gynecologic Diseases and Sexual Disorders in Women and Men

G. Willy Davila, Angela Gentili,
Thomas Mulligan, and Barbara Resnick

Most older women generally do not seek regular gynecologic care as they no longer need to have Pap tests done, and may not be actively engaged in sexual activity and do not need birth control. They may, however, have problems associated with their gynecological system and/or sexual disorders that need to be evaluated and managed to improve their overall health and quality of life.

HISTORY AND PHYSICAL EXAMINATION

Older women should be asked about gynecologic-related issues including involuntary loss of urine or feces, sexual behavior patterns, potential exposure to sexually transmitted diseases, and use of alternative medical treatments (e.g., for sexual drive or vaginal dryness). The history related to sexual activity is the most important part of the evaluation of sexual function; careful questioning can detect problems that the individual might not otherwise volunteer. It is important to provide a comfortable atmosphere and privacy. Ask the woman about her interest in sexual activity (i.e., sex drive), dyspareunia (i.e., painful sexual activity) if she is sexually active, lack of vaginal lubrication, and any negative experiences such as current negative or abusive interactions with a spouse or significant other (particularly if she is a caregiver or in a dependent situation receiving care).

Nongynecologic medical problems that can have significant gynecologic effects should be noted. For example, women who have had breast cancer therapy may have severe vaginal atrophy (i.e., thinning and inflammation of the vaginal walls due to a decline in estrogen). Women with significant osteoporosis and curvature of the spine may be more likely to have genital prolapse, which occurs when the pelvic organs (uterus, bladder, rectum) slip down from their normal position and either protrude into or press against the wall of the vagina. Previous obstetrical events may have damaged the pelvic floor causing urinary incontinence and genital prolapse. History taking should also include inquiry about abdominal distention (a sign of ovarian cancer) and abnormal vaginal discharge or bleeding (signs of endometrial, cervical, or vaginal cancer), and a history of estrogen use. Positioning of the woman to ideally visualize the vaginal area may be a challenge. To examine the woman in bed, which is often the most practical, position her on an inverted bedpan placed under the sacrum in order to elevate the pelvis. As an alternative position the woman can be positioned in the left lateral decubitus position: the woman lies on her left side, with knees flexed.

A simple pelvic examination of an older woman includes the following:

- Examination of the vulva for abnormal pigmentation, erythema, or raised lesions.
- Evidence of atrophy: vaginal dryness, pale vaginal mucosa. This is easily seen just by looking at the inside of the lips of the vagina.
- Instruct the woman to perform the Valsalva maneuver to evaluate for pelvic organ prolapse and urinary incontinence: take a deep breath and then forcibly exhale against pursed lips or a closed airway. Observe if tissues protrude from the vaginal opening or if there is leakage of urine (see Chapter 26, "Urinary Incontinence").

Older women are at risk for ovarian cancer and should be seen by their primary health care provider if there are any signs of this problem: abdominal distension or pain, urinary retention. Normally, the ovaries become smaller with age; a referral can further examine the woman and determine if there are abnormal changes. Further testing usually involves abdominal or pelvic ultrasound.

TREATMENT OF MENOPAUSAL SYMPTOMS

Estrogen is labeled by the U.S. Food and Drug Administration (FDA) for the treatment of menopausal symptoms, urogenital dryness, and for prevention of osteoporosis. Although there are many benefits to estrogen use, there are risks as well.

The average age of menopause is 51 among White women living in the United States. With a life expectancy of 78 years, the average woman is postmenopausal one-third of her life. Many women and their health care providers choose to treat or prevent the side effects of estrogen deficiency in menopause, although the popularity of this therapy is waning in response to the recent findings of the Women's Health Initiative (WHI) trial, which showed that the risk of stroke and breast cancer are greater among those who take estrogen. Vasomotor symptoms or hot flashes are the most common symptom of menopause, occurring in up to 80% of perimenopausal women. Symptoms persist beyond 5 years in 25% of women and are lifelong in a small minority. Although the cause of the vasomotor response remains unknown, vasomotor symptoms are usually relieved with estrogen treatment. When estrogen is contraindicated (history of breast cancer) or not tolerated because of swelling (most commonly of the feet and hands), breast tenderness, or weight gain, then antidepressant medications such as selective serotonin reuptake inhibitors or progestins can be used. Herbal remedies such as yams and black cohosh have also been tried, although there is little evidence to support their use. Some individuals find some benefit from phytoestrogens—an estrogenlike substance found in some plants and plant products. The chemical structure of these natural products, such as soy, resemble the body's estrogen and allows them to weakly bind to an estrogen receptor, potentially blocking excess estrogen, or, when estrogen is low, quieting the system's need for estrogen.

TREATMENT OF UROGENITAL SYMPTOMS

Urogenital Atrophy

Urogenital atrophy occurs in all postmenopausal women. The cells of the vagina depend on estrogen stimulation, but there is less available following menopause. Consequently, these tissues become dry, pale, smoother, and thinner; there may be inflammation and tenderness due to these changes. The changes are readily reversed with the administration of local (topical) estrogen: one half an applicator (1 to 2 g) of intravaginal use of estrogen cream, as infrequently as two nights per week, provides topical estrogen therapy with minimal (if any) absorption into the body. Alternatively, an estrogen ring may be used (3 months per ring) or vaginal tablets used twice weekly. Estrogen cream is also an excellent lubricant for use during intercourse or for pessary insertion (see the section "Pessaries" later in this chapter).

Vaginal Infection and Inflammation

Postmenopausal women are susceptible to a broad range of vaginal infections. Fungal infections are common, particularly in diabetic and obese older women who have chronic moisture and irritation in the vaginal area. The resident or caregiver may notice an odorless, white cheeselike drainage from the vagina; the labia may be red; pain and burning with urination or any sexual activity might be reported. Fungal infections are easily treated with oral, intravaginal, and topical antifungal agents that are now sold over-the-counter. The woman will likely need help to insert a vaginal applicator or suppository. If she is willing to try and learn to do this independently, instruct her to do this while standing with a wide-based stance and holding on with one hand to the bathroom sink or grab bar. Alternatively, lying on her back with her knees flexed may also facilitate insertion. Vaginal infections common in reproductive-age women such as trichomonas and *Gardnerella* vaginosis are less common in elderly women. It is likely that this is because of the higher vaginal pH of older women. The presence of Gardnerella vaginosis is noted by complaint of gray, yellow, or white drainage with a fishy odor, pain, burning, irritation, and redness. It is treated with an oral antibiotic.

DISORDERS OF THE VULVA

With aging, the skin of the vulva loses elasticity; the underlying fat and connective tissues undergo degeneration resulting in loss of collagen and thinning of the epithelial layer. Consequently, postmenopausal women who are not on estrogen therapy are predisposed to a variety of dermatologic disorders and symptoms. Vulvar skin irritation occurs from a variety of agents and causes burning, itching, and edema; vulvar excoriation can result from scratching an inflamed vulva. Hygiene products used for urinary or fecal incontinence may lead to chemical dermatitis, as does urine itself. Treatment of incontinence is important to solving this problem. Local (topical) corticosteroids such as hydrocortisone 1% ointment applied daily, sitz baths, or routine washing with warm soapy water and drying the area well can help alleviate vulvar irritation. Any growth (e.g., warts) noted on the vulva should be noted and the primary health care provider informed.

DISORDERS OF PELVIC FLOOR SUPPORT

Child bearing, constipation, chronic coughing, and heavy lifting increase intra-abdominal pressure and can cause progressive weakening of the connective tissue and muscular supports of the genital organs, thus leading to *genital prolapse.* Common symptoms of prolapse include pelvic pressure (pressure in the lower abdomen), lower back pain, urinary or fecal incontinence, difficulty with rectal emptying, or a palpable mass. Vaginal prolapse can include *rectocele,* protrusion of rectum against the posterior vaginal wall, or *cystocele,* descent (i.e., dropping down) of the anterior vaginal wall. *Urethrocele,* which is when part of the urethra protrudes into the anterior wall of the vagina, can occur with a cystocele. These conditions are visible by asking the woman to bear down or cough while standing or lying on her back. It is important to check whether or not any of these conditions have been previously evaluated. Treatment generally starts with Kegel's exercises to strengthen the pelvic floor musculature (see Chapter 26, "Urinary Incontinence"). Alternatively, a pessary can be used to hold in place or prevent the prolapse from occurring.

Treatments

Pessaries

Pessaries are commonly used in an effort to delay or avoid surgery. Their use in older women may be indicated in order to provide comfort and restore bladder function when comorbid illness makes surgery undesirable or untenable. Pessaries are made from rubber, plastic, or silicone and come in a variety of shapes and sizes: doughnuts, rings, cubes, inflatable balls, and foldable models. They are usually fit by a gynecologist; follow-up care will vary. Most older women will either have this done by the gynecologist on a regular basis or require some nursing care to help with pessary changes and cleaning. All women with pessaries should be instructed to report any unusual discharge, bleeding, or discomfort, and any changes in bladder or bowel function. All users should have a pelvic examination once or twice a year. If discomfort is present or the device becomes uncomfortable, a different size or type should be tried.

Surgery for Prolapse

Surgical treatment of vaginal prolapse can be classified as either reconstructive or obliterative. Reconstructive procedures are designed to restore normal anatomy, whereas obliterative procedures result in closure, or sewing up, of the vaginal canal. The decision to do an obliterative procedure should be made carefully as it would mean no sexual interactions that included penile penetration.

POSTMENOPAUSAL VAGINAL BLEEDING

Postmenopausal bleeding, defined as bleeding after 1 year of amenorrhea (i.e., no menses), occurs in a significant number of older women. Hormone replacement with estrogen or other medications such as selective estrogen receptor modulating agents (e.g., tamoxifen), aromatase (Arimidex), or progesterone drugs (Megace) are common causes of postmenopausal vaginal bleeding. Stopping these medications can resolve the bleeding. The woman should be evaluated, as well, for signs of tissue trauma such as open sores from scratching, or irritation of clothing, or from a pessary. If no immediate cause of the bleeding is noted, further evaluation is needed.

FEMALE SEXUALITY

Age-Associated Changes

Many factors are important in the sexual responsiveness of older women, including changes that occur with menopause, cultural expectations, relationship problems, previous sexual experiences, chronic illnesses, and depression. In the United States, women live about 29 years after menopause and outlive their spouses by an average of 8 years. Although the frequency of intercourse decreases with aging, sexuality remains important for some older women. Lack of sexual activity among women may be because they have no partner. For women with partners, lack of sexual activity is reportedly due the woman's disinterest in intercourse (43%), the man's disinterest (24%), or the man's illness or erectile dysfunction (29%).

The female sexual response cycle changes with aging; many of the changes are thought to be due to a decline in serum estrogen concentration after menopause. During the excitement phase, the clitoris may require longer direct stimulation; genital engorgement (i.e., increased blood flow to the vagina and labia) is reduced. Decreased blood flow during the excitement phase contributes to the reduced vaginal lubrication that occurs with aging, although with increased foreplay and gentle stimulation, lubrication is usually adequate for intercourse. During orgasm, fewer and weaker contractions occur, although older women can still achieve multiple orgasms.

Female Sexual Dysfunction

For the most part, menopause is accompanied by decreased sexual function and decreased sexual interest. In addition, there is an increase in urogenital symptoms such as urinary urgency, dysuria, frequency, urinary incontinence, vaginal itching, vaginal dryness, and painful intercourse. Dyspareunia, defined as pain with intercourse, can be due to physical or psychological factors, or a combination of the two. The most common cause of dyspareunia is atrophic vaginitis due to estrogen deficiency. Other causes include localized vaginal infections, bladder infections, pelvic tumors, excessive penile thrusting, or improper angle of penile entry.

Estrogen replacement can improve vaginal lubrication and sense of well-being with regard to pleasurable sexual activity, but it has little effect on libido (i.e., sex drive that is thought to be dependent on testosterone, even in women, rather than on estrogen). The ovaries and adrenal glands are the main sources of androgens in women. It is possible that there is a female androgen deficiency syndrome, with impaired sexual function, loss of energy, depression, and serum total testosterone concentrations in the lower end of normal for women (< 15 ng/dL), but there is no well-substantiated evidence or definition.

Older women commonly have multiple medical problems that may also affect sexual desire. Women with diabetes mellitus report decreased libido and lubrication, and longer time to reach orgasm. Rheumatic diseases affect sexuality because of functional disability. After mastectomy for breast cancer, 20% to 40% of women experience sexual dysfunction, possibly because of disruption of body image, marital and family problems, spousal reaction, therapy for the cancer, or the psychological impact of a breast cancer diagnosis. Some drugs can adversely affect sexual function, including antihistamines, antihypertensives, antidepressants, antipsychotics, antiestrogens, central nervous system stimulants, narcotics, alcohol, and anticholinergic drugs.

Psychosocial factors have an important role in sexual dysfunction. Women commonly marry men older than themselves and live longer than men. Consequently, heterosexual older women are likely to spend the last years of their lives alone. Even when a partner is available, he might have erectile dysfunction. Finally, lack of privacy may be a problem when the older couple live in a community with caregivers coming in and out of the room.

Treatment

Dyspareunia due to atrophic vaginitis and decreased lubrication responds well to topical or systemic estrogen therapy. However, it is important to explain to the woman that complete restoration of vaginal tissue function may take up to 2 years. If the resident is not a candidate for or does not want to use estrogen, water-soluble vaginal lubricants (e.g., Replens, Astroglide, K-Y Jelly) are beneficial. Importantly, local stimulation through regular intercourse helps maintain a healthy vaginal mucosa. Longer foreplay allows more time for vaginal lubrication, just as older men often need longer and more direct stimulation to achieve an adequate erection. Decreased libido may respond to testosterone, but no androgen preparation is approved by the FDA for female sexual desire disorders. There has been some use of sildenafil (Viagra) for female sexual dysfunction, although the results are conflicting. The older woman should also receive education about male sexual aging in addition to female sexual aging. Otherwise, she might mistakenly attribute her partner's diminished erection and need for more genital stimulation to her own inability to arouse her partner. Other psychological issues, including depression, history of sexual abuse, and relationship problems, should be addressed and treated in coordination with the woman's primary health care provider.

MALE SEXUALITY

Age-Associated Changes

As men age their sex interests and activities likewise change. The frequency of sexual intercourse and the prevalence of engaging in any sexual activity decreases. Among men 60 to 70 years old, 50% to 80% engage in any sexual activity, a prevalence rate that declines to 15% to 25% among those age 80 years and older. However, sexual interest often persists despite decreased activity. The man's level of sexual activity, interest, and enjoyment in younger years often determines his sexual behavior with aging. Factors contributing to a man's decreased sexual activity include poor health, social issues, partner availability, decreased libido, and erectile dysfunction.

Aging is associated not only with changes in sexual behavior but also with changes in the stages of sexual response. During the excitement phase, there is a delay in erection, decreased response by the scrotal sac, and loss of testicular elevation. Orgasm is diminished in duration and intensity, with decreased quantity and force of seminal fluid emission. During the resolution phase, there is rapid detumescence (i.e., decrease in the swelling of the penis) and testicular descent. The refractory period between erections is also prolonged.

Erectile Dysfunction

Erectile dysfunction is the inability to achieve or maintain an erection adequate for sexual intercourse. The prevalence of erectile dysfunction increases with age; by age 70, 67% of men have erectile dysfunction. The causes of sexual dysfunction in men are summarized in Table 46.1.

The most common cause of erectile dysfunction in older men is vascular disease. The risk for vascular erectile dysfunction increases with traditional vascular risk factors such as diabetes mellitus, hypertension, hyperlipidemia, Parkinson's disease, stroke, and smoking. The second most common cause of erectile dysfunction in older men is neurologic disease. Disorders that affect nerve innervation to the penis prevent vasodilation (i.e., widening of the blood vessels in the penis), necessary for an erection to occur. In patients with spinal cord injury, the extent of erectile dysfunction largely depends on the completeness and level of the spinal injury; those who have complete lesions or injury to the sacral spinal cord are more likely to have loss of erectile function. Surgical procedures such as a radical prostatectomy commonly disrupt the nerve innervation to the penis, resulting in postoperative erectile dysfunction.

Many commonly used medications are associated with erectile dysfunction. Medications with anticholinergic effects, such as antidepressants, antipsychotics, and antihistamines, may cause erectile dysfunction by blocking parasympathetic-mediated penile artery vasodilatation and trabecular smooth muscle relaxation.

Almost all antihypertensive agents have been associated with erectile dysfunction; of these, β-blockers, clonidine, and thiazide diuretics have higher incidence rates. One reason for the dysfunction may be that the medication lowers the blood pressure below the critical threshold needed to maintain sufficient blood flow for penile erection, especially in those men who already have penile arterial disease. Over-the-counter medications such as cimetidine and ranitidine may also cause erectile dysfunction.

The prevalence of psychogenic erectile dysfunction correlates inversely with age, actually being less of a problem in older men when compared to younger men. Common causes of psychogenic erectile dysfunction include relationship conflicts, performance anxiety, childhood sexual abuse, and fear of sexually transmitted diseases. Older men, however, may have widower's syndrome, in which the man involved in a new relationship feels guilt as a defense against subconscious unfaithfulness to his deceased spouse.

The role of androgens in erection is unclear. Overall, testosterone appears to play a minor role in erectile function and a larger role in libido. Hyperthyroidism, hypothyroidism, and hyperprolactinemia have been associated with erectile dysfunction. Prolactin is a peptide hormone produced by the anterior pituitary gland primarily associated with lactation (i.e., making breast milk). However, less than 5% of erectile dysfunction is caused by endocrine abnormalities.

46.1 | Causes of Sexual Dysfunction in Older Men

CAUSES (IN DESCENDING ORDER OF PREVALENCE)	CHARACTERISTICS
Vascular disease	■ Gradual onset ■ Vascular risk factors: diabetes mellitus, hypertension, hyperlipidemia, tobacco use
Neurologic disease (e.g., spinal cord injury, autonomic dysfunction, surgical procedures)	■ Gradual onset ■ Neurologic risk factors: diabetes mellitus, history of pelvic injury, surgery or irradiation, spinal injury or surgery, Parkinson's disease, multiple sclerosis, or alcoholism
Medications (e.g., anticholinergics, antihypertensives, cimetidine, antidepressants)	■ Sudden onset ■ Lack of sleep-associated erections or lack of erections with masturbation ■ Association of starting the new medication with sexual dysfunction
Psychogenic (e.g., relationship conflicts, performance anxiety, childhood sexual abuse, fear of sexually transmitted diseases, widower's syndrome)	■ Sudden onset ■ Sleep-associated erections or erections with masturbation continue to occur
Hypogonadism	■ Gradual onset ■ Decreased libido more than erectile dysfunction ■ Small testes, gynecomastia (enlarged breasts) ■ Low serum testosterone levels
Endocrine (e.g., hypothyroidism, hyperthyroidism)	■ Rare, < 5% of cases of erectile dysfunction

Treatment of Erectile Dysfunction

Multiple effective therapeutic options are now available for the treatment of erectile dysfunction. Treatment should be individualized and based on cause, personal preference, partner issues, cost, and practicality of the treatment.

Medication therapy for erectile dysfunction consists of sildenafil, vardenafil, or tadalafil—all of which are phosphodiesterase inhibitors that help to increase the penile response to sexual stimulation. They are effective in improving the rigidity and duration of erection.

The drugs should be taken 1 hour before sexual activity and will not have any effect until sexual stimulation occurs. All three of these agents are contraindicated if the man is on a nitrate drug, since the combination can produce fatal hypotension. Injection of vasoactive drugs such as papaverine, phentolamine, and alprostadil into the penis are also effective in producing erections adequate for sexual activity. Potential side effects are bruising, ecchymoses or hematoma, local pain, fibrosis from repeated injections, and priapism (i.e., persistent erection). Testosterone supplementation increases libido and may improve erectile dysfunction in men with true deficiencies in testosterone. It is available as an intramuscular injection (testosterone enanthate or cypionate) or topical transdermal patch and gel. Possible side effects associated with testosterone include polycythemia, increase in prostate size, gynecomastia, and fluid retention.

An external device, such as vacuum tumescence, is another effective treatment for erectile dysfunction. The apparatus consists of a plastic cylinder with an open end into which the penis is inserted. A vacuum device attached to the cylinder creates negative pressure within the cylinder, and blood flows into the penis to produce penile rigidity. A penile constriction ring placed at the base of the penis then traps the blood in the corpora cavernosa to maintain an erection for about 30 minutes. The vacuum device is effective for psychogenic, neurogenic, and venogenic erectile dysfunction, but it requires manual dexterity. Local pain, swelling, bruising, coolness of the penile tip, and painful ejaculation are potential side effects. It is important to remove the constriction ring after 30 minutes. Surgical implantation of a penile prosthesis is another therapeutic option but mechanical failure, infection, device erosion, and fibrosis are possible complications.

Inappropriate Sexual Behavior

Unfortunately, it is possible that the sexual behavior exhibited by an assisted living community resident may be inappropriate. Individuals with Alzheimer's disease or some type of cognitive impairment (associated with head trauma, delirium, or other types of dementias) may experience sharply increased sexual interest (in 7%–25% of men) or acting out, known as hypersexuality. Problem behaviors commonly seen include jealous accusations that a spouse is having an affair, sexual overtures to a nonspouse, or masturbation in public. These behaviors are more commonly seen in elderly men than women. Generally the behaviors are believed to be due to changes in the frontal lobe, temporolimbic system, striatum, and the hypothalamus. The behaviors are commonly grouped as sex talk, sexual acts, and implied sexual acts.

Sex talk, the most common of the behaviors, is the use of inappropriate language, usually not consistent with the individual previously. Sexual acts include such behaviors as touching, grabbing, exposing oneself, or masturbating in public or excessively in private. Implied sexual acts involve inappropriate reading of pornographic materials or requesting or demanding inappropriate care for the purpose of genital stimulation (e.g., cleaning the penis, rectal examinations).

Behavioral Interventions

The first approach to management should be a behavioral intervention. As shown in Exhibit 46.1, these include such activities as avoiding embarrassing or yelling at the individual, attempting to redirect the inappropriate behavior, and ultimately avoiding any situations that stimulate the inappropriate behavior. For some older adults, bathing creates an opportunity for inappropriate sexual activity such as touching the caregiver inappropriately or making inappropriate comments. Bathing by a same-sex caregiver may help in these situations. Alternatively, certain clothes may facilitate inappropriate behaviors. For example, clothing in which a male can easily access his penis to masturbate in public places should be avoided. Ongoing education of all caregivers and family can help to manage the situation and avoid discomfort on the part of the resident, family, or caregivers.

When behavioral interventions are not effective, more aggressive interventions, including medication management, may be needed. Urgent intervention is needed if the person becomes physically aggressive or

46.1 | Behavioral Management of Inappropriate Sexual Behavior

1. Avoid becoming angry at, arguing with, or embarrassing the person.

2. Approach the resident with a gentle and calm demeanor.

3. Seek a reason for the behavior; it is possible the individual is removing clothes because he or she is tired, warm, or uncomfortable.

4. Gently inform the individual that the behavior where he or she is sitting is inappropriate and best done in a private area; help him or her get to that private area.

5. Distract or redirect the individual toward another activity such as eating.

6. Increase the level of appropriate physical contact: hugging, stroking the hair, massage.

7. Provide clothing that is difficult to remove easily.

8. Avoid activities that seem to initiate the behaviors.

violent. Have a plan of action in place that indicates whom to call for help (e.g., family members, friends, or the police). Major concerns include avoiding any sexual exploitation and abuse or assault on staff or another resident, especially if that person is unable to give meaningful consent to participation in a sexual act with another individual.

Pharmacological Interventions

The goal of a *stepped approach* to medication management of inappropriate sexual behavior is to use drugs that may eliminate not only the inappropriate behavior but other associated symptoms or disease states. In situations of inappropriate sexual behavior when there is evidence of cognitive impairment, the first line of therapy recommended is a cholinesterase inhibitor with memantine. These drugs may help the behavior as well as the underlying cognitive problems. If this treatment is ineffective, and there is evidence of hypersexuality and psychotic behavior, an antipsychotic medication may be useful. If there is hypersexuality with manic or impulsive behavior, a mood stabilizer anticonvulsant will be helpful. In the event that the individual exhibited inappropriate sexual behavior and is also depressed, then the first line of treatment may more appropriately include a selective serotonin reuptake inhibitor. These drugs are also helpful if the individual has some obsessive/compulsive behaviors as well. Alternatively, other antidepressants such as trazadone may be effective. In situations in which the individual does not respond to these treatments, alternative options include drugs such as cimetidine, normally used for the treatment of indigestion; it is effective for inappropriate sexual behavior because of its antiandrogen effects. Pindolol, a cardiac medication, may help reduce inappropriate sexual behavior by decreasing adrenergic drive, thus decreasing agitation, aggression, and all inappropriate behaviors. When all other treatment options fail, hormonal agents can be initiated that result in chemical castration and thus a decrease in testosterone and subsequent behaviors and sexual abilities. These medications are not without side effects and residents should be treated with the lowest possible dose to ensure the necessary response.

RESOURCES

Lindau, S.T., Schumm, L.P., Laumann, E.O., Levinson, W., O'Muircheartaigh, C.A., & Waite, L.J. (2007). A study of sexuality and health among older adults in the United States. *New England Journal of Medicine, 357*(8), 762–774.

Ozkan, B., Wilkins, K., Muralee, S., & Tampi, R.R. (2008). Pharmacotherapy for inappropriate sexual behaviors in dementia: A systematic review of literature. *American Journal of Alzheimer's Disease and Other Dementias, 23*(4), 344–354.

Thorson, A.I. (2003). Sexual activity and the cardiac patient. *American Journal of Geriatric Cardiology, 12*(1), 38–40.

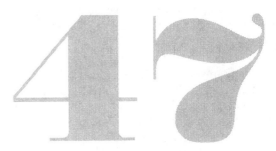

Prostate Diseases and Disorders

Lisa J. Granville and Susan Avillo Scherr

With advancing age, the prevalence of prostate diseases increases dramatically. The three most common conditions are benign prostatic hypertrophy (BPH), prostate cancer, and prostatitis. Self-reported prostate disease affects about 3 million Americans. BPH develops in over half the men age 65 years and older and affects the overwhelming majority of men after age 85 years. Prostate cancer is the second leading cause of cancer death. However, many men have asymptomatic or low-grade tumors that cause few or no health problems and are not the direct cause of death. The prevalence of prostatitis is similar to that of ischemic heart disease or diabetes mellitus in men.

BENIGN PROSTATIC HYPERPLASIA

Epidemiology

BPH is a noncancerous enlargement of the epithelial and fibromuscular tissues of the prostate gland. Epithelial tissues comprise 20% to 30% of prostate volume and contribute to the seminal fluid. Fibromuscular tissue comprises 70% to 80% of the prostate and is responsible for expressing prostatic fluid during ejaculation. Age and long-term androgen (e.g., testosterone) stimulation cause the development of BPH. Microscopic appearance of BPH may occur as early as age 30, is present in 50% of men by age 60, and is in 90% of men by age 85. In half of these cases, microscopic BPH develops into palpable macroscopic BPH. Of those with macroscopic BPH, only half develop into clinically significant disease (i.e., symptoms) that is brought to medical attention. BPH is one of the most common conditions in aging men; in the United States it accounts for more than 1.7 million office visits and 250,000 surgical procedures annually.

Prostatism or Lower Urinary Tract Symptoms

Given that the symptoms of BPH are nonspecific, other diseases can produce identical symptoms. BPH blocks urine flow and results in lower urinary tract symptoms including irritation such as frequency, urgency, nocturia, hesitancy, intermittency, weak stream, and incomplete emptying. Symptom severity is not related to prostate size, urine flow rates, or postvoid residual volume. The primary effect of symptoms is on quality of life related to urinary incontinence, although complications such as recurrent urinary tract infection, bladder stones, urinary retention, chronic renal insufficiency, and hematuria can develop.

Treatment Approaches

BPH therapy is patient-dependent and driven by the impact of symptoms on the resident's quality of life. All residents should be educated regarding lifestyle modification: fluid adjustments (e.g., avoid caffeine) and avoidance of medications (especially anticholinergics) that aggravate symptoms. Residents with mild to moderate symptoms may be satisfied with lifestyle modification only rather than more aggressive intervention. Medication is usually the first approach. Indications for surgical treatment include resident's preference, dissatisfaction with medication, and persistent urinary retention, as well as renal damage, bladder stones, recurrent urinary tract infections, or hematuria *if* these are clearly due to prostatic obstruction.

Medical Treatment

The two main pharmacologic approaches are α-adrenergic antagonists and 5-alpha reductase inhibitors. α-adrenergic antagonists, or α-blockers, are directed at the dynamic component of urethral obstruction. Smooth muscle of the prostate and bladder neck has a resting tone mediated by α-adrenergic innervation. α-blockers relax the smooth muscle in the hyperplastic prostate tissue, prostate capsule, and bladder neck, thus decreasing resistance to urinary flow. The most common adverse effects of α_1 agents are dizziness, mild asthenia (fatigue or weakness), and headaches. Postural hypotension occurs infrequently and can be minimized by careful dose titration.

The enzyme 5-alpha reductase is required for the conversion of the hormone testosterone to the more active dihydrotestosterone. Finasteride is an inhibitor of this enzyme and reduces tissue levels of dihydrotestosterone, thus reducing prostate gland size. Improvements in symptoms and urine flow rates may not be evident for up to 6 months. Finasteride is most effective in men with larger prostates (i.e., > 40 g, about the size of a plum). When used together over years, the combination of α-adrenergic antagonists with 5-alpha reductase inhibitors is safe and can reduce the clinical progression of BPH better than either agent alone. Benefits include lower risk of urinary retention, urinary incontinence, renal insufficiency, and recurrent bladder infections. A number of trials consistently demonstrate that the herbal preparation *Serenoa repens,* or saw palmetto, improves urinary symptoms and flow measures in men with BPH similar to those associated with finasteride treatment and with fewer reported adverse effects.

Surgical Treatment

Surgical management includes transurethral resection of the prostate (i.e., going through the urethra), transurethral incision of the prostate, prostatectomy, transurethral vaporization of the prostate, and device insertion such as stent placement. Surgical approaches offer the best chance for symptom improvement but also have the highest rates of complications. The benefits of surgical treatments are generally considered equivalent, but complication rates differ. Transurethral resection of the prostate is the standard of care to which other BPH treatments are compared and has an 80% likelihood of successful outcome in properly selected residents. Usually performed under spinal anesthesia, a transurethral resection of the prostate involves the passage of an endoscope through the urethra to remove surgically the inner portion of the prostate. Long-term complications may include retrograde ejaculation (ejaculation back into the bladder), urethral stricture, bladder neck contracture, incontinence, and impotence. Transurethral incision of the prostate is an endoscopic procedure via the urethra to make one to two cuts in the prostate and prostate capsule, relieving urethral constriction.

PROSTATE CANCER

Incidence and Epidemiology

Cancer of the prostate is the most common noncutaneous cancer and the second leading cause of cancer deaths among men in the United States. It was estimated that in 2005, 232,090 men would be diagnosed and 30,350 men would die from prostate cancer. The incidence increases with age and is rare in men younger than 40 years. Incidence varies according to race, with African Americans having the highest risk worldwide. Among Black men, cancer of the prostate occurs at an earlier age, has a higher mortality rate, and tends to be at a more advanced stage of disease at time of diagnosis. Family history is a contributing risk factor. Men with one first-degree relative (the parents, brothers, sisters, or children of an individual) affected have more than a twofold increased risk; with two first-degree relatives affected, there is more than an eightfold increased risk. Androgens are necessary for prostate cancer pathogenesis; the disease does not occur in men castrated before puberty. Diets high in total fat consumption are associated with increased risk. The association between cancer of the prostate and early onset of sexual activity, sexually transmitted disease, or vasectomy is inconclusive.

Symptoms

The majority of residents, especially those with early-stage potentially curable disease, are asymptomatic.

When the cancer spreads to other areas of the body, symptoms such as bone pain are reported. Extension of disease to adjacent nerves may cause impotence and pelvic pain. Spread to lymph nodes (particularly the nodes in the groin) may cause a blockage in the urethra. Leg edema may develop from lymphatic obstruction. Metastasis to the bone may cause severe local pain, anemia, pathologic fractures, and spinal cord compression.

Screening Controversy

The benefit of early detection and the best approach to treatment of prostate cancer are controversial. At the heart of the screening debate is the fact that no direct evidence exists to show that early detection decreases prostate cancer mortality rates. The majority of men with prostate cancer die with the disease, not from it. The well-recognized burden of progressive cancer of the prostate is the impetus for early detection and management. The American Urological Association and the American Cancer Society recommend annual screening by the prostate-specific antigen (PSA) test and digital rectal exam (DRE) beginning at age 50 for men with at least a 10-year life expectancy and earlier (age 40) for men at high risk (Black men, first-degree relative affected). Groups that use explicit criteria to develop evidence-based practice guidelines (e.g., U.S. Preventive Services Task Force, American College of Physicians, and Canadian Task Force on the Periodic Health Examination) recommend against routine PSA screening for cancer of the prostate. Guidelines of all these clinical groups agree, however, that the controversy surrounding screening should be discussed with residents in order to achieve individualized, informed courses of action. The effectiveness of PSA screening is particularly questionable in elderly men (i.e., > 65).

Screening and Diagnostic Tests

DRE is done to palpate the prostate gland, particularly the posterior surfaces of the lateral lobes, where cancer most often begins. Cancer characteristically is hard, nodular, and irregular. The value of DRE is that it can detect some cancers in men with a normal PSA level. However, DRE is inherently inaccurate because parts of the prostate gland cannot be reached, or clinicians may think they feel an abnormality when it is not actually a cancer. Despite its limitations, DRE remains important for screening and staging.

The serum PSA test is not specific for cancer of the prostate. PSA elevations occur in benign conditions of the prostate, namely, BPH and prostatitis, and following ejaculation and prostatic massage (e.g., after a prostate exam). The sensitivity of the PSA test is also imperfect. Declines in PSA values have been associated with acute hospitalization and use of medications such as finasteride and saw palmetto. Normal PSA levels are found in 30% to 40% of men with cancer confined to the prostate (false-negative tests). Abnormal DRE or PSA tests lead to further testing, which usually involves a transrectal ultrasound–guided biopsy of the prostate for pathologic diagnosis. The Gleason grading system is then used to evaluate the extent of cancer involvement: range is from 1, or well differentiated, to 5, poorly differentiated. Well-differentiated tumors have a favorable prognosis; poorly differentiated tumors have an unfavorable prognosis. Most clinically detected tumors are moderately differentiated.

Common Management Interventions for Localized Prostate Cancer

Three approaches to localized prostate cancer are routinely recommended: watchful waiting, radical prostatectomy, and radiation therapy. Watchful waiting (also called *expectant* or *conservative management* or *surveillance*) is the approach offered most commonly to men with less than a 10-year life expectancy, who have significant medical comorbidities, or whose tumor is small and well to moderately differentiated. Because most men with cancer of the prostate are asymptomatic, watchful waiting spares these men the burden of unnecessary treatment.

Radical prostatectomy is surgical removal of the entire prostate gland and the seminal vesicles. It can be performed through a perineal incision near the rectum or with a retropubic (lower abdominal) incision. The major sequelae associated with this treatment are urinary incontinence and erectile dysfunction. Men following radical prostatectomy are more likely to experience stress incontinence, with symptoms ranging from occasional leakage to no urinary control. Bladder neck contractures also occur and cause urinary retention. Both sexual dysfunction and urinary symptoms have a negative impact on quality of life. This treatment is generally offered to men with locally confined disease, with greater than a 10-year life expectancy, and without contraindications to surgical intervention.

Radiation therapy, the third option, is provided through external beam radiation or through implantation of radioactive sources (known as *brachytherapy*). Pelvic lymph nodes can be radiated as well. Proctitis and urethritis are common acute side effects associated with radiation. Chronic complications include erectile dysfunction, urinary incontinence, and chronic proctitis. The incidence of urinary stress incontinence after radiation therapy is significantly less than with surgery, but the presence of irritative voiding dysfunction is greater. Bowel dysfunction commonly occurs after radiation and includes diarrhea, rectal urgency, and fecal soiling.

Management of Locally Advanced Prostate Cancer

Locally advanced prostate cancer extends deeper into the prostate tissue and includes the seminal vesicle. Radiation therapy and medication that will result in androgen deprivation is the recommended treatment. Unfortunately, androgen deprivation therapy can cause significant negative impact on quality-of-life: loss of stamina, increased fatigue, hot flashes, diminished muscle mass, and premature osteoporosis. Men should therefore be given the choice if they want to start androgen deprivation treatment or watch and wait for symptoms and evidence of recurrent disease following radiation without androgen deprivation.

Management of Advanced Disease

Advanced disease is treated with androgen ablation and symptom-specific approaches, such as direct radiation therapy to painful bone metastasis. Androgen ablation aims to eliminate all testosterone by orchiectomy (i.e., removal of the testes) or use of luteinizing hormone-releasing hormone (LHRH) agonists with anti-androgens.

PROSTATITIS

Etiology

Prostatitis is an inflammatory condition of the prostate that may indicate acute bacterial, chronic bacterial, or nonbacterial causes. The most common sources of acute or chronic infection are urine backup in the urethra, an indwelling Foley catheter, or spread of bacteria from the rectum. More than 80% of patients with prostatitis have no identifiable infectious agent.

Diagnosis

Acute bacterial prostatitis is characterized by fever, chills, dysuria, and a tense or boggy, extremely tender prostate. Because bacteremia (the spread of the bacteria into the blood system) may result from manipulation of the inflamed gland, minimal rectal examination is indicated. A urine specimen is generally used to help providers make this diagnosis.

Treatment

Acute bacterial prostatitis is treated with antibiotics. Antibiotics are less effective for chronic bacterial prostatitis because of poor penetration of the prostate by most of these drugs. Prolonged therapy of 6 to 16 weeks is common.

RESOURCES

AUA Practice Guidelines Committee. (2003). AUA guideline on management of benign prostatic hyperplasia (2003). Chapter 1: Diagnosis and treatment recommendations. *Journal of Urology, 170*(2 Pt. 1), 530–547.

Crawford, E. D., Pinsky, P. F., Chia, D., Kramer, B. S., Fagerstrom, R. M., Andriole, G., et al. (2006). Prostate specific antigen changes as related to the initial prostate specific antigen: Data from the prostate, lung, colorectal and ovarian cancer screening trial. *Journal of Urology, 175*(4), 1286–1290.

Murphy, G. D., Byron, D. P., & Pasquale, D. (2003). Underutilization of digital rectal examination when screening for prostate cancer. *Archives of Internal Medicine, 164*, 313–316.

O'Rourke, M. E. (2006). The older adult with prostate cancer. In D. G. Cope & A. M. Reb (Eds.), *An evidence-based approach to the treatment and care of the older adult with cancer* (pp. 225–249). Pittsburgh, PA: Oncology Nursing Society.

Stamey, T. A. (2004). The era of serum prostate specific antigen as a marker for biopsy of the prostate and detecting prostate cancer is now over in the USA. *British Journal of Urology International, 94*(7), 963–964.

Surveillance Epidemiology and End Results (SEER) Program. (2007). *SEER*Stat Database: Incidence—SEER 17 regs limited-use, Nov 2006 sub (1973–2004 varying)*. Bethesda, MD: National Cancer Institute, DCCPS, Surveillance Research Program, Cancer Statistics Branch.

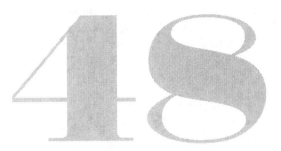

Musculoskeletal Diseases and Disorders

John W. Rachow and Barbara Resnick

Musculoskeletal complaints are among the most common reasons that older adults have pain and seek the help of a health care provider. Among those age 65 and older, osteoarthritis (OA) is the most prevalent articular disease. Nearly 70% of those age 70 and older have radiographic evidence of OA; almost half of these people develop symptoms. The back, weight-bearing joints such as the knees and the hips, and foot problems lead to some of the most distressing symptoms and disabling conditions affecting older adults.

MUSCULOSKELETAL DISEASE

True joint disease (i.e., *arthritis*) is characterized by symptoms and physical examination findings localized to the joints. A resident's history of joint swelling is strong evidence from the outset that true joint involvement is present. History of pain in a joint with motion or weight bearing is suggestive of arthritis. Alternatively, musculoskeletal symptoms may include problems in the surrounding muscles, nerves, and even general metabolism of the individual. These more involved disorders include chronic postural strain, acute muscular and ligamentous strain, bursitis, fibromyalgia, and neuropathies. Pain complaints in these disorders often involve anatomic regions, such as the shoulder area, or a whole extremity, and rarely include a history

of joint swelling; the resident commonly cannot clearly indicate which joint is involved.

When symptoms of pain and fatigue are generalized and not specifically focused on an individual joint, it is important to explore if there are any signs or symptoms of inflammation. In the inflammatory disorders there may also be a rash, fever, stomatitis (i.e., sore mouth), dysphagia (i.e., difficulty swallowing), Raynaud's phenomenon (poor circulation in the hands that causes pain or tingling), or true muscle weakness. All of these findings suggest that there may be some type of autoimmune disorder. The absence of such symptoms make generalized conditions such as fibromyalgia or regional conditions such as chronic postural strain more likely.

The Role of Exercise in Treatment

Regardless of the underlying cause of the musculoskeletal problem, exercise is the most appropriate intervention. Exercise helps preserve muscle and bone mass, reverses the increased fat-to-muscle ratio associated with aging, and preserves physical function. The specific amount of exercise needed to achieve the desired benefit varies based on individual goals and capabilities. Combined guidelines from the American College of Sports Medicine, the Centers for Disease Control and Prevention (CDC), and the National Institutes of Health (NIH) generally recommend that older adults engage in

30 minutes of physical activity most days of the week. This activity should incorporate aerobic activity (i.e., walking, dancing, swimming, biking), resistance training (lifting weights or using resistive exercise bands), and flexibility training. Exercises can be done individually or in a group setting depending on the individual's preference, cognitive ability, and motivational level.

Given the many benefits of physical activity and the relatively low risk of serious adverse events associated with low- and moderate-intensity physical activity, a consensus group from the American Heart Association and the American College of Cardiology (Berg, 2004) no longer recommends routine stress testing for those initiating a physical activity. For sedentary older people who are asymptomatic, low-intensity physical activity can be safely initiated regardless of whether or not an older adult has had a recent medical evaluation. Screening of some type, however, is recommended for older adults to help assure them of the safety of exercise and to provide direction as to the appropriate exercise program in which to engage. The EASY screening tool (http://www.easyforyou.info) can be used by the older adult's primary health care provider to identify the appropriate physical activity program given underlying chronic medical problems. This tool consists of six simple questions that, depending on responses, identify appropriate exercise programs (see Chapter 18, "Physical Activity").

SOFT-TISSUE RHEUMATISM

The variety and number of conditions that present with musculoskeletal symptoms is impressive. This section describes some of these common problems, their presentation, and how they are managed in older adults.

Fibromyalgia

Fibromyalgia is a generalized pain syndrome that occurs at nearly all ages; prevalence rates of 2% to 10% are similar around the world, independent of nationality or ethnicity and cultural factors. Although there is no known underlying cause of this disease, the uniform worldwide incidence is so high that it is believed to be a true clinical problem. The average age of onset is around 45 years and afflicts adults well into their 80s; most sufferers are female. Research indicates that the distress experienced by fibromyalgia patients diminishes with advancing age, suggesting that management in older adults may be less challenging. Mainstays of treatment have changed little in recent years. Aerobic exercise is recommended, as are analgesics (see Chapter 21, "Chronic Pain and Persistent Pain").

Rotator Cuff Disease

The shoulder rotator cuff is formed by tendons that hold the humeral head and humerus in place and allow this joint to work in a circular motion. Individuals with this condition might not be able to recall a specific event that contributed or caused the rotator cuff disease. Some may recall a recent fall or an episode in which the shoulder was used such as pulling on a rope or lifting a heavy object. Unfortunately, damage to the rotator cuff can occur just from changes in the bones associated with chronic arthritis and poor circulation to the tendons and shoulder joint. Complete loss of the rotator cuff makes it particularly difficult to raise the arm to the side (i.e., abduction). Partial tear in a ligament that holds the shoulder (head of the humerus) in place may elicit pain when the resident is asked to raise the arm above the head or to try and comb hair or brush teeth. Treatment should include avoidance of activities that cause acute pain but should encourage continued use of the shoulder in routine daily activities such as reaching things on a shelf. Lack of use can result in decline in functional movement of the shoulder joint and ultimately cause the individual even more pain. Surgery is usually an intervention of last resort in the treatment of rotator cuff disorder (see Figure 48.1).

Frozen Shoulder Syndrome (Adhesive Capsulitis)

Frozen shoulder is an acute process that involves inflammation of the shoulder joint. The condition can follow other shoulder disorders or injury and usually involves just one side. Complaints include shoulder pain and tenderness and severely restricted range of motion, both active (i.e., the resident moves the shoulder/arm independently) or passive (i.e., an assistant tries to move the shoulder/arm). Early intervention with aggressive range-of-motion exercises combined with pain medication, particularly anti-inflammatory agents, are important to preserve future shoulder motion and reduce inflammation. Adhesive capsulitis usually follows a course of several months that includes three phases: freezing, frozen, and thawing. With timely treatment, the outcome should be good, but physical therapy needs to extend well beyond the thawing phase so that the individual continues to work on moving the shoulder and regaining function.

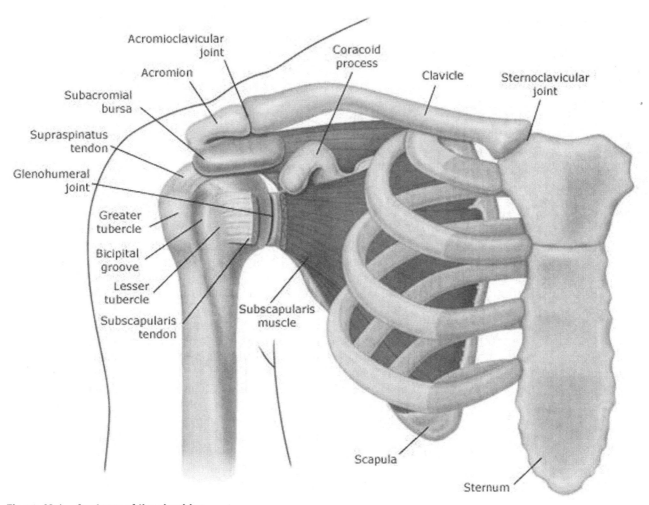

Figure 48.1 Anatomy of the shoulder.

Olecranon Bursitis

The olecranon bursa is the elbow and the sac around it that allows for lubrication and movement of the joint. Enlargement with marked swelling due to an accumulation of fluid with or without inflammation and surrounding cellulitis (i.e., skin infection) is common in older adults. Infection of the bursa is also common, usually with staphylococci. Antibiotic treatment is often needed; the course of recovery can be long, with frequent relapses and inflammation of the elbow. Alternatively, noninfectious olecranon bursitis can be due to trauma. This can occur, for example, in older adults who lean on their elbows while sitting in a wheelchair. Counseling, education, and repositioning (with padding) are important to avoid the activity that causes the inflammation to prevent further trauma.

Carpal Tunnel Syndrome

Carpal tunnel syndrome occurs when the median nerve, which runs from the forearm into the hand, becomes pressed or squeezed at the wrist. The median nerve controls sensations to the palm side of the thumb and fingers (although not the little finger), as well as impulses to some small muscles in the hand that allow the fingers and thumb to move. The carpal tunnel—a narrow, rigid passageway of ligament and bones at the base of the hand—houses the median nerve and tendons. Sometimes, thickening from irritated tendons or other swelling narrows the tunnel and causes the median nerve to be compressed. Entrapment of the median nerve where it passes through the carpal tunnel of the wrist is one of the most common nerve-entrapment syndromes in older adults. The most common cause is repetitive trauma. Individuals with carpal tunnel syndrome commonly complain of nighttime hand pain, tingling, and numbness that can radiate up the arm. Pain during the day, even with radiation proximally to the shoulder, is occasionally reported. Evaluation should include activities in the resident's day that could exacerbate carpal tunnel disease. A cock-up wrist splint provides some support for the wrist; worn at night, it can lessen symptoms. Surgical release of the ligament can relieve symptoms when other conservative measures fail.

Popliteal Cyst (Baker Cyst)

A popliteal cyst may develop at any age. Knee arthritis is generally believed to be the underlying cause. A symptomatic cyst can present with knee pain and pressure in the posterior aspect of the knee. In addition to pain, the cyst can become a space-occupying growth and can prevent deep venous return from the lower leg, causing swelling in the entire leg. A popliteal cyst can rupture spontaneously or with exertion. The result can be dramatic: acute pain, swelling, warmth, and erythema (redness) of the lower leg that mimics all the signs of deep-vein thrombosis (i.e., blood clot). In a few days bruising may be noticed in the lower leg and above the ankle. Treatment in older adults usually focuses on pain management and control of the underlying arthritis. Local injections with a steroid may be used to decrease inflammation (see Chapter 21, "Chronic Pain and Persistent Pain," for management).

JOINT DISEASE

Osteoarthritis

OA is the most common joint disease among older adults and is the major cause of knee, hip, and back pain. It is not, by definition, inflammatory, although inflammation can occur from an accumulation of fluid around the joint. In OA there are progressive changes in the bone such that eventually there is boney proliferation or overgrowth visible on X-rays as boney enlargement of the joints of the hand. Pain and reduced joint motion are also the hallmarks of OA, with associated wasting of the muscles around the bones. The presence of OA in weight-bearing joints is associated with gait abnormalities and increases the risk for falling and injury. Disability can be profound.

Once diagnosed, a wide variety of treatment modalities can be used to treat osteoarthritis. Treatment can be separated into three different categories: nonpharmacological, pharmacological, and surgical. Nonpharmacological interventions include weight loss, physical therapy to strengthen surrounding muscles, and exercise programs to maintain strength and function. Braces and neoprene sleeves can reduce pain and improve function. A neoprene sleeve is a soft pull-on support that provides compression around the joint and helps improve circulation and decrease inflammation.

Early interventions to strengthen atrophied muscles related to the diseased joint and improve joint motion are critical. This includes referral to a physical therapist for evaluation and design of a set of exercises the resident can do daily at home or participation in exercise programs for older adults with arthritis (see http://www.easyforyou.info). With OA of the weight-bearing joints, especially the knees, an ongoing walking exercise program may result in progressive functional improvement and reduction in pain rather than the often feared inevitable deterioration of the affected joints. Weight reduction can help reduce pain and improve function, especially if the lumbar spine or weight-bearing joints are involved.

Pharmacological management is targeted toward symptomatic relief and includes use of analgesics, nonsteroidal anti-inflammatory drugs (NSAIDs), intraocular steroid injections (i.e., steroid injections into the joint), and viscosupplementation (i.e., lubrication injected directly into the joint). In addition, colchicine, topical NSAIDs, acupuncture, and nutraceuticals (i.e., extracts of foods claimed to have a medicinal effect on human health) have also been used effectively. The most common nutraceuticals include glucosamine and chondroitin; support for their effectiveness in pain management and reducing joint space narrowing at dosages of 1,500 mg/day of glucosamine and 800 mg/day of chondroitin are reported. Arthroscopic interventions, surgical interventions done in an outpatient surgical setting, are primarily recommended for situations in which there is known inflammation and when other noninvasive interventions have failed. Likewise, joint replacement should be reserved for individuals with severe symptomatic disease who do not respond to more conservative interventions. Optimal management often involves the use of multiple treatment modalities, and the best combination of treatments will vary from person to person.

Recommendations about which analgesics to use for OA have changed over the past decade. Research shows that acetaminophen is often as effective as any of the NSAIDs or opioids. Significant gastrointestinal and renal toxicity can be associated with NSAID use in older adults. The American College of Rheumatology and the American Geriatrics Society recommend that acetaminophen should be the first analgesic chosen in treating OA. Clinical studies suggest an emerging consensus that NSAIDs may be slightly more effective in treating OA of the knee, especially when analgesia is still required after 3 to 6 months of treatment.

If acetaminophen is initially ineffective, nonacetylated salicylates such as salsalate or magnesium choline salicylate, which have lower gastrointestinal toxicity than most older NSAIDs, can be given. The selective cyclooxygenase-2 enzyme (COX-2) inhibitors are more expensive and have the same risk of unwanted renal effects as the NSAIDs. They may also be associated with increased risk of myocardial infarction. The COX-2 inhibitors are further discussed in the section "Rheumatoid Arthritis" later in the chapter. Hyaluronic acid is a major component of the synovial fluid and lubricates the joint. An injection of hyaluronic acid given once a week for three weeks can relieve knee pain for up to 6 months.

Gout

Gout is perhaps the oldest recognized form of arthritis. It often presents as acute pain usually of the first metatarsal phalangeal joint, mid-foot, or ankle. With subsequent attacks, the knee, elbow, or wrist can be involved. Later in the course of untreated disease, attacks tend to be less intense, last longer, and may feature simultaneous involvement of more than one joint. In addition, chronic low-grade inflammation in multiple joints appears and tophi (i.e., deposits of uric acid under the skin on hands and other surfaces) develop.

Treatment consists of two different phases: management of the acute problem and then long-term management to prevent gout attacks. The acute episode is best managed with a short course of an NSAID. The choice of the NSAID is not critical, as the risk of gastrointestinal toxicity is less likely to emerge during the 10 to 21 days needed for an acute attack to respond. Drugs such as allopurinol or probenecid, which can acutely lower uric acid levels, should not be used in the management of acute gout, as lowering of uric acid level during the acute stage will intensify and prolong an acute gout attack. Once the acute attack is resolved, attention turns to correcting the underlying problem of high uric acid levels that caused the attack. Urate accumulation in body tissues can be due to uric acid overproduction in the body, reduced kidney elimination, or a combination of both. Drugs, for example, probenecid, that promote renal uric acid excretion can correct hyperuricemia (i.e.,

high uric acid levels) in young adults who have normal kidney function. In older adults, reduced kidney function makes these drugs less effective. The most effective treatment for uric acid reduction, colchicine, can also be effective for prevention of gout in older adults, although it should be used cautiously in residents with liver and kidney disease and commonly causes diarrhea.

INFLAMMATORY DISORDERS

Polymyalgia Rheumatica

Polymyalgia rheumatica (PMR) is a distinct syndrome that occurs in older adults, as early as age 50 but predominantly after age 60. Onset tends to be insidious, with corresponding delays in diagnosis. The classic symptom of PMR is stiffness and aching pain upon arising in the morning often around the hips or shoulders. Erythrocyte sedimentation rate (ESR) is so often markedly elevated that a high ESR is one of the essential diagnostic criteria. The syndrome may be accompanied by fatigue, low-grade fever, weight loss, and variable expression of synovitis of proximal joints of the upper, more than the lower, extremities. Recent studies of PMR have confirmed the presence of synovitis identical to that seen in rheumatoid arthritis (RA), with synovial thickening, effusions, and lymphocytic synovial infiltration. Progression of PMR can lead to chronic polyarthritis that fulfills criteria for RA. Of more immediate clinical importance is the common coexistence of PMR with giant cell arteritis (GCA), a more serious, potentially life-threatening disease. (This relationship is discussed in the next section.) Treatment of uncomplicated PMR with corticosteroids is associated with significant iatrogenic long-term morbidity, including diabetes mellitus, osteoporotic fracture, muscle atrophy, hypertension, glaucoma, acceleration of cataracts and skin atrophy. The cause of PMR is unknown. Studies for infectious agents responsible for triggering the syndrome have been inconclusive. Type II HLA gene associations have been found, but associations differ from those for RA.

The standard treatment of PMR is oral prednisone beginning at 15 mg daily. Dramatic improvement is so likely that some clinicians have suggested that low-dose corticosteroid responsiveness confirms the diagnosis of PMR. Normalization of the ESR corresponds to initial symptomatic improvement. Prednisone dose can be tapered over succeeding months on the basis of control of symptoms. Running a course of 2 to 3 years, many individuals are able to discontinue prednisone treatment for PMR by that time. Unfortunately, mean time to the first adverse event on corticosteroid therapy for PMR is about 1.6 years. Occasionally individuals with PMR respond to NSAIDs. Though long-term prednisone has significant toxicity, prednisone may be safer than NSAIDs in older adults, provided the prednisone dose can be minimized and parallel efforts are made to protect bone mass. A randomized clinical trial of methylprednisolone acetate, at a dosage of 120 mg intramuscular every 3 to 4 weeks, controlled PMR with fewer fractures, less weight gain, and lower cumulative dose than a daily oral prednisone regimen.

Giant Cell Arteritis

GCA is the most common form of *vasculitis* to affect older adults. This form of vasculitis predominantly affects proximal branches of the aorta. Therefore, inflammatory and ischemic manifestations are primarily seen in the head and upper extremities. Occasionally, gross inflammation with tender, nodular swelling and erythema of the temporal arteries can be seen. In the absence of gross findings, symptoms of temporal headache, jaw and tongue claudication (pain in the jaw and tongue when chewing or talking), and sudden vision loss may be reported. Diagnosis can be confirmed by biopsy of a temporal artery, thus the often-used synonym, *temporal arteritis*. The American College of Rheumatology criteria for the diagnosis of GCA are available on their Web site (American College of Rheumatology, 2009). Recognition of GCA is often preceded by several months of a nonspecific systemic illness that includes weight loss, fever, and muscle aching that is indistinguishable from PMR. This condition can also present with sudden blindness with no prior systemic illness or with upper-extremity limb claudication. Other manifestations can include stroke, ischemic necrosis of tongue or scalp, or, rarely, myocardial infarction. Aortic aneurysm, predominantly thoracic, is a late manifestation of GCA even when GCA was previously appropriately treated. The incidence of aneurysm in GCA is about 10%, with thoracic and abdominal aneurysm discovery 5.9 and 2.5 years, respectively, after GCA diagnosis.

The cause of GCA is unknown. Infectious agents have long been suspected, but none has yet been confirmed as causative. Recent studies of biopsy material revealed the presence of parvovirus B19 DNA. In another study, serum IgM antibodies (i.e., implying recent infection or re-infection) against type I parainfluenza virus was well correlated with biopsy-positive GCA.

The diagnosis of GCA may require a high index of suspicion combined with the finding of an otherwise unexplained elevated ESR above 40 mm/hour. Combined elevation of ESR and C-reactive protein is more specific (97%) than elevated ESR alone for biopsy-positive GCA. Because of the risk of sudden blindness, most clinicians start high-dose oral prednisone as soon as the possibility of GCA is seriously considered, and then proceed to biopsy. Administration of prednisone does not change arterial histology for weeks. Diagnosis can sometimes even be established or reestablished after a few years of prednisone treatment. Arterial involvement is patchy, and diagnostic histological changes can be missed by biopsy. This oversight can be minimized by biopsy of the symptomatic side and by obtaining a several centimeters length of artery. Multiple longitudinal sections as well as cross-sections of artery are examined by a pathologist. Yet, on occasion, biopsies are negative in cases where suspicion remains high. Biopsy of the opposite side is recommended by some clinicians. However, in a study of bilateral temporal artery biopsy in 150 patients suspected of GCA, results from the two sides agreed in 97% of cases.

Since 25% of cases of GCA are associated with PMR, there is a longstanding controversy as to which individual with PMR should undergo temporal artery biopsy. There are no clear data to guide decision making in this situation. One reasonable criterion would be to obtain temporal artery biopsies in cases of PMR in which there are symptoms or physical findings suggestive of arteritis (i.e., temporal headache; visual changes; tongue, jaw, or limb claudication; neck or chest pain; or neurological changes suggestive of central nervous system ischemia). The temporal artery can also be involved with other forms of systemic vasculitis. Vasculitides other than GCA should be considered whenever the temporal artery biopsy shows necrotizing vasculitis but an absence of giant cells.

Treatment of GCA requires high-dose prednisone initially. No other treatment has been so clearly proven to be effective. Clinicians differ on the definition of high dose, with some recommending starting dosages as high as 120 mg daily. There are no data that show dosages above 40 mg daily to be more effective. Older adults are highly susceptible to corticosteroid toxicity, and toxicity increases markedly with total dose. The use of higher doses should be individualized and considered when there is resistance to initial treatment or disease is unusually severe. Response is confirmed when ESR falls rapidly over the first month of therapy. Tapering of the steroid should begin at the rate of 10% to 20% of the total dose per month as soon as the ESR is normalized. Published studies of methotrexate as a steroid-sparing agent have not consistently proven methotrexate to be effective.

Rheumatoid Arthritis

Late-onset RA appears to be clinically different from the same disease with onset earlier in life. The condition in the older adult is more likely to be of rapid onset, involve fewer and more proximal joints, and to be rheumatoid-factor negative. Nodules are less likely, and joint destruction may be less severe. Overall prognosis may be better than with earlier-onset, seropositive, nodular, erosive disease. Nevertheless, RA is a chronic disease that persists indefinitely, with high risk for progressive joint damage and functional impairment. Recent reviews confirm that late-onset RA is still a serious disease. Signs and symptoms of RA are listed in Exhibit 48.1.

Treatment is almost always indicated; therapeutic options have increased since 1998 with the introduction of a variety of entirely new drugs for the management of RA. In more severe cases, consultation with a rheumatologist is indicated. NSAIDs are often recommended as first-line medications for symptom control

in RA. The older nonselective NSAIDs, such as ibuprofen, naproxen, diclofenac, and several others, nonspecifically inhibit both cyclooxygenase isoenzymes. Celecoxib was approved in late 1998 as the first of a new class of NSAIDs, the selective COX-2 inhibitors. Rofecoxib was approved in mid-1999 for OA and pain and more recently for RA. Valdecoxib was the third COX-2 inhibitor to become available for RA and was approved for marketing in late 2001.

The hope for the selective COX-2 inhibitors was that they would be substantially free of antiplatelet effects, gastric toxicity, and renal toxicity. Clinical studies have confirmed that the incidence of serious gastric toxicity was about half that of nonselective COX NSAIDs. However, if COX-2 inhibitors are used concomitantly with mini-dose aspirin, the risk of gastric toxicity becomes similar to that of older NSAIDs. Renal toxicity, unfortunately, has proved to be as serious with the COX-2 inhibitors as with older NSAIDs.

In 2004, reports emerged that there was an increased risk of myocardial infarction during the first 6 weeks after starting rofecoxib. Subsequent studies of rofecoxib for prevention of adenomatous polyps confirmed an increased risk of stroke and myocardial infarction with long-term use of rofecoxib versus placebo. These reports led to the withdrawal of rofecoxib from the market in late 2004. Valdecoxib was voluntarily withdrawn from the market by the manufacturer in early 2005. Celecoxib is still marketed. The mechanism of increased cardiovascular adverse effects from COX-2 inhibitors is uncertain. Lack of inhibition of platelet function could be a partial explanation, as older NSAIDs at least reversibly inhibit platelet aggregation.

As such, NSAIDs can no longer be considered first-line therapy for arthritis or other chronic, painful conditions. Alternatives to old NSAIDs and selective COX-2 inhibitors might include the relatively selective COX-2 inhibitors: nabumetone, etodolac, and meloxicam. Nabumetone and etodolac were introduced prior to celecoxib, and meloxicam was introduced in 2004. These three agents have generally lower serious gastric adverse effects than older NSAIDs and have less renal toxicity than either older NSAIDs or the selective COX-2 inhibitors. At this time, they are not known to cause an increased risk of stroke and myocardial infarction with long-term use. Therapy with a low-dose corticosteroid such as prednisone may be a preferable option, provided doses can be limited to 5 mg daily and precautions are taken to preserve bone density. The nonacetylated salicylate, salsalate, has minimal gastric mucosal toxicity yet has preserved anti-inflammatory activity.

48.1 | Signs and Symptoms of Rheumatoid Arthritis

- Morning stiffness for at least 6 weeks

- Arthritis of three or more joint areas for at least 6 weeks

- Arthritis of the hand joints for at least 6 weeks

- Symmetric arthritis for at least 6 weeks

- Subcutaneous rheumatoid nodules

- Elevated serum rheumatoid factor and/or sedimentation rate

- X-rays that show erosions or breakdown of the bone and joint inflammation and deformities

- Symmetrical (both right and left side of the body) inflammation of the small joints of the hands, wrists, feet, and knees

- Fatigue, lack of appetite, low-grade fever are present when there is active disease

RA is a lifelong systemic disease associated with progressive joint and extra-articular organ involvement that leads to functional decline and shortened longevity. Mere symptomatic treatment is no longer considered appropriate. Disease-modifying drugs should be considered for treating all cases of RA. Longitudinal studies confirm the preservation of function when disease-modifying drugs are instituted early and maintained over the long term.

Parenteral gold, penicillamine, azathioprine, and cyclophosphamide use has markedly declined in the past decade because of the availability of safer effective drugs. Methotrexate has been approved for use in RA for more than a decade and is the disease-modifying agent of choice. However, when given daily, methotrexate can cause hepatic injury, with cirrhosis and end-stage liver failure. Low-dose, weekly, treatment with methotrexate dramatically reduced the risk of hepatic toxicity, and ethanol intake must be completely avoided. Methotrexate can be used in combination with other immunosuppressive agents to yield proven additive or synergistic benefit. Since 1991, more than 100 cases of lymphoproliferative disease have been reported in patients with RA who are under treatment with methotrexate. Usually, the lesion is extranodal non-Hodgkin's lymphoma; remission is often seen when methotrexate is stopped. At least one population-defined study did not find excess cancer in RA patients treated with methotrexate in comparison with RA patients who never received methotrexate.

Randomized controlled studies confirm that minocycline 100 mg twice daily is effective in treating RA with minimal toxicity. Minocycline[OL] would be a good choice for mild disease or when there is a need to start therapy even when the initial phase of diagnostic uncertainty has not passed. Similarly, hydroxychloroquine is well tolerated and does not require blood-test monitoring for toxicity. When dosages are limited to 5 mg/kg/day, the risk of retinal toxicity is very low. Weekly oral methotrexate is well tolerated by the older adult and can be added if hydroxychloroquine alone is ineffective. Sulfasalazine (only the enteric coated tablets are approved for RA) is more effective than hydroxychloroquine but requires divided daily dosing, has a high incidence of gastrointestinal intolerance, and cannot be given in the presence of sulfa allergy.

Cyclosporine is approved for use in severe RA alone or in combination with methotrexate. Toxicity remains a concern; the role of cyclosporine in treating RA is still evolving. Leflunomide, approved in 1998, is the first disease-modifying antirheumatic drug introduced for over a decade and is the first such drug approved both for symptomatic improvement of RA and to prevent radiographic progression in joint damage. It has relatively fast onset of action (about 4 weeks) in comparison with older disease-modifying drugs. Etanercept was approved in late 1998 for use in treating RA that had failed at least one other disease-modifying agent. Etanercept is a tumor necrosis factor receptor blocker produced by recombinant DNA techniques. It is given in twice-weekly subcutaneous injections and is expensive. Clinical benefit is seen within 1 to 12 weeks, and it must be given indefinitely to maintain benefit. The major risk of etanercept is the development of serious granulomatous infections (see discussion of infliximab in the following paragraph). Headache is a common, less severe adverse effect.

Infliximab was approved in late 1999 in combination with methotrexate for treatment of RA. This drug is a monoclonal antibody that prevents interaction of tumor necrosis factor alpha with its receptor. It must be given by intravenous infusion. Clinical trials show marked initial response to a single infusion, but continued response to bimonthly infusions requires concomitant administration of oral methotrexate. Both etanercept (0.07%) and infliximab (0.24%) are associated with an increased incidence of granulomatous infections with organisms such as tuberculosis, atypical mycobacterium, yeast, listeria, and nocardia. Other adverse effects associated with infliximab include systemic postinfusion reactions of fever, chills, headache, chest pain, and dyspnea. Antibody formation is common but reduced by the concurrent use of methotrexate.

Adalimumab was approved in 2002. It is similar to infliximab except that this therapeutic antibody is entirely human. It is given by subcutaneous injection every other week and does not require concomitant methotrexate therapy. Serious infections similar to those seen with infliximab have been reported, but data about relative incidence are not available. Anakinra was introduced in 2001 as a recombinant form of the human interleukin-1 receptor antagonist IL-1Ra. It is administered as daily subcutaneous injections. Treatment can continue as long as the individual is responding positively in terms of symptom control and is not having side effects. Infections during anakinra therapy are mostly bacterial respiratory tract infections with no opportunistic infections.

Systemic Lupus Erythematosus (SLE)

Thought of as a disease in younger women with a higher prevalence among Black women, SLE can present in later life. It is a multisystem disorder with a wide variety of presentations and predominant organ system involvement at any age. Diagnosis with high specificity is confirmed when any 4 or more of 11 criteria are documented singly or together at any time during the person's life (for a detailed description of the American College of Rheumatology criteria, see American College of Rheumatology, 2009). Criteria include malar rash, photosensitivity, stomatitis, nonerosive arthritis, serositis (i.e., pleurisy or pericarditis), seizure, nephropathy (i.e., urinary casts or heavy proteinuria), cytopenias (i.e., leukopenia, hemolytic anemia, or thrombocytopenia), positive antinuclear antibody, and any one of other immunologic abnormalities (i.e., anti-double stranded DNA, anti-SM, or false positive test for syphilis). Fever, Raynaud's phenomenon, alopecia, migraine, antiphospholipid syndrome, and Sjögren's syndrome (see the section "Sjögren's Syndrome and Sjögren's Disease") are also often seen in SLE.

It is not surprising that patterns of organ involvement in SLE are different in older adults. Numerous studies suggest that late-onset SLE affects women and men more equally (3:1 in older adults versus 10:1 in young adults); relatively more White than Black older adults are affected. Late-onset SLE is less likely to present with rash, arthritis, Raynaud's phenomenon, nephropathy, and the involvement of the central nervous system and more likely to present with serositis, Sjögren's syndrome, and positive rheumatoid factor. In older adults, SLE onset may be more insidious, involve fewer organ systems, and have fewer relapses. As nephropathy and central nervous system involvement are related to mortality in younger women, late-onset lupus has been sometimes thought of as a milder disease. Despite the impression of milder disease in older adults, immunosuppressive and cytotoxic medications are required as often in managing late-onset SLE.

Hormonal factors may be partly responsible for the differences between early- and late-onset SLE. Estrogens are suspected of being an aggravating factor in young women. Studies of the administration of postmenopausal estrogen for 2 years or more in women are associated with a fivefold increase in SLE risk. The increased risk is somewhat lower if estrogen is combined with a progestational agent. In a population-based study, SLE in women was found to be associated with a doubled overall incidence of cancer.

Treatment of SLE in older adults is similar to treatment given in early-onset disease. Corticosteroids are less well tolerated by the older adult and should be reserved as much as possible for organ- or life-threatening SLE flare-ups. Hydroxychloroquine is of benefit in SLE skin involvement and in reducing the overall number of disease relapses in younger adults. Hydroxychloroquine is well tolerated and has few serious adverse effects in dosages of 5 mg/kg/day or less. Dapsone, azathioprine, and weekly oral methotrexate are used by some clinicians as alternatives to corticosteroids or as corticosteroid-sparing agents. Monthly intravenous pulse cyclophosphamide is reserved for severe or life-threatening disease.

Sjögren's Syndrome and Sjögren's Disease

Sjögren's syndrome with xerostomia and keratoconjunctivitis sicca has been long recognized as occasionally complicating RA. The incidence of Sjögren's syndrome in other connective-tissue diseases is also increased. Dry eye and dry mouth (i.e., sicca) symptoms without confirmation of Sjögren's syndrome occur in almost 40% of older adults who do not have a connective-tissue disease; these symptoms are undoubtedly contributed to by many of the medications often prescribed to older adults. The treatment of sicca symptoms and uncomplicated Sjögren's syndrome is targeted to the sufferer's complaints and includes artificial tears, artificial saliva, and ophthalmologic and dental preventive care. Pilocarpine 5 mg three times a day can help stimulate saliva flow.

Sjögren's disease (SD) is a systemic, multiorgan chronic disease that features lymphocytic infiltration of exocrine glands throughout the body, including lacrimal, salivary, respiratory tree, intestinal tract, pancreatic, hepatic, renal, and vaginal glands. In addition, cutaneous vasculitis and central nervous system involvement are often seen. The involvement of salivary and lacrimal glands is responsible for the sicca symptoms seen in Sjögren's syndrome that are associated with other connective-tissue diseases. The peak onset of SD is in midlife to early late life.

There is no single diagnostic test for SD. Unexplained interstitial lung disease, renal impairment, hepatic dysfunction, esophageal dysfunction, malabsorption, or central nervous system disease resembling multiple sclerosis should raise the suspicion of SD. Antinuclear, anti-SSA, and anti-SSB antibodies are usually present. Rheumatoid factor and a variety of autoantibodies against gastric parietal cells, mitochondria, smooth muscle, and thyroid are often seen. An ophthalmologic examination can confirm the presence of keratoconjunctivitis, and biopsy of a lip or lacrimal gland can confirm the presence of characteristic lymphocytic infiltration. Biopsy of a rash can verify the presence of cutaneous vasculitis.

Symptomatic and preventive treatment is indicated for sicca symptoms, as previously described. Trial therapy with hydroxychloroquine may help stabilize disease activity, as in SLE. Dapsone may be effective for cutaneous vasculitis. Corticosteroids and other cytotoxic drugs should be reserved for organ- or life-threatening disease.

Polymyositis and Dermatomyositis

Polymyositis (PM) is a heterogeneous group of inflammatory diseases of striated muscle that are not unique to older adults; however, late-onset PM is evaluated and treated somewhat differently in older adults. The onset of PM is often insidious. The cardinal symptom is muscle weakness, most marked in proximal muscle groups. Muscle tenderness is usually not prominent. Exercise tolerance is reduced, and an inability to perform simple tasks such as reaching above the head or ascending stairs may be present. Other system involvement is common in PM and reminiscent of other connective-tissue diseases, including rash, arthritis, esophageal dysmotility, and Raynaud's phenomenon. Cardiac involvement is not rare and usually presents with dysrhythmias. Rash may involve the eyelids (heliotrope) or the nose and malar areas, or be more generalized. Rash with dorsal thickening over the interphalangeal joints (i.e., Gottron's papules) are distinctly different from the dorsal phalangeal rash of systemic lupus that spares the interphalangeal joints. When rash is present, PM is referred to as dermatomyositis (DM).

In contrast to childhood PM, adult-onset PM affects women more often than men, and Blacks more often than Whites. Also, esophageal involvement and respiratory failure complicated with bacterial pneumonia are more likely in older PM adults. Up to 50% of cases of late-onset PM, and especially DM, are associated with underlying malignancy. No one cancer type seems most strongly associated: colon, lung, breast, prostate, uterus, and ovary are all well represented with PM and DM. Ovarian cancer is the most commonly associated gynecologic cancer underlying PM and DM. Mortality in adult PM and DM is usually associated with esophageal disease, respiratory failure with bacterial pneumonia, and malignancy.

Serum levels of muscle enzymes are usually markedly elevated in PM. Electromyography reveals changes consistent with myositis, provided that the affected muscle is tested. Paraspinal muscle involvement is typical and should be included in the muscles tested. Diagnosis is confirmed with muscle biopsy that reveals inflammatory cellular infiltrates. The diagnosis of PM or DM in older adults also entails a search for underlying malignancy. Minimum evaluation would include chest radiography and colon examination. In women, a pelvic examination and imaging plus mammography is recommended; in men, a prostate examination and prostate-specific antigen testing is recommended. Therapy is generally directed at the inflammatory process itself. Corticosteroids are almost always the first drug of choice.

RESOURCES

American College of Rheumatology. (2009). *Classification criteria for rheumatic diseases*. Retrieved April 23, 2009, from http://www.rheumatology.org/publications/classification

Berg, A.O., Allan, J.D., Calonge, N., Frame, P., Garcia, J., Harris, R.P., et al. (2004). Screening for coronary heart disease: Recommendation statement *Annals of Internal Medicine, 140*, 569–572.

Blumstein, H., & Gorevic, P.D. (2005). Rheumatologic illnesses: Treatment strategies for older adults. *Geriatrics, 60*(6), 28–35.

Ene-Stroescu, D., & Gorbien, M.J. (2005). Gouty arthritis. A primer on late-onset gout. *Geriatrics, 60*(7), 24–31.

Hoskison, K.T., & Wortmann, R.L. (2007). Management of gout in older adults: Barriers to optimal control. *Drugs and Aging, 24*(1), 21–36.

Porcheret, M., Jordan, K., Croft, P., & Primary Care Rheumatology Society. (2007). Treatment of knee pain in older adults in primary care: Development of an evidence-based model of care. *Rheumatology, 46*(4), 638–648.

Reid, M.C., Papaleontiou, M., Ong, A., Breckman, R., Wethington, E., & Pillemer, K. (2008). Self-management strategies to reduce pain and improve function among older adults in community settings: A review of the evidence. *Pain Medicine, 9*(4), 409–424.

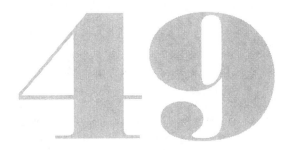

Neurologic Diseases and Disorders

Coleman O. Martin, Harold P. Adams, Jr., and Joan Gleba Carpenter

The number of disorders that affect the nervous system increases rapidly with advancing age. The goal of the nurse is to assess baseline status and be sensitive to changes in neurological function.

CEREBROVASCULAR DISEASE

Ischemic Stroke

Stroke is a leading cause of disability and death among older adults. The incidence of stroke increases with advancing age, approximately doubling with each decade after 60 years of age. Overall, men are at higher risk of stroke until age 84, when women become at higher risk.

Hypertension is the most prevalent risk factor for stroke; its treatment results in a substantial reduction in risk of stroke. Treatment of isolated systolic hypertension in older adults reduces the risk of stroke by nearly 40% (see Chapter 43, "Hypertension"). Heart disease is also an important risk factor for stroke, including atherosclerotic coronary heart disease, left ventricular hypertrophy, valvular heart disease, valve replacement, and valvular and nonvalvular atrial fibrillation (see Chapter 42, "Cardiovascular Diseases and Disorders"). Cigarette smoking independently increases the risk of stroke as much as threefold. The incidence of stroke declines significantly even after 2 years of cessation of smoking; after 5 years, the level of risk returns to that of nonsmokers. Elevated blood lipids and alcohol use are also important risk factors for stroke (see Chapter 37, "Substance Abuse").

Signs and symptoms of stroke include sudden weakness and/or loss of sensation or movement on one side of the body (typically), confusion, difficulty speaking and/or swallowing, visual changes, and balance changes and can progress to a complete lack of responsiveness. The nurse should assess the onset and duration of symptoms. Initial examination of a person with signs and symptoms of stroke should focus on vital signs, level of consciousness, orientation, ability to speak and understand language, facial paresis, muscle strength, and coordination.

In contrast to a stroke, a *transient ischemic attack* (TIA) typically lasts several minutes to several hours, with all symptoms resolving within 24 hours. This temporary disruption in blood flow in the brain causes slurred or garbled speech or difficulty understanding others, sudden blindness in one or both eyes or double vision, dizziness, loss of balance, or loss of coordination. Testing to determine if the episode was a stroke or TIA may be based on symptoms and progression of the problem. To make a definite diagnosis, the resident will generally undergo computed tomography (CT) and/or magnetic resonance imagery (MRI) tests among others. Treatment will depend on the extent of brain damage, location in the brain, and the underlying cause of the stroke.

Aspirin is the mainstay of antiplatelet therapy for atherosclerotic stroke prevention (i.e., prevention of the progressive narrowing and hardening of the arteries over time). Aspirin, which is low in cost and generally well tolerated in low dosages, prevents the accumulation of plaque in the arteries and thereby prevents the narrowing that causes blockages. Many clinicians routinely prescribe 81 to 325 mg per day; however, even the lower dosage (i.e., baby aspirin) may cause gastrointestinal irritation and blood loss. Clopidogrel 75 mg once daily is an alternative for individuals who cannot tolerate aspirin. Warfarin is reserved for primary or secondary stroke prevention when the individual is at risk for developing a blood clot from underlying problems such as atrial fibrillation or severe valvular disease.

Intracerebral Hemorrhage (Acute Bleed)

Intracerebral hemorrhage accounts for 15% to 20% of all strokes. Approximately 80% occur between the ages of 40 and 70. A racial distribution suggests that Black Americans and Asian Americans may be at slightly higher risk than White Americans. The most common risk factor for intracerebral hemorrhage is hypertension, present in 75% to 80% of the cases. Excessive use of alcohol is also associated with a higher incidence.

The signs and symptoms of an intracerebral bleed may include a sudden headache, often during activity. However, headache may be mild or absent in the older person. Loss of consciousness is common, often within a few seconds or minutes. Nausea, vomiting, delirium, and seizure may be part of the presentation. Neurologic changes are usually sudden and progressive. The observed physical findings are based on where the bleeding is occurring. When located in the left side of the brain, paralysis will occur on the right side of the body. Bleeding in the posterior fossa causes cerebellar or brain stem deficits (e.g., decreased movement of the eye, labored breathing, pinpoint pupils, coma). Large hemorrhages can be fatal within a few days in about 49% of older adults. For some survivors, consciousness may return and the neurologic deficits will gradually diminish as the blood is reabsorbed.

STROKE PREVENTION

Stroke prevention includes control of risk factors through diet and exercise and adherence to medications for hypertension, hyperlipidemia, diabetes, and atrial fibrillation. Before and after a stroke, smoking cessation should be encouraged, and drinking alcohol should be limited to moderate intake. Moderate drinking is defined as not more than one standard drink per day: one 12-ounce can of beer; one 5-ounce glass of wine; or a mixed drink containing 1.5 ounces of 80-proof spirits.

STROKE MANAGEMENT

- Optimize the physical function and independence of the individual via participation in therapy and exercise activities as appropriate.
- Prevent falls: Encourage participation in physical therapy, occupational therapy, and speech language pathology; evaluate and optimize the resident's ability to manage in his or her environment.
- Manage complications following stroke; control constipation; manage urinary incontinence or retention; prevent contractures and skin breakdown; continually evaluate and optimize environmental safety; follow swallowing precautions, as necessary.
- Stroke support group: depression may occur in post-stroke individuals because of some loss of independence and usual quality of life.

SUBDURAL HEMATOMA

A subdural hematoma is the collection of blood between the dura and the arachnoid and is usually due to head trauma (that can be mild, particularly in older adults).

Perhaps most relevant for older adults is *chronic subdural hematoma,* the symptoms of which are headache, slight or severe impairment in cognition, and hemiparesis. Some older adults may have seizures, and focal neurologic signs (e.g., weakness, sensory loss, and change in sensation) may be present.

Treatment of the hematoma varies depending on whether or not any symptoms are present. If symptomatic, and particularly if the individual's condition is worsening, then surgical removal of the hematoma may be attempted. If asymptomatic, or if the resident's condition is improving, then it is likely that the resident will just be monitored for any further changes.

HEADACHES

Prevalence of headaches diminishes with age; only 2% of all sufferers of an initial migraine are over 50 years of age. A resident who complains of a headache, however, should be carefully evaluated for the following: complaints of severe pain described as the worst headache ever, onset of pain with exertion or cough, associated loss of balance, sensory loss, unequal or nonreactive pupils, and neck rigidity. These symptoms are cause to contact the primary care clinician for immediate evaluation.

Many commonly used medications can cause dull, diffuse, and nondescript headaches. These include vasodilators (e.g., nitrates), antihypertensives (e.g., reserpine, atenolol, and methyldopa), antiparkinsonian agents, and stimulants (e.g., Ritalin).

One cause of headache commonly found among older adults is *giant cell (temporal) arteritis*. Pain may be centered at the temporal or occipital areas of the brain. The person may complain of visual changes, generalized aching, and may have a low-grade fever. Diagnosis is made by biopsy of the artery. Prompt evaluation is necessary to prevent the development of blindness, as the inflammation can spread to the optic nerve.

MOVEMENT DISORDERS

A movement disorder may be defined simply as abnormal involuntary movements. These movements are not the result of weakness or sensory deficits; they are the result of dysfunction of the basal ganglia or the extrapyramidal motor system.

Parkinson's Disease

Parkinson's disease is a progressive neurodegenerative disease in which cell death in the substantia nigra consequently reduces dopamine levels in the brain. This results in a constellation of signs, including tremor at rest, bradykinesia (i.e., slowness of movement), rigidity, and postural instability or poor balance with a tendency to retropulse (i.e., lean backwards). Incidence of Parkinson's disease increases dramatically with age and is likely due to the combined effects of genetic and environmental factors (e.g., pesticides).

The clinical findings include tremor, usually in one hand but sometimes in both, classically involving the fingers in a pill-rolling motion. The tremor is present at rest and usually decreases with active, purposeful movement (e.g., picking up a glass). Muscular rigidity with stiff, jerky movement is noted when attempting to move the individual's elbow, for example, through range of motion. *Bradykinesia* refers to slowness in initiating movement. *Freezing* is a term used to describe the sudden interruption of movement noted in persons with Parkinson's disease, especially if they

come to a challenging area in the environment such as a doorway. The person's face can become masklike, may lack expression, and have diminished eye blinking. Mood abnormalities, usually depression or anxiety, are common, as are cognitive impairment and dementia.

Nonpharmacological Treatment and Symptom Management

Treatment programs must be individualized. Nonpharmacologic therapy includes a regular exercise program. Attention to symptoms associated with the disease, or treatment of the disease, includes such things as managing the constipation (see Chapter 45, "Gastrointestinal Diseases and Disorders"), orthostatic hypotension (see Chapter 42, "Cardiovascular Diseases and Disorders"; Chapter 24, "Dizziness"), and insomnia (see Chapter 32, "Sleep Disorders").

Pharmacological Treatment

See Table 49.1 for an overview of medication used in treatment of Parkinson's disease. Levodopa (in the form of levodopa/carbidopa) provides the most improvement in the motor manifestations of Parkinson's disease. Specifically, levodopa helps alleviate the symptoms of bradykinesia and rigidity. It is less successful in treating tremor and problems with balance, and it does not prevent progression of the disease. After 2 to 5 years, more than 50% of individuals with Parkinson's disease experience an unpredictable phenomenon referred to as an on-off effect, making it difficult to anticipate when they will freeze. Increasing the dosage of the levodopa may help, but this increases the risk of major side effects including involuntary movements (called dyskinesias) such as twitching, nodding, and jerking, sudden psychosis and hallucinations, nausea, abdominal cramping, orthostatic hypotension, and confusion.

Surgical options are increasingly being utilized for Parkinson's disease patients with symptoms that are uncontrollable by medical therapies. Depending on a resident's most troubling symptoms, brain stimulators or stereotactic lesioning may be considered. Generally, the morbidity of these procedures is low among individuals in otherwise fair to good health who do not have dementia.

Chorea

Choreiform movements, known as *senile chorea*, sometimes occur as an isolated symptom in persons 60 years and older. Involuntary complex movements of the face,

49.1 | Overview of Medications Used to Treat Parkinson's Disease

DRUG	DESCRIPTION
Levodopa-carbidopa (Sinemet)	Converted by nerve cells into dopamine, the neurotransmitter that is deficient in Parkinson's disease. Carbidopa allows more levodopa to get to the brain by preventing it from being metabolized (i.e., broken down) elsewhere in the body.
Selegiline (e.g., deprenyl, eldepryl)	Selegiline given with levodopa enhances and prolongs the response.
Amantadine (Symmetrel)	An antiviral drug that also reduces the symptoms of Parkinson's disease. It is often used in combination with levodopa or anticholinergics. After several months, its effectiveness wears off in one-third to one-half of the patients taking it.
Anticholinergics (e.g., Benadryl, Artane, and Cogentine)	Help control the symptoms of tremor and rigidity. While effective, these drugs can have side effects such as dry mouth, blurred vision, urinary retention, and constipation that limit their use in older adults.
Dopamine agonists, for example, bromocriptine, (Pergolide); apomorphine (Apokyn); bromocriptine (Parlodel); pergolide (Permax); pramipexole (Mirapex); popinirole (Requip)	These drugs enter the brain directly at the dopamine receptor sites. They are less effective than levodopa and are often prescribed in conjunction with Sinemet to prolong the duration of action of each dose of levodopa. They may also reduce the involuntary movements associated with levodopa.
COMT (catechol-0-methyl-transterase) inhibitors: Comtan	COMT inhibitors block the COMT enzyme, which results in greater and more sustained availability of the prescribed levodopa/carbidopa.
Propargylamine monoamine oxidase type B (MAO-B) inhibitors: rasagiline (Azilect) and Zydis Selegiline (Zelapar)	Use of these drugs is associated with less functional decline over time. Rasagiline is useful as an adjunctive agent when added to levodopa to reduce off time in advanced Parkinson's disease.

mouth, and tongue may occur alone or with unilateral or bilateral limb movements. Neither mental disturbance nor family history of Huntington's chorea is associated with senile chorea. Chorea can be treated with medications.

Essential Tremor

Essential tremor is the most common form of abnormal tremor. It is an action tremor that is present when the limbs are in active use (e.g., while writing or holding a cup). The tremor most commonly involves the arms, head, and voice. Other areas of the body may include the chin, tongue, and legs. The tremor is often slightly worse in one arm than in the other. Functionally, the tremor may interfere with many daily activities, such as eating, writing, or fastening buttons. Stress or anxiety can exacerbate the tremor.

The prevalence of essential tremor increases with advancing age, affecting as many as 1% to 5% of persons age 60 years and older. There is likely a familial component to this disorder. Main indications for treatment are embarrassment and disability; difficulty performing certain tasks (e.g., eating and writing). Initial therapy includes β-blocking agents (e.g., propranolol, atenolol[OL]), primidone[OL], phenobarbital[OL], diazepam[OL], and newer agents, including gabapentin[OL] and clozapine[OL]. Response to these agents is variable (i.e., some individual's experience moderate improvement, whereas others experience none), and the tremor is rarely eliminated. Some patients with severe, medically refractory tremor may undergo deep brain (thalamic) stimulator surgery that is effective in controlling the tremor.

Prevention

Prevention of the negative outcomes of movement disorders lies in preventing injury, usually from falling.

- Many older adults benefit from a course of physical therapy aimed at restoring their confidence in walking and maintaining balance.
- Physical and occupational therapists can teach simple tricks to manage unpredictable and disabling episodes and can help select an appropriate size, weight, and type of cane or walker.
- An occupational therapist home visit can advise about the appropriate placement of wall rails, grab bars, and other assistive devices to reduce the possibility of falling.
- Maintenance of adequate hydration will help avoid aggravating postural hypotension.

EPILEPSY

A seizure is a paroxysmal excessive or hypersynchronous cerebral neuronal discharge, or both, that results in a transient change in motor function, sensation, or mental state. Recurrent seizures are the defining feature of epilepsy. Seizures are broadly classified as *partial* or *generalized*. Partial seizures are subdivided on the basis of whether or not the seizure is associated with impairment of consciousness. Simple partial seizures do not impair consciousness and most often are associated with rhythmic motor twitching (e.g., twitching of the face). Complex partial seizures are associated with alterations of consciousness and amnesia for the event. Automatisms (i.e., motor or verbal behaviors repeated inappropriately) and other motor manifestations may occur with complex partial seizures. Verbal automatisms range from simple vo-

calizations, such as moaning, to swearing inappropriately and repeatedly.

Generalized seizures in older adults are almost invariably convulsive (i.e., grand mal). Common causes of generalized seizures include vascular disease, space-occupying lesions, brain trauma, alcohol withdrawal, and neurodegenerative diseases. When describing a seizure, focus on the movements during the seizure, any loss or change of consciousness, and the person's actions during and after the episode (e.g., thrashing his or her arms and legs, complaining of severe headache, and/or falling asleep after the event). This information can be helpful to the primary health care provider in making a diagnosis or managing the seizure disorder. Each state has laws regarding seizure disorder and driving; this is a crucial area of counseling for the older adult with a seizure disorder.

Treatment of epilepsy involves the use of antiepileptic drugs (AEDs). Older adults may be particularly sensitive to the side effects of these drugs. For example, AEDs may intensify an underlying dementia or exacerbate mild cognitive decline. There are a variety of AEDs; most must be started slowly and the dose increased gradually. Reduction in seizure frequency and severity and the onset of side effects are monitored to determine if the person is on the correct dosage. Description and documentation and report of any seizure activity observed in the resident is critically important.

During a seizure: assist the resident to a safe position (i.e., lying on a comfortable surface) and prevent trauma (e.g., prevention of biting the tongue or hitting limbs on hard surfaces).

MOTOR NEURON DISEASE

Amyotrophic lateral sclerosis (ALS) is a neurodegenerative condition involving both upper and lower motor neuron cell bodies; it is characterized clinically by progressive weakness and wasting of skeletal muscles, and can eventually cause respiratory failure. Incidence increases with age but plateaus in the 60s. Older adults with ALS commonly present with gait disturbance, falls, foot drop, weakness in grip, dysphagia, or dysarthria. Prognosis is poor; treatment is mostly supportive; average survival is 2 to 3 years.

MYELOPATHY

Myelopathy means that there is something wrong with the spinal cord. The person will complain of difficulty walking because of generalized weakness or problems with balance and coordination. Myelopathy occurs commonly in older adults and is generally due to spinal stenosis, a progressive narrowing of the spinal canal. Bone spurs and arthritic changes reduce the space available for the spinal cord within the spinal canal. The bone spurs may begin to press on the spinal cord and the nerve roots; this pressure interferes with how the nerves function normally.

Many people with myelopathy will begin to have difficulty with things that require a fair amount of coordination, such as walking up and down stairs or fastening buttons. MRIs can provide diagnostic proof. Treatment is generally conservative and involves optimizing function, managing pain, and protecting the joint (e.g., a cervical collar).

RADICULOPATHY

Radiculopathy results from compression of a spinal root as it exits the spinal cord. In the spaces between the vertebrae, sensory nerves (i.e., nerves conducting sensory information toward the brain) and motor nerves (i.e., nerves conducting commands from the brain to muscles) connect to the spinal cord. Smaller, separate nerve bundles, called the roots of the nerve, are located at that entry/exit point. Damage to the spinal nerve roots can lead to pain, numbness, weakness, and paresthesia (i.e., abnormal sensations that occur without any cause).

Pain may be in the cervical (neck), thoracic (middle back), and lumbar (lower back) areas of the spine. Lumbar radiculopathy is also known as *sciatica*. Radiculopathy is different from myelopathy. Myelopathy involves pathological changes in, or functional problems with, the spinal cord itself, rather than the nerve roots. Radiculopathy is problems with the nerve roots and can result in pain, altered reflexes, weakness, and nerve-conduction abnormalities (i.e., impaired transmission of messages between the nerves and the muscles).

PERIPHERAL NEUROPATHY

The prevalence of peripheral neuropathy in older adults is estimated to be as high as 20%. In its most common form, it causes pain and numbness in hands and feet. The pain is typically described as tingling or burning, while the loss of sensation is often compared to the feeling of wearing a thin stocking or glove.

The most common cause of peripheral neuropathy is diabetes. Other common causes are medications (e.g., amiodarone, colchicine, phenytoin, lithium, vincristine, isoniazid), alcohol abuse, and nutritional deficiencies (e.g., vitamins B_6 and B_{12} deficiency, as well as deficiencies of thiamine, folate, and niacin), renal disease (i.e., uremia), monoclonal gammopathy (e.g., multiple myeloma), and neoplasm (e.g., infiltration of peripheral nerves by malignant cells, paraneoplastic syndromes associated with oat cell carcinoma of the lung, breast cancer, ovarian cancer, renal cell carcinoma, and prostate cancer).

Peripheral neuropathy usually begins in the feet with complaints of numbness and tingling, and may then spread from the feet to the hands and then up the legs and arms. There may also be sharp burning pain, extreme sensitivity to touch, lack of coordination, and muscle weakness or paralysis.

Treatment depends on the cause, ranging from withdrawal of the causative agent (e.g., alcohol, medications) to nutritional supplementation (for nutritional deficiency) or treatment of the primary cancer (neoplastic neuropathy). There is some evidence that optimizing glucose control may lessen the severity of diabetic neuropathy. Treatment of neuropathic pain includes the use of tricyclic antidepressants, anticonvulsant medications (e.g., carbamazepine[OL], gabapentin[OL]), and selective serotonin reuptake inhibitors. Topical agents include capsaicin cream and local anesthetic medications.

RESTLESS LEGS SYNDROME

Although classified as a neurologic disease, restless leg syndrome (RLS) is covered in Chapter 32, "Sleep Disorders."

RESOURCES

Backer, J.H. (2006). The symptom experience of patients with Parkinson's disease. *Journal of Neuroscience Nursing, 38*(1), 51–57.

Sethi, N.K., & Harden, C.L. (2008). Epilepsy in older women. *Menopause International, 14*(2), 85–87.

Stang, P.E., Carson, A.P., Rose, K.M., Mo, J., Ephross, S.A., Shahar, E., et al. (2005). Headache, cerebrovascular symptoms, and stroke: The Atherosclerosis Risk in Communities Study. *Neurology, 64*(9), 1573–1577.

Vacca, V. (2007). Diagnosis and treatment of idiopathic normal pressure hydrocephalus. *Journal of Neuroscience Nursing, 39*(2), 107–111.

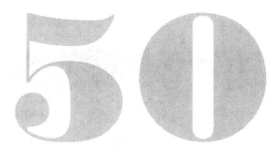

Hematologic Diseases and Disorders

Gurkamal Chatta, David A. Lipschitz, and Barbara Resnick

Hematopoiesis is the formation of blood cellular components. All cellular blood components are derived from hematopoietic stem cells (HSCs). Approximately 10^{11}–10^{12} new blood cells are produced daily. HSCs reside in the bone marrow and have the unique ability to give rise to all of the different mature blood cell types (e.g., red blood cells [RBCs], white blood cells, and platelets). In a healthy person, a red blood cell survives 90 to 120 days (on average) in the circulation; therefore, about 1% of red blood cells break down each day. The spleen (part of the reticulo-endothelial system) is the main organ that removes old and damaged RBCs from circulation. In healthy individuals, the breakdown and removal of RBCs from circulation is matched by the production of new RBCs in the bone marrow. With age, the body does not respond as quickly to stresses of blood loss or infection. That is, the body cannot as quickly or as efficiently make new red blood cells or increase the number of white blood cells to respond to infection when compared to a younger individual. In addition, hematological diseases are more common with age.

ANEMIA

Anemia is the most common age-related hematologic abnormality occurring in both men and women. In the general adult population, the annual incidence of anemia is estimated to be 1% to 2%. In comparison, the incidence of anemia among older adults (> 65 years of age) is four- to sixfold higher. Using World Health Organization criteria, anemia is present if hemoglobin concentrations drop below 12 g/dL (7.5 mmol/L) in women or below 13 g/dL (8.1 mmol/L) in men. In several studies, the prevalence rate of anemia before age 80 is 8% to 10% in women and 12% to 14% in men. In the over-80 cohort, the prevalence of anemia is 12% to 16% in women and 18% to 22% in men.

Presentation of Anemia

The presence of multiple chronic illnesses in older adults often makes it difficult to evaluate anemia. Health care providers often do not assess older adults for anemia, mistakenly believing that anemia is a consequence of the aging process rather than of disease. Anemia may develop slowly, with few specific symptoms or signs appearing until late in the course of the illness. Many symptoms of anemia mimic those of other conditions (e.g., functional decline, increase in cognitive problems, increase in falls, worsening heart disease). Caregivers and health care providers sometimes assume that nonspecific symptoms such as fatigue, weakness, and lack of stamina are normal signs of aging. Table 50.1 provides an overview of the signs and symptoms of anemia.

Not uncommonly, older adults adjust to the symptoms of anemia and do not complain. However, it is important to identify and treat anemia to prevent the

50.1 | Signs and Symptoms of Anemia

MILD ANEMIA	MODERATE ANEMIA	SEVERE ANEMIA
■ Bleeding gums	■ Increased heart rate	■ Angina
■ Complaints of being tired all the time	■ Mild fatigue	■ Exercise intolerance
■ Complaints of chest pain	■ Palpitation	■ Palpitations
■ Complaints of dizziness	■ Shortness of breath on exertion	■ Severe fatigue
■ Decreased ability to participate in exercises		■ Shortness of breath at rest
■ Decreased activity level		
■ Decreased appetite		
■ Functional decline		
■ Increase in falls		
■ Increased confusion		
■ Increased irritability		
■ Jaundice		
■ Labored breathing, especially with exertion		
■ Pale or cool skin		
■ Sleep problems		

development of complications associated with anemia (Exhibit 50.1). Treatment may, in fact, improve the function and quality of life of the resident.

The various types of anemia seen in older adults are summarized in Table 50.2. The diagnosis is always made by checking a blood count. Table 50.3 provides an overview of the blood indices used to evaluate for anemia.

Iron Deficiency Anemia

Iron is the only nutrient that limits the rate of erythropoiesis (i.e., the process by which red blood cells are made in the bone marrow) and is the most common cause of anemia in older adults. It is diagnosed by lab data reporting decreased serum iron and reduced transferrin saturation (i.e., serum iron divided by the total iron-binding capacity, or TIBC, expressed as a percentage). The ferritin level (i.e., indication of iron stores in the body) will be low (less than 100 ng/mL). Nutritional iron deficiency is very rare in older adults as the body tends to conserve iron, and stores of iron may actually improve with age. When unexplained iron deficiency does occur, it is almost exclusively due to blood loss from the gastrointestinal tract. Other common causes

50.1 | Complications Associated With Anemia

Increased mortality

Cardiac complications (congestive heart failure, left ventricular hypertrophy, myocardial infarction)

Cognitive impairment

Depression

Falls

Functional impairment

of blood loss, however, can be from multiple falls and hematomas (bruises), blood loss from the bladder that occurs chronically and just accumulates over time, or after any type of surgical procedure.

Anemia of Chronic Disease

The pathophysiology of anemia of chronic disease is complex. It is due to the inability of the body to free up the iron that is stored in the body so that it can be used to make red blood cells. As a consequence, serum iron falls and, as with blood-loss anemia, there is inadequate iron supply for erythropoiesis. In contrast to blood-loss anemia, in which iron stores are absent, in anemia of chronic disease the iron stores are normal or increased. Laboratory results show a low serum iron, low transferrin saturation, and normal to increased iron stores (ferritin > 100 ng/mL). The term *anemia of chronic disease* is often used to explain an anemia associated with some other major disease process such as cancer, collagen vascular disorders, rheumatoid arthritis, and inflammatory bowel disease.

Anemia of Chronic Kidney Disease (CKD)

Erythropoiten, together with iron, is needed to develop red blood cells. Anemia associated with CKD is due to decreased erythropoiten production in the kidney. Typically, erythropoiten is recommended for hemoglobin levels below 12 g/dL. Blood counts and iron levels should be monitored regularly. It is particularly important to make sure the individual has sufficient iron

when starting and being treated with an erythropoiten or red blood cells cannot be made.

Aplastic Anemia (Bone Marrow Failure)

Bone marrow failure is generally associated with suppression of all marrow elements, red blood cells, white blood cells, and platelets. Common causes include drugs, an autoimmune disorder, or a cancer. Testing is necessary to hopefully treat the underlying cause of the aplastic anemia.

Vitamin B$_{12}$ and Folate Deficiency

Vitamin B$_{12}$ and folate deficiency increases among older adults. Low blood levels of both B$_{12}$ and folate are also accompanied by increased levels of homocysteine and methylmalonic acid (MMA). Therefore older adults with low normal (< 350 pg/mL) B$_{12}$ levels may also need to have the level of MMA or homocysteine checked to further evaluate the individual for B$_{12}$ deficiency. If MMA or homocysteine level is elevated, it is an indication that there is a true B$_{12}$ deficiency, even though the resident may not have any symptoms at this time.

Vitamin B$_{12}$ deficiency, also know as *pernicious anemia*, is due to decreased absorption of vitamin B$_{12}$ in the stomach. Often this is due to an age associated decrease in intrinsic factor, needed to facilitate the absorption of B$_{12}$. In these situations the B$_{12}$ is replaced, either via high dosages of oral supplement or through injections. Folate deficiency of sufficient severity to cause anemia in older adults is less common and is usually associated with long-term and/or excessive alcohol use. Replacement of folate can be easily done with oral supplements.

The Myelodysplastic Syndromes

The myelodysplastic syndromes (MDS) are a group of disorders characterized by impairment in the body's ability to make red blood cells at the level of the bone marrow. Individuals with MDS usually have a macrocytic anemia and a reduced white blood cell count. Platelets are generally normal or increased. Treatment of MDS in the older adult tends to be supportive with monitoring of the progression of the anemia and changes in the white blood cell count.

Hemolytic Anemia

The causes of hemolytic anemia in older adults are generally due to a lymphoproliferative disorder (such as non-Hodgkin's lymphoma or chronic lymphocytic leukemia),

50.2 | Physiologic Classification of Anemia

HYPOPROLIFERATIVE (RESIDENT DOESN'T MAKE ENOUGH BLOOD CELLS)	HEMOLYTIC (RESIDENT DESTROYS HIS OR HER OWN RED BLOOD CELLS)
Iron-deficient anemia (microcytic anemia)	Caused by an autoimmune disorder
Diseases in the bone marrow where blood cells are made (normocytic anemia)	Caused by medications or toxins in the environment
Disease in the kidney where erythropoietin is made	
Vitamin B_{12} deficiency (macrocytic anemia)	
Folate deficiency (macrocytic anemia)	

Key definitions: Microcytic anemia: Blood cells viewed under the microscope are pale (*hypochromic*) and abnormally small (*microcytic*). Macrocytic anemia: Blood cells viewed under the microscope are abnormally large (*macrocytic*).

50.3 | Normal Laboratory Values for Tests for Anemia

HEMATOLOGY TESTS	NORMAL RESULTS
Hematocrit (Hct)	40%–52% (male)
	37%–46% (female)
Hemoglobin (Hgb)	13.2–16.2 gm/dL (male)
	12.0–15.2 gm/dL (female)
Red blood cell count (RBC)	4.3–6.2 × 10^6/μL (male)
	3.8–5.5 × 10^6/μL (female)
	3.8–5.5 × 10^6/μL (infant/child)
White blood cell count (WBC)	4.1–10.9 × 10^3/μL
Platelet count (Plt)	140–450 × 10^3/μL
RBC mean cell volume (MCV)	82–102 fL (male)
	78–101 fL (female)

(continued)

50.3 | Normal Laboratory Values for Tests for Anemia *(continued)*

HEMATOLOGY TESTS	NORMAL RESULTS
Reticulocyte	0.5%–1.5% (adult)
Iron studies	
Total serum iron (TSI)	76–198 µg/dL (male)
	26–170 µg/dL (female)
Total iron-binding capacity (TIBC)	262–474 µg/dL
Transferrin	204–360 mg/dL
Ferritin	18–250 ng/mL (male)
	12–160 ng/mL (female)

collagen vascular disease, or drug ingestion. Corticosteroids and splenectomy are usually effective treatments.

PLATELETS AND COAGULATION

Platelet count does not change with aging, but concentrations of a large number of coagulation enzymes (i.e., enzymes needed to facilitate development of blood clots) increase with age. Consequently, it is believed that older adults have increased hypercoagulability (i.e., they develop blood clots more readily than do younger individuals when in bed or sitting for extended periods of time). Evidence of bleeding under the skin is not uncommon in older adults. Unexplained bruises, repeated nosebleeds, gastrointestinal losses, or excessive blood loss during surgery or following dental extraction are common presentations. In these individuals, it may be recommended that platelet counts be evaluated. *Thrombocytopenia,* or a platelet count of less than 150,000 ml, can occur, although it is not certain how low the platelet count must be before there is evidence of bleeding.

Common causes of thrombocytopenia include decreased production of platelets in the bone marrow, disorders of the spleen, and increased destruction of platelets as they are circulating. Decreased production of platelets occurs in older adults with leukemia or other bone marrow problems, or this may be due to drugs that suppress platelet production. Increased destruction of platelets is due to autoimmune disorders. Treatment of thrombocytopenia depends on the cause.

RESOURCES

Dharmarajan, T.S. (2008). Anemia and response to epoetin alfa: The cause of anemia matters! *Journal of the American Geriatrics Society, 56*(8), 1574–1575.

Dharmarajan, T.S., & Widjaja, D. (2008). Adverse consequences with use of erythropoiesis-stimulating agents in anemia prompt release of guidelines to ensure safe use and maximize benefit. *Geriatrics, 63*(6), 13–29.

Montané, E., Ibáñez, L., Vidal, X., Ballarín, E., Puig, R., García, N., et al. (2008). Catalan Group for Study of Agranulocytosis and Aplastic Anemia. Epidemiology of aplastic anemia: A prospective multicenter study. *Haematologica, 93*(4), 518–523.

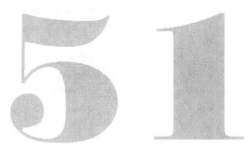

Oncology

Susan Avillo Scherr, William B. Ershler, and Dan L. Longo

Prevalence studies indicate that cancer is primarily a burden for geriatric populations. In fact, the median age for cancer in the United States is 70 years. Although cancer has long been recognized as a disease of older adults, emphasis on geriatric issues and cancer is a recent development.

Three questions form the underpinnings of this new emphasis.

- Why are tumors more common in older adults?
- Is there a difference in tumor aggressiveness with advancing age?
- Should treatment be different for the older adult?

Experimental data and clinical experience indicate that tumors are not resistant to treatment by virtue of age alone. However, age is associated with slight reductions in certain organ functions, and these deficiencies in physiologic reserve might be magnified by comorbid conditions. Cancer treatments, especially chemotherapy, may therefore be associated with an increase in adverse events. Hence, treatment should be tailored to the individual, taking into consideration potential increased toxicities and balancing this with expectations of survival in the context of comorbidities.

The National Cancer Institute's Surveillance, Epidemiology and End Results (SEER) data reveal that more than 50% of all cancers are diagnosed in older adults age 65 years and older, and this older adult population incurs more than 60% of all cancer deaths. The data

also reveal important trends. Whereas between 1968 and 1985 cancer mortality decreased 23% in individuals younger than 55 years (primarily reflecting advances in the therapy of acute leukemias, Hodgkin's disease, non-Hodgkin's lymphomas, and testicular cancers), cancer mortality for those age 55 years and older increased by 17%. Thus, the older population is faced with an increasingly prevalent disease for which modern therapies have not improved overall survival. There is much to learn about providing optimal management of cancer in older adults, but an emphasis on disease prevention and screening remains a logical priority.

CANCER BIOLOGY AND AGING

Explaining the Increased Prevalence of Cancer With Age

The four most frequently occurring cancers in adults over age 50 are prostate, breast, lung, and colorectal. There are at least three reasons for the increased prevalence of cancer with age. First, cancers are thought to develop over a long period, perhaps decades. This is best exemplified by the current understanding of colon cancer, which has been shown to develop because of an accumulation of several damaging genetic events occurring over time. These events, also known as *mutations*, are changes in DNA that are caused by carcinogens. If mutations are acquired at a constant rate, older people are more likely to live long enough to develop the 8 to 10 genetic lesions that it takes to develop a malignancy.

A second reason for the greater prevalence of cancer with advancing age is that DNA repair mechanisms are thought to decline with age. As a consequence, cells may accumulate damage. Normally, a dividing cell pauses in G1 (i.e., the gap following mitosis [M] and before DNA replication [S]) and in G2 (i.e., the gap following S, or DNA replication and before M, mitosis) to take inventory and repair any damage before proceeding to the next phase. These are the G1 and G2 checkpoints. Older cells may fail to detect or repair damage and fail to control DNA replication accurately. This leads to *aneuploidy* and to uncontrolled proliferation. In younger people, these aberrations may trigger the death of the cell; in older people, the errors may be tolerated and fail to signal cell death. Cells without functioning checkpoints are vulnerable to loss of growth control.

A third contribution to increased cancer incidence in older people may be a decline in the function of the immune system, particularly in cellular immunity. A number of findings suggest that the immune system can recognize and control certain cancers. A decline in immune function may lead to the emergence of a cancer in an older person that was controlled when that person was younger. However, no direct link currently exists between the decline in immune function and the increase in cancer incidence in older adults.

The Different Characteristics of Cancer With Age

A long-held but incompletely documented clinical dogma holds that cancers in older adults are less aggressive or slower growing. However, epidemiologic data from tumor registries or large clinical trials do not support this notion. Such data may be confounded by geriatric problems that shorten survival independently of the cancer (e.g., comorbidity, multiple medications, physician or family bias regarding diagnosis and treatment in elderly persons, and age-associated life stresses). These factors may counter any primary influence that aging might have on tumor aggressiveness. There is experimental support, however, for the contention that there is reduced tumor aggressiveness with age. Despite this data, it remains difficult to know in any given individual whether the course of the disease will be characterized by an indolent or aggressive pattern of growth. Additional study is necessary to document age-associated differences in tumor cell biology.

Ethnic Differences in Cancer Incidence and Mortality

As the demographics of the U.S. population change, additional information is needed on incidence and natural history differences in cancers occurring in different ethnic and racial groups. The U.S. Census Bureau estimates that by 2050, Hispanic Americans will account for nearly 25% of the population, and Black Americans, Asian Americans, and Native Americans will combine to total another 25%. Overall, Black Americans have the highest cancer incidence and mortality rates; it is 10% higher than among White Americans, 50% to 60% higher than among Hispanic Americans and Asian Americans, and more than twice as high as among Native Americans. The cancer death rate for Black Americans is about 30% higher than for White Americans and more than twice as high as for Hispanic Americans, Asian Americans, and Native Americans. From 1992 to 1998, 5-year survival for all cancers was 64% for White Americans and 53% for Black Americans.

Factors contributing to the ethnic differences are not defined. However, certain data suggest that when the quality of the health care delivered to White and Black Americans is similar, disease outcomes in the two groups are comparable. Specific incidence, diagnosis, and survival data for common cancers in different ethnic groups are provided in Table 51.1 and Table 51.2.

PRINCIPLES OF CANCER MANAGEMENT

Current forms of cancer treatment include surgery, radiation, cytotoxic chemotherapy, hormone manipulation, and biologic therapy. Age alone does not preclude any of these approaches, but because of normal changes with age in certain organs and also age-associated conditions (i.e., comorbidities), special considerations are warranted.

Randomized clinical trials are the most reliable methodology to study medical intervention; treatment decisions are best founded on the results of such work. However, despite efforts from the cooperative oncology groups, individuals entered into trials are by and large younger and presumably healthier than the typical geriatric person with the same disorder. Furthermore, common end points of these trials are length of survival (for therapeutic interventions) or disease-specific deaths (for prevention studies), and these end points are not always the most appropriate outcomes for older adults

51.1 | Ethnic and Racial Differences in Cancer Incidence

SITE	WHITE AMERICANS		BLACK AMERICANS		HISPANIC AMERICANS		ASIAN AMERICANS	
	MALE	FEMALE	MALE	FEMALE	MALE	FEMALE	MALE	FEMALE
All	555.9	431.8	696.8	406.3	419.3	312.2	392.0	306.9
Breast	—	140.8	—	121.7	—	89.8	—	97.2
Colon	64.1	46.2	72.4	56.2	49.8	32.9	57.2	38.8
Lung	79.4	51.9	120.4	54.8	46.1	24.4	62.1	28.4
Prostate	164.3	—	272.1	—	137.2	—	100.0	—

51.2 | Racial Differences in Cancer Diagnosis and Survival

SITE	ADVANCED DISEASE AT DIAGNOSIS (%)		5-YEAR SURVIVAL (%)	
	WHITE AMERICANS	BLACK AMERICANS	WHITE AMERICANS	BLACK AMERICANS
Breast	33	43	88	74
Colon	19	24	63	53
Lung	38	40	15	12
Head and neck	55	73	60	36
Bladder	21	35	83	64
Endometrial	22	39	86	60

(because of their inherently limited life expectancies on the basis of age alone).

Clinical researchers are beginning to address issues of geriatric oncology. More geriatrics-oriented trials focus more on symptom reduction and quality-of-life outcomes than on life expectancy. Surveys indicate that older adults, when fully informed, most often choose life-extending treatments, even at the risk of toxicity. It is the physician and the resident's family that are most focused on quality-of-life issues. For the most part, tumors are not more resistant to treatment in older adults.

It is also commonly appreciated that acute toxicities (e.g., nausea, vomiting, hair loss) are less prominent in older adults. Thus, although quality of life remains a primary treatment consideration, efforts at extending life should not be denied older adults on the basis of their age alone.

Cancer Screening

Screening is designed to detect disease in asymptomatic individuals with the hope that early-stage disease is more readily curable. Screening for colon cancer, cervical cancer, and probably breast cancer saves lives. Controlled prospective randomized trials are the only method of documenting the value of screening. The study populations must be followed for many years to document the cancer cause-specific survival advantage to the screened group.

A screening test is evaluated on the basis of its capacity to distinguish people with disease from those without disease. Screening is of greatest value when the disease being sought is common in the population being screened and the test being used is highly specific. The use of weakly specific tests in populations with low disease prevalence does not save lives. In some instances, more harm is done through morbidities and mortality associated with the diagnostic evaluation of positive screening tests than the good associated with early detection of cancer. Current screening guidelines essentially indicate that women 65 years of age, particularly if sexually inactive and if they have had prior negative testing, do not need to continue to have Pap tests. Screening for breast, bowel, and prostate cancers continue to vary based on the organization establishing the guidelines. The general recommendation is to take a life expectancy approach such that those with a 5- to 10-year life expectancy may not benefit from screening. Given the range of recommendations and the fact that, regardless of age, screening is a reimbursable service for older individuals, an individualized approach should be taken. Residents and/or their licensed authorized representatives should be given information as to the benefit and potential risks to screening.

Chemotherapy

Older adults, in light of normal age changes and chronic illnesses, may be at increased risk of toxicity associated with chemotherapy (see Table 51.3). Toxicities include such things as worsening of renal function and myelosuppression (e.g., anemia, low white counts, and low platelet counts). It is important for purposes of comfort and reassurance that the resident, family, and staff are familiar with the expected side effects of chemotherapeutic agents. Contact with the oncologist to gain this information is an appropriate nursing intervention.

Hormonal Therapy

Hormonal treatment is effective in cancers of the breast, prostate, and endometrium. Tamoxifen, a selective estrogen receptor modulator, has antagonistic and partial agonistic effects. It is a useful therapy in adjuvant treatment of breast cancer and also has estrogenlike positive effects on cardiovascular risk factors and bone disease. Other more selective drugs in this category, such as raloxifene, are in clinical testing. Although inactive as a single agent, tamoxifen is synergistic with chemotherapy in the management of malignant melanoma. Currently used hormonal agents are listed in Table 51.4. Most of these are well tolerated by older persons and commonly are the treatment of choice in this age group.

Biologic Therapy

Modulation of immune response is a particularly attractive option in treating the older adult whose natural defenses against cancer may be impaired by immune senescence. Only a limited number of options are clinically available, and these are clearly inadequate to restore a normal immune response in the older person. Recombinant α-interferon at moderate doses (e.g., 3 million units, three times weekly) is reasonably well tolerated by individuals of all ages. At higher doses, α-interferon causes myelodepression, severe fatigue, flulike illness, malaise, fever, neuropathy, and abnormalities of liver enzymes. There are reports of delirium, depression, and dementia following α-interferon use in persons aged 65 and older. This is particularly important because interferon is an effective therapy for chronic myeloid leukemia, hairy cell leukemia, and multiple myeloma—hematologic malignancies that occur more commonly among older adults.

Interleukin-2 is used to treat metastatic melanoma and renal cancer. It can produce severe dose-related toxicity, including capillary leak syndrome, hypotension, adult respiratory distress syndrome, cardiac arrhythmias, peripheral edema, renal failure (i.e., prerenal), cholestatic liver dysfunction, skin rashes, and thrombocytopenia. These complications tend to appear gradually in less severe form; generally, individuals do not suddenly deteriorate. The toxicities reverse completely within a few days of stopping the drug. Among clinicians, the impression is that interleukin-2 toxicities are less severe and develop later in older adults.

Monoclonal antibodies directed against CD20 (rituximab) are useful to treat B-cell lymphomas and work against HER-2/*neu* (trastuzumab) to treat breast cancer. In most individuals, the antibodies are given just before combination chemotherapy; the antibodies appear to augment the response to the drugs. These humanized antibodies generally have mild toxicities. Residents may develop hypotension or shortness of breath with the first infusion because of the release of antibodies

51.3 | Chemotherapy Issues in Geriatric Oncology

ISSUE	COMMENTS
General	Comorbidities and multiple medications add complexity
Pharmacokinetic changes	Progressive delay in elimination of renally excreted drugs, due to a reduction in glomerular filtration rate, may account, in part, for more severe toxicity
Pharmacodynamic changes	Possible enhanced resistance with age to antitumor agents Increased expression of the multidrug resistance gene has been reported in some older adults Other proteins that result in drug efflux have been shown to have prognostic importance, but age-associated changes have not been described Increased tumor hypoxia with age has been observed in a marine model
Toxicity	Mucositis, cardiotoxicity, and peripheral and central neurotoxicity become more common and more severe with aging Cardiotoxicity is a complication of anthracyclines and anthraquinone, mitomycin C, and high-dose cyclophosphamide; the incidence of cardiotoxicity also increases with age Peripheral neurotoxicity with vincristine is more common and more severe in older adults The incidence of cerebellar toxicity from high-dose cytosine arabinoside increases with age
Myelotoxicity	Chemotherapy-related myelotoxicity may become more severe and more prolonged with aging, but moderately toxic treatment regimens, such as CMF (cyclophosphamide, methotrexate, fluorouracil), cisplatin and fluorouracil, and cisplatin and etoposide are tolerated by many older adults aged 70 and older without life-threatening neutropenia or thrombocytopenia Infections are markedly increased among older acute leukemia adults undergoing intensive induction treatment. In these cases, it is possible that the disease itself, rather than an age-associated change in marrow reserve, is responsible for the depletion of hematopoietic stem cells
Recent advances	Granulocyte colony-stimulating factor and granulocyte-macrophage colony-stimulating factor have reduced the incidence of neutropenic infections in patients receiving intensive treatment; effectiveness does not appear to be diminished with advanced patient age Certain new drugs or new formulations may be particularly suitable to the older adult, for example, oral etoposide and fludarabine, gemcitabine, vinorelbine, capecitabine, paclitaxel protein-bound particles, and liposomal doxorubicin

and antigens. Symptoms clear when the infusion rate is slowed down, and such symptoms rarely recur. Other antibodies against cancers are in development.

Radiation Therapy

Radiation therapy provides palliation for virtually all cancers, and it may be part of a treatment plan for lymphomas and cancers of the prostate, bladder, cervix, esophagus, breast, and head and neck area. Since the early 1960s, the trend has been to use radiation therapy as an alternative to surgery in poor surgical candidates, mainly older adults age 65 and older, with the implied expectation that such an approach is less toxic. Side effects include fatigue, mucositis (i.e., sores and inflammation in the mouth), thinning of the skin, cough and hoarseness, breast pain and swelling, dysuria, hot flashes, and diarrhea.

51.4 | Hormonal Agents Commonly Used in Treating Cancer

SITE	HORMONAL AGENTS
Breast	Antiestrogens: tamoxifen, toremifene
	Progestational agents: medroxyprogesterone acetate
	Aromatase inhibitors: aminoglutethimide, letrozole, anastrozole, exemestane
Prostate	Luteinizing hormone analogs: goserelin, leuprolide
	Estrogens: diethylstilbestrol
	Antiandrogens: flutamide, bicalutamide
Endometrium	Progestational agents
	Antiestrogens

Surgery

Concerns related to cancer surgery in the older adult are safety and rehabilitative potential. Several reports indicate that age itself is not a risk factor for elective cancer surgery, but the length of hospital stay and the time to full recovery become more prolonged with older adults (i.e., > 75).

Advances in anesthesia and surgery have benefited the older adult. Included among these are new endoscopic procedures that provide valuable palliation for the many tumors of the gastrointestinal tract, and the more widespread use of spinal anesthesia for major abdominal interventions, with a substantial decline in perioperative complications and mortality. More widespread use of laparoscopic surgical techniques and application of laser and photodynamic therapy is also broadening the surgical armamentarium and providing more older adults with potential palliation and cure.

The trend to manage cancer without deforming surgery may preclude the need for complex rehabilitation and may be of special value for older adults. Organ preservation without compromising treatment outcome is a reality for cancers of the anus and of the larynx, and is being studied for cancers of the oropharynx, esophagus, bladder, and vulva. Also, initial chemotherapy before primary surgery is effective in patients with large primary breast and lung cancers. Such an approach results in less extensive and potentially more curative surgical procedures.

Quality-of-Life Issues

Several studies have determined that perception of quality of life is highly subjective. Early assessments of quality of life focused on functional status and freedom from pain, but these factors, although important, are inadequate to evaluate far-reaching consequences of serious disease in all domains of life. There are many assessment tools used to evaluate quality of life in older adults, but there is no specific gold standard. It may be best to explore with the individual resident what is important to him or her, what he or she values, to help the resident determine how the cancer and treatment can be best managed to optimize quality of life.

SPECIFIC CANCERS

Many cancers, including breast, lung, colorectal, prostate, cervical, and pancreatic peak in incidence among older adults. Older adults do not survive long with cancer, with deaths occurring within the first 30 months of diagnosis. This is particularly true among those 85 years of age and older. Older adults with cancer deserve special considerations, and care and treatment must be individualized based on underlying comorbidities and the specific risks and benefits to treatment for the individual.

Breast Cancer

Breast cancer is one of the most prevalent cancers among older women. Fortunately, however, the course of the disease is more indolent (i.e., slower in progression) in older individuals. This is because of the higher prevalence of a well-differentiated hormone-receptor rich, slowly proliferating tumor and the relative lack of estrogen noted in older versus younger women. Controversy surrounds several critical issues in the management of this most common malignancy in older women. These issues include the following.

Postoperative Irradiation Following Lumpectomy

Although irradiation following lumpectomy is safe in women aged 65 and older, it may be a source of significant inconvenience. The value of postoperative irradiation has been questioned because the local recurrence rate of breast cancer may decrease with age, and the inconvenience of daily radiation treatment protocols may outweigh the limited benefits for some.

Need for Axillary Lymphadenectomy (Lymph Node Removal)

Given the benefits, regardless of if there is any spread of the cancer to the lymph nodes, of adjuvant tamoxifen in all postmenopausal women with estrogen-receptor positive breast cancer, removal of the lymph node in the axilla (under the arm) may add unnecessary morbidity for the older woman. This is particularly true if the procedure requires general anesthesia. However, proponents of lymphadenectomy claim that the procedure not only has a staging function but may also improve the curability of breast cancer or reduce the duration of tamoxifen treatment. Axillary dissection has generally been replaced by biopsy of the sentinel node, the first lymph node draining the area of the breast that harbors the cancer.

Adjuvant Hormonal Treatment

Many studies have established that adjuvant treatment for breast cancer with tamoxifen for at least 2 years pro-

longs both the disease-free survival and the overall survival of postmenopausal women. The benefits and risks of more prolonged treatment, especially for women over 70, are still controversial. Aromatase inhibitors were initially licensed as second-line hormonal treatment for patients who have progressed on tamoxifen. Increasingly, however, these drugs are recommended as first-line treatment in postmenopausal women with early-stage breast cancer that is hormone-receptor-positive, estrogen-receptor-positive, progesterone-receptor-positive, or both.

Initial Management of Metastatic Breast Cancer

Women age 65 and older with metastatic, hormone receptor-positive breast cancer are likely to have effective palliation with hormonal therapy, such as tamoxifen. Hormonal and chemotherapeutic treatments benefit older adults with hormone receptor–poor tumors. Chemotherapy is safe and effective in this group of older adults, as well.

Lung Cancer

Lung cancer is becoming increasingly common in older women for reasons that are not completely understood. The increase may in part be due to more widespread smoking among women. In addition, some data suggest that women are at greater risk of developing lung cancer per unit of tobacco exposure. Lung cancer currently is the leading cause of cancer death in men and women. Early recognition and surgical resection remain the best chance for cure. For patients with lesions in a location that precludes surgery, localized radiation may result in improving outcomes. Chemotherapy also produces clinical responses and provides effective palliation for some individuals with metastatic disease. New chemotherapeutic agents, such as vinorelbine and gemcitabine, and more established agents such as paclitaxel or docetaxel used in lower-dose weekly schedules, are effective treatments for older adults with lung cancer.

Colon Cancer

Two-thirds of colon cancer cases occur in persons age 65 years and over. With advancing age, there is greater likelihood of right-sided lesions and presentations with anemia rather than pain. Colonoscopy is the mainstay of diagnosis, primarily because it enables the gastro-enterologist to directly visualize and biopsy the large colon and part of the small colon. Surgical excision may be adequate for lesions confined to the colon, but if extension to regional nodes is observed, postoperative adjuvant chemotherapy (usually 5-fluorouracil plus leucovorin) reduces recurrence by 40% to 50%. Survival of patients with disease metastatic to liver or other organs remains poor, despite the availability of some new drug options.

Prostate Cancer

See Chapter 47, "Prostate Diseases and Disorders."

Hematologic Malignancies

Leukemias

Acute myeloid leukemia (AML) following myelodysplastic syndromes (i.e., changes in the bone marrow that cause alterations in the development of red blood cells) usually progresses quite slowly and does not require aggressive treatment.

Chronic Lymphocytic Leukemia

Chronic lymphocytic leukemia (CLL) is the most common form of leukemia in the Western world; about 12,500 cases are diagnosed each year in the United States. Median age at diagnosis is 61 years. The diagnosis is most often made incidentally when a peripheral white blood cell count reveals leukocytosis with a small lymphocyte count above 4,000/μL. Treatment is generally withheld until it is required to control a life-threatening or symptomatic complication such as infection and bone marrow failure. About 25% of patients will develop autoimmune anemia (i.e., they will destroy their own red blood cells) or thrombocytopenia some time in the course of the disease. Autoimmune mechanisms can be treated with glucocorticoids (e.g., prednisone) or splenectomy. Once anemia or thrombocytopenia develop as a consequence of marrow failure, median survival is about 18 months.

Non-Hodgkin's Lymphoma

The prognosis of low- and intermediate-grade non-Hodgkin's lymphoma worsens with age, but the explanation remains unclear. Treatment of older persons with intermediate-grade large cell lymphoma is controversial. As many as 30% of such patients obtain a durable com-plete remission with standard treatment (CHOP regimen, which includes cyclophosphamide, doxorubicin, vincristine, and prednisone). Administration of lower-than-normal doses results in a poorer outcome.

Hodgkin's Disease

Hodgkin's disease, although generally believed to be more common in young adults, has a curious peak in incidence rates for those late in life. Aggressive chemotherapy (e.g., doxorubicin, bleomycin, vinblastine, dacarbazine) is an effective treatment.

Multiple Myeloma

Multiple myeloma is diagnosed in about 14,400 people each year in the United States. Median age at diagnosis is 68 years; it is rare in people younger than 40 years. Black Americans have twice the incidence of White Americans. Classic signs and symptoms of myeloma include changes in the blood count, lytic bone lesions (e.g., fractures that are due to cancer in the bone), and a serum or urine electrophoresis that shows monoclonal gammopathy (i.e., higher-than-normal level of a protein called M protein in the blood). Patients with myeloma require treatment when the lytic bone lesions become symptomatic or progressive, infections are recurrent, or serum paraprotein increases. Standard treatment consists of oral chemotherapy, bisphosphonates (e.g., alendronate) to decrease bone breakdown, medications to build red blood cell counts such as erythropoietins, radiation, and pain management as needed.

PRINCIPLES OF MANAGEMENT

Both the incidence and prevalence of cancer increase with age; older adults more often present with advanced-stage disease. Screening the older population for common cancers (such as colon, breast, and prostate) before they experience symptoms are likely to discover earlier and more curable lesions. As with screening, residents should be provided with information about the pros and cons of treatment and participate in making decisions around treatment choices.

See also Chapter 38, "Dermatologic Diseases and Disorders," for the diagnosis and treatment of skin cancers, Chapter 22, "Chronic Pain and Persistent Pain," and Chapter 17, "The Continuum of Care," for discussion of palliative and end-of-life care.

RESOURCES

Bach, P. B., Schrag, D., Brawley, O. W., Galaznik, A., Yarken, S., & Begg, C. B. (2002). Survival of Blacks and Whites after a cancer diagnosis. *Journal of the American Medical Association, 287*(16), 2106–2113.

Balducci, L., Lyman, G. H., Ershler, W. B., Balducci, L. Lyman, G. H., & Ershler, W. B. (Eds.). (2004). *Comprehensive geriatric oncology* (2nd ed.). Philadelphia, PA: Lippincott Williams and Wilkins.

Cope, D. G. (2006). Cancer and the aging population. In D. G. Cope & A. M. Reb (Eds.), *An evidence-based approach to the treatment and care of the older adult with cancer* (pp. 1–11). Pittsburgh, PA: Oncology Nursing Society.

Haas, M. L. (2006). The older adult receiving radiation therapy. In D. G. Cope & A. M. Reb (Eds.), *An evidence-based approach to the treatment and care of the older adult with cancer* (pp. 311–324). Pittsburgh, PA: Oncology Nursing Society.

Muss, H. B., & Longo, D. L. (Eds.). (2004). Cancer in the elderly. *Seminars Oncology, 31,* 125–296.

Web Site Resources for the Care of Older Adults

MISSION/GOAL	ORGANIZATION/RESOURCE	WEB ADDRESS
Public policy and information	Administration on Aging	http://www.aoa.gov/
Elder abuse and mistreatment	Adult Protective Services	http://www.apsnetwork.org
Locate a Medicare certified home health agency	AgeNet Eldercare Network (public service of Administration on Aging)	http://www.eldercare.org
Alzheimer's disease (dementia)	Alzheimer's Association	http://www.alz.org/
Assisted living nursing: information, certification, state chapters	American Assisted Living Nurses Association (AALNA)	http://www.alnursing.org
Pain management	American Academy of Pain Medicine	http://www.painmed.org
Not-for-profit long-term care provider association	American Association of Homes and Services for the Aging	http://www.aahsa.org
Advocacy and information	AARP	http://www.aarp.org/
Information regarding advance directives, wills, elder law, and so forth	American Bar Association	http://www.abanet.org http://www.abanet.org/publiced/practical/healthcare_directives.html
Guidelines for anticoagulation	American College of Chest Physicians, 2008 Guidelines	http://www.arixtra.com/chestphysicians.html
Diabetes information	American Diabetes Association	http://www.diabetes.org
Interdisciplinary educational resources and guidelines	American Geriatrics Society	http://www.americangeriatrics.org/
For-profit long-term care provider association	American Health Care Association	http://www.ahca.org/

(continued)

Web Site Resources for the Care of Older Adults *(continued)*

MISSION/GOAL	ORGANIZATION/RESOURCE	WEB ADDRESS
Educational material for residents and families; support groups; research promotion	American Insomnia Association (AIA)	http://www.american insomniaassociation.org
Standards of practice	American Nurses Association	http://www.nursingworld.org/MainMenu/ThePractic ofProfessionalNursing/ EthicsStandards/ CodeofEthics.aspx
Information about macular degeneration	American Macular Degeneration Foundation	www.macular.org/
Guide to assessing and counseling older drivers	*The Physician's Guide to Assessing and Counseling Older Drivers* American Medical Association	http://www.ama-assn.org/ama/pub/category/10791.html.
Interdisciplinary clinical and policy information about long-term care (nursing homes and assisted living)	American Medical Directors Association	http://www.amda.com/
Pain management	American Pain Society	http://www.ampainsoc.org/
Educational material for residents and families; support groups; research promotion; advice for traveling with continuous positive airway pressure (CPAP)	American Sleep Apnea Association.	http://www.sleepapnea.org.
Interdisciplinary resources on aging issues focused on community-dwelling older adults	American Society on Aging	http://www.asaging.org
Ethics	American Society for Bioethics and Humanities	http://www.asbh.org
Medication management policy and clinical practice	American Society of Consultant Pharmacists	http://www.ascp.com/
Exercise and physical therapy information and resources	American Association of Physical Therapy	http://www.aapt.com/
Questions and answers	Americans With Disabilities Act	http://www.ada.gov
Description of arthritis and treatment options	Arthritis Foundation	http://www.arthritis.org/
Inpatient and outpatient rehab facility accreditation	Commission on Accreditation of Rehabilitation Facilities (CARF)	http://www.carf.org

(continued)

Web Site Resources for the Care of Older Adults *(continued)*

MISSION/GOAL	ORGANIZATION/RESOURCE	WEB ADDRESS
Prophylaxis (e.g., immunization) and management of infectious disease	Centers for Disease Control and Prevention (CDC)	http://www.cdc.gov/
Nationally relevant information about assisted living	Center for Excellence in Assisted Living	http://www.theceal.com
Resources for assessment and management of older adults across all settings	ConsultGeriRN	http://www.hartfordign.org/Resources/clinical/
Eldercare locator: a public service of the Administration on Aging	Eldercare Organization	http://www.eldercare.org
Clinical and practice information across all settings	Gerontological Advanced Practice Nurses Association	http://www.ncgnp.org/
Interdisciplinary information focused on policy, social, and clinical issues in aging	Gerontological Society of America	http://www.geron.org/
Quality improvement; culture of safety	Institute for Healthcare Improvement	http://www.ihi.org
Standards of care; survey; accreditation	Joint Commission (formerly Joint Commission for Accreditation of Healthcare Organizations [JCAHO])	http://www.jointcommission.org
Medicare information	Medicare	http://www.medicare.gov/
Links to different data fields and reports for Nursing Home information	Medicare	http://www.medicare.gov/NHCompare/home.asp
Activities for people with dementia	*Meet Me at the Moma* Museum of Modern Art	http://www.moma.org/education/alzheimers.html
Bowel and bladder information and guidelines	National Association for Continence	http://www.nafc.org/
To locate a Medicare certified home health care agency	National Association for Home Care	http://www.nahc.org
Aging resources	National Association of Area Agencies on Aging	http://www.n4a.org
Nursing administration across all settings	National Association of Directors of Nursing Administration	http://www.nadona.org/
Information	National Center for Creative Aging (NCCA)	http://www.creativeaging.org

(continued)

Web Site Resources for the Care of Older Adults *(continued)*

MISSION/GOAL	ORGANIZATION/RESOURCE	WEB ADDRESS
Trade organization and information	National Center for Assisted Living	http://www.ncal.org/
Includes a chat room as well as education resources and so forth	National Center for Sleep Disorders Research (NIH) Restless Legs Syndrome Foundation	http://www.rls.org.
The basics: major types of elder abuse	National Center on Elder Abuse	http://www.elderabuse center.org.
Nurse practice acts; explanations of delegation, license revocation, and so forth	National Council of State Boards of Nursing	http://www.ncsbn.org
Nonprofessional caregiving advice, policy, and so forth.	National Family Caregivers Association	http://www.nfcares.org
Geriatric nursing resources for all nurses	National Gerontological Nurses Association	http://www.ngna.org/
Basics of Older Americans Act	National Health Policy Forum	http://www.nhpf.org/ pdfs_basics/Basics_Older AmericansAct_04-21-08.pdf
Nursing home ratings for providers and consumers	Nursing Home Compare	http://www.medicare.gov/ nhcompare/home.asp
Hospice: end of life philosophy and management; locate a certified hospice provider	National Hospice and Palliative Care Association	http://www.nhpco.org
Aging resources for patients and providers	National Institute on Aging	http://www.nih.gov/nia
For sleep information, assessment tools, treatment, and so forth	National Institutes of Health (NIH) National Heart, Lung, and Blood Institute	http://www.nhlbi.nih/ gov/health/public/sleep/ index/htm
For workplace rights	National Labor Relations Board	http://www.nlrb.gov/ Workplace_Rights
Information	Society for Creative Aging	http://www.s4ca.org
Elder mistreatment	Try This	http://www.hartfordign.org
Assessment tools	Try This: and How to Try This Series Assessment Tools on the Care of Older Adults	http://www.hartfordign. org/Resources/Try_This_ Series/

(continued)

Web Site Resources for the Care of Older Adults *(continued)*

MISSION/GOAL	ORGANIZATION/RESOURCE	WEB ADDRESS
Information regarding sleep	Pittsburg Sleep Quality Index (PSQI) Try This 6.1	http://www.hartfordign.org
Sleep scale	Epworth Sleepiness Scale (ESS) Try This 6.2	http://www.hartfordign.org.
Questionnaire for sleep apnea risk	University of Maryland Medical Center Sleep Disorders Center	http://http://www.umm. edu/sleep/apnea_risk.htm
Locate a Medicare certified home health agency	Visiting Nurses Association National Association for Home Care Eldercare Locator	http://www.vnaa.org http://www.nahc.org http://www.edlerdcare.org